"An invaluable resource for clinicians wishing to make evidence-based treatment accessible to patients in a wide range of settings. Drs Bailey-Straebler and Sproch provide a well written, easy to use, detailed guide to the use of one of the best evidence-supported treatments for eating disorders, CBT-E, in group format."

Zafra Cooper, DPhil, DClinPsych, *Professor of Psychiatry (Adjunct), Department of Psychiatry, Yale School of Medicine, US; Professor Emeritus of Clinical Psychology, Department of Psychiatry, Oxford University, UK*

"This book is a crucial resource for clinicians and researchers working with eating disorders. It introduces, for the first time, the implementation of 'enhanced cognitive behavior therapy' (CBT-E) adapted for group delivery. The text provides comprehensive guidance on adapting group CBT sequentially for outpatient treatment and modularly/non-sequentially for higher levels of care. Including therapist insight boxes and approximately 70 handouts—comprising worksheets for patients and informational sheets—this book equips therapists to deliver the treatment well and address challenges they might face. I am eager to recommend this exceptional resource to all my students and colleagues."

Riccardo Dalle Grave, MD, *Director, Department of Eating and Weight Disorders, Villa Garda Hospital Garda (VR), Italy*

"Drs. Bailey-Straebler and Sproch's treatment guide for Group CBT-E make it possible for the evidence-based CBT-E to be delivered effectively in treatment programs that rely on group-based interventions. The manual is well written, user-friendly and has already become an essential resource for clinicians who want to assure that eating disorder group treatments offer effective recovery-focused strategies."

Evelyn Attia, MD, *Suzanne Crosby Murphy Professor of Psychiatry, Columbia University Medical Center; Director, Center for Eating Disorders New York Presbyterian Hospital, US*

Group Cognitive Behavior Therapy for Eating Disorders

This treatment guide equips therapists with the necessary tools to implement the leading recommended treatment for eating disorders, "enhanced" cognitive behavior therapy (CBT-E), in a group format.

Group CBT-E is a structured treatment designed to help patients make critical changes to their eating, dieting, and other eating disorder symptoms. It aims to engage patients in identifying and addressing over-evaluation of shape and weight, managing stressful events and emotions without eating disorder behaviors, and developing relapse prevention skills. The treatment guide includes detailed session agendas and outlines, practical tips, advice on addressing sensitive topics, and numerous reproducible handouts that patients can personalize for their treatment needs. Group CBT-E empowers patients to actively engage in their recovery journey and emphasizes the valuable support found in group therapy settings, where shared experiences foster learning, encouragement, and a sense of understanding. The treatment's structured and individualized approach not only enhances patient outcomes, but also boosts therapist confidence.

This book is a vital resource for therapists seeking clear guidance on implementing CBT-E in group format. Its practical components, such as clinical examples, therapist insights, patient handouts, and detailed CBT-E formulation guidance, are useful for all CBT-E therapists.

Suzanne Bailey-Straebler, PhD, PMH-BC, is the Clinical Director of the Center for Eating Disorders Partial Hospital Program and Outpatient Specialty Clinic at Weill Cornell Medicine, New York Presbyterian Hospital.

Laura Sproch, PhD, CED-S, is a clinical psychologist who specializes in the treatment of eating disorders through her work as a therapist, supervisor, researcher, and administrator.

Group Cognitive Behavior Therapy for Eating Disorders

Suzanne Bailey-Straebler and Laura Sproch

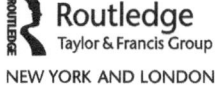

Routledge
Taylor & Francis Group

NEW YORK AND LONDON

Designed cover image: © cover Image by Sophie Chu-O'Neil

First published 2025
by Routledge
605 Third Avenue, New York, NY 10158

and by Routledge
4 Park Square, Milton Park, Abingdon, Oxon, OX14 4RN

Routledge is an imprint of the Taylor & Francis Group, an informa business

ISBN: 978-1-032-58624-3 (hbk)
ISBN: 978-1-032-58623-6 (pbk)
ISBN: 978-1-003-45084-9 (ebk)

DOI: 10.4324/9781003450849

Typeset in Times New Roman
by SPi Technologies India Pvt Ltd (Straive)

To my parents, Mary Ellen and Chuck.
And to my loves, Christian and Alexander.

S.B-S.

To Winston, Beatrix, and the rest of your generation. May you grow up to make the world a better place, each in your own unique and magnificent ways.

L.S.

Contents

Tables

Figures

Authors

Suzanne Bailey-Straebler, PhD, PMH-BC, is the Clinical Director of the Center for Eating Disorders Partial Hospital Program and Outpatient Specialty Clinic at Weill Cornell Medicine, New York Presbyterian Hospital. She holds academic appointments as an Associate Professor of clinical nursing at Columbia University Medical Center and as a Research Associate in psychiatry at Weill Cornell Medicine. She is a lead trainer for the CBT-E training group and has trained and supervised therapists around the world. For over a decade Dr Bailey-Straebler was a Senior Research Clinician at the Centre for Research on Eating Disorders at Oxford (CREDO) headed by Professors Christopher Fairburn and Zafra Cooper. While there, she received extensive clinical training, was a contributing author of the CBT-E treatment manual, assisted in the creation of a web-based CBT-E training program, and completed her doctoral thesis on improving therapist training in evidence-based treatments.

Laura Sproch, PhD, CEDS-C, has had the privilege of working in a variety of eating disorder-specialized treatment centers across the country, applying CBT and CBT-E in individual and modified group formats at all levels of care, as well as supervising, training, consulting, and developing programs based on these interventions. She is the former Program Director of the New England Eating Disorders Program at Sweetser, a leading eating disorder treatment program in the state of Maine, where she led the partial hospitalization, intensive outpatient, and outpatient programs. Prior to that position, Dr Sproch managed the research program and developed and implemented outpatient group therapy protocols at the Center for Eating Disorders at Sheppard Pratt in Baltimore, one of the top psychiatric hospitals in the United States. She has presented on eating disorders and evidence-based treatment at conferences and trainings across the country. Dr Sproch opened her private practice, Vibrant Psychology, in 2023.

Acknowledgments

This book would not be possible without the pioneering work of Christopher Fairburn, Zafra Cooper, Roz Shafran, and Riccardo Dalle Grave. So many have benefited from your unparalleled expertise and wisdom.

We also extend our gratitude to our multidisciplinary team of readers for their useful insights, astute comments, and thought-provoking questions. Your collective contributions not only enhanced the quality of this book but also enriched its depth and clarity. Specifically, we thank Samantha Berlow, Melissa Cemel, Laura Cordella, Lydia Crafts, Sara Fruchter, Fayrisa Greenwald, Melissa Klein, Jennifer Panitz, Dominique White, and Rachel Zambrowicz. We greatly appreciate the cover artwork created by Sophie Chu-O'Neil, whose talent and creativity brought to life the inclusive image we envisioned for this book.

SB-S: I am extremely grateful to my CBT-E mentors, Christopher Fairburn and Zafra Cooper. And my CBT-E companion, Rebecca Murphy. What an incredible journey it has been. Thank you to my family for their never-ending love and support, especially CB and AB.

LS: I would like to recognize a career's worth of dedicated mental health providers and scholars that I have worked alongside and learned from, including my colleagues, staff, supervisors, teachers, trainees, administrators, and mentors. In particular, I would like to acknowledge Dr Steven Crawford, whose confidence in my work helped to shape my professional path, and Dr Kimberly Anderson, my CBT advisor and mentor, who truly exemplifies how to be a resilient, balanced, and brilliant female leader in this field. Thank you to my very supportive family, especially Will, for everything, always.

Finally, we express our heartfelt thanks to the patients who participated in various iterations of these groups, offering invaluable feedback and perspectives. You have all been instrumental in shaping the content of this book, and we are deeply grateful to you.

Chapter 1

An Introduction to This Book

We are delighted that you have picked up this Group CBT-E treatment guide. As therapists who have devoted our careers to implementing effective therapies for individuals with eating disorders, we have personally experienced how exceptionally rewarding conducting such treatment can be. We are also aware that treating these conditions can feel daunting and intimidating. We designed this treatment guide as an easy-to-use resource with clear direction and many clinical tips to ease the process of treating these complex disorders. We hope that you find the application of Group CBT-E to be both valuable for you and significantly beneficial for the patients in your care.

Why Group CBT-E?

Cognitive behavior therapy (CBT) is one type of psychological treatment that can effectively treat many psychological conditions, including eating disorders. CBT-E, described in detail in Chapter 2, is a well-researched and recommended specific form of CBT for eating disorders. This book presents Group CBT-E, which is closely modeled on the individual format. Group CBT-E follows the treatment stages of Individual CBT-E and provides the main treatment interventions adapted for group delivery.

There are several reasons we decided to create this group format version of CBT-E:

1. To increase access to effective treatment for individuals with eating disorders.
2. To increase treatment adherence and reduce therapist drift, ensuring that patients receive all the active ingredients of treatment.
3. To provide clear treatment guidance for therapists implementing groups at higher levels of care.
4. To offer patients the benefits of group treatment delivery.

Increasing Access to Effective Treatment

To date, Individual CBT-E has the most robust evidence for reducing eating disorder symptoms for patients with a wide range of eating disorders, and yet few patients receive this treatment. One way of increasing treatment access is to offer treatments that are scalable.

DOI: 10.4324/9781003450849-1

Scalable treatments (e.g., group therapy, self-help, and guided self-help treatment, digital (app-based) treatment, and single-session interventions) can be more efficiently delivered to a greater number of patients at once than one-on-one individual treatment sessions. Group CBT-E can greatly increase treatment access. Depending on the size of the group, group therapy offers the opportunity to see between 6 and 8 patients at once, compared to a single patient in individual therapy. With more group therapy interventions, not only would more patients receive treatment, but waitlists could also be dramatically reduced. This is critical as reduced waitlist time is associated with shorter duration of illness and possibly improved treatment response.

We could compare treatment scalability for a therapist who provides four 50-minute individual therapy sessions (for a total of 3 hours, 20 minutes) to a therapist that runs three one-hour group therapy sessions (for a total of 3 hours). The individual therapist will have provided treatment to four patients, while the group therapist will have reached 18–24 patients in a relatively similar period of time.

Increasing Treatment Adherence and Reducing Therapist Drift

We have written this protocol to be very user friendly and have been careful to structure the presentation of this treatment in a way that supports treatment adherence. As you will see, Group CBT-E provides almost 70 patient handouts. These include worksheets for patients to fill in and information sheets. The handouts serve several purposes, not least of which is that they assist therapists in implementing all treatment components (i.e., treatment adherence). By implementing all components each session, therapist drift (i.e., when a therapist is no longer delivering the treatment in the way it was intended) is reduced. Improving treatment adherence and reducing therapist drift is important for ensuring that patients receive the treatment most likely to improve their symptoms.

Guidance at Higher Levels of Care

Group therapy is the main mode of treatment delivery at HLOC, including inpatient psychiatric units, residential centers, partial hospital programs, and intensive outpatient programs. However, protocols or guides on how to implement specific group therapies for eating disorders, including CBT-E, are lacking. Over the years, we have frequently received requests to produce such a guide, and what follows in this book contains much of the 'in-house' guidance we developed and have used at our respective centers.

The Benefits of Group-delivered Therapies for Patients

Group-based therapeutic interventions are effective in symptom reduction, and overall functional enhancement, as well as providing non-specific benefits related to group cohesion. Participating in groups offers individuals an opportunity to share in a collective understanding of their eating disorder experience. This shared space reduces the sense of isolation often associated with eating disorders. Moreover, it allows for supporting others, which at times, particularly initially, can feel more manageable than supporting oneself. Over time, this support of others can gradually shift toward support for oneself.

As long time CBT-E therapists, we have observed how beneficial group delivery of the same individual treatment components can be for patients. We have countless examples of times when support from a peer with shared lived experience in the group made the messaging more engaging and meaningful to another group member.

Additionally, groups offer a supportive space to openly share behaviors and thoughts that may be scary to say aloud. Being able to share with others who "get it" has the double benefit of stripping the eating disorder of secrecy and removing some of the shame that often accompanies it.

> We often hear peer support like this: "I totally understand what you are going through in those painful moments right after eating a feared food. It's rotten, I know. All I can say is that it felt impossible at first and then, it just got better for me over time and now I'm not so scared of the food." This type of support from a peer with lived experience just sounds different than from a therapist, and is so frequently gratefully received.

What You Can Expect in This Guide

Scripts

As CBT-E supervisors, one of the main questions we are asked is: "How do you say it?" We have provided suggested scripts throughout the book. These are ideas about how we might introduce or explain a topic and are there to guide you. The words you ultimately use in the group should be your own, influenced by the needs of the group members. Although CBT-E is a guided treatment, it is designed to be individualized or tailored to meet the needs of your individual patients. The goal is to provide patients with all the necessary ingredients (i.e., skills) to make a long-lasting recovery, but the exact way you present these skills will vary to some degree.

Samples and Examples

In addition to the scripts, you will find samples and examples of all group work. These samples will give an idea of what a collaboratively created list (i.e., a list that was created with both the therapist and group members) might look like for each skill or intervention. Similar to the scripts, the samples are there to guide you but are not intended to be replicated exactly. You will blend the samples with your clinical judgment about what will work best for the individuals in your group. The important aspect is to deliver all the treatment components in a personalized way to meet the needs of your patients.

Therapist Insights

Throughout the guide, you will see 'Therapist Insight' boxes. Here you will find tips and suggestions from our clinical experience of applying Group CBT-E. Many of the insights are a combination of trial and error when implementing earlier versions of this treatment in real-world settings and were created with feedback and input from patients engaged in these groups.

Handouts

Fellow therapists frequently ask if handouts exist for certain skills and interventions. To answer this request, we have made Group CBT-E rich with these tools. In addition to their benefits in aiding therapist adherence, handouts provide the following benefits:

- They allow for a group-based treatment to be more individualized. Individual CBT-E is a highly bespoke treatment that is guided by the needs and challenges of the single patient in the room. A group does not allow for this level of personalization. Handouts help to solve this difficulty by allowing each patient to engage with the group content in an individualized way. Used in this way, the treatment is more patient-led than therapist-led.

- They are useful aids to help keep information organized and allow information to be shared both verbally and in writing. This potentially reduces anxiety for some patients who find it comforting to know that they do not need to remember everything from the session. It is hoped that at the end of the treatment, patients will have a complete workbook of handouts to aid with long-term relapse prevention.

Resource-Rich Appendices

At the end of the book, you will find an extensive appendix section filled with many useful extras. These cover topics such as: an in-depth exploration of the CBT-E transdiagnostic formulation; a pre-treatment screening tool; and special considerations for running and implementing groups.

Simple, Clear, and Inclusive Language

The language in this book is intended to be accessible to all therapists, and by extension, to all patients participating in Group CBT-E. We have avoided the use of jargon, idioms, and other linguistic tools such as analogies, metaphors, or similes. We have also attempted to be as inclusive as possible in our language throughout the book, recognizing that we hold our own implicit biases that may have inadvertently affected our writing. We have attempted to use language that is intentionally respectful and culturally sensitive, aiming to avoid biases and expressions of discrimination. Eating disorders can affect all individuals regardless of shape, weight, age, culture, disability, ethnicity, gender, gender identity, income, neurodiversity, race, sexual orientation, and more. Likewise, therapists represent a diverse and varied group of individuals. Therefore, it is important that this guide feels usable by all. We recognize that we have missed opportunities to further improve the inclusivity of this text and encourage readers to contact us so that subsequent editions can be updated and modified.

Chapter 2

Eating Disorders and Enhanced Cognitive Behavior Therapy

Eating Disorders: Current Classification

There are eight recognized feeding and eating disorders in the *Diagnostic and Statistical Manual of Mental Disorders* (5th ed. text revision; DSM–5-TR; American Psychiatric Association, 2022): pica, rumination disorder, avoidant/restrictive food intake disorder (ARFID), anorexia nervosa (AN), binge eating disorder (BED), bulimia nervosa (BN), other specified feeding and eating disorder (OSFED), and unspecified feeding and eating disorder. The characteristics of each vary, but all share a disturbance of eating behavior and often high levels of psychosocial distress. Individuals frequently report significant isolation, withdrawal, loss of friendships and relationships, and feelings of hopelessness related to the disordered eating.

The most commonly recognized eating disorders are BED, BN, AN, and their related disorders, which typically fall under the category of OSFED.

BED and BED of Low Frequency or Limited Duration

BED and subthreshold BED are defined by recurrent distressing episodes of binge eating without compensatory behaviors. Binge eating episodes are defined as eating objectively large amounts of food in a period of no longer than two hours, coupled with feeling a loss of control. For the diagnosis of BED to be met, binges must be associated with three or more of the following: eating more rapidly than considered normal; eating until feeling uncomfortably full; eating large amounts of food when not feeling physically hungry; eating alone due to feelings of embarrassment over binge eating; and feeling disgust, sadness, or guilt after the binge episode (APA, 2022). Debate exists in the field regarding the presence of weight and shape concerns in individuals with BED. Diagnostically, this criterion is not required. However, studies have found that many individuals with BED do, in fact, have weight and shape concerns (Grilo, 2013; Wang et al., 2019), as well as endorse body image distress levels as severe as those with AN and BN.

BN and BN of Low Frequency or Limited Duration

BN and subthreshold BN are characterized by recurrent episodes of binge eating and inappropriate compensatory behaviors (e.g., self-induced vomiting, fasting, driven exercise or

DOI: 10.4324/9781003450849-2

the misuse of laxatives, diuretics, or other medications) to prevent weight gain. Individuals with BN and subthreshold BN base their self-evaluation primarily on their shape and weight. The symptoms of subthreshold BN are identical to those of BN apart from the frequency of binge eating and/or the recency of symptom onset.

Anorexia Nervosa (AN) and Atypical Anorexia Nervosa (AAN)

AN and AAN are both characterized by severe food restriction resulting in significant weight loss. Individuals with AN/AAN often have an intense fear of weight gain, an over-evaluation of shape and weight as a means to define self, and an inability to recognize the seriousness of being at such a low weight. There are two subtypes for AN: AN-restricting and AN-binge/purge. Individuals with a binge/purge subtype engage in binge eating and/or in compensatory behaviors. Individuals with AN are considered medically underweight. Those with AAN are considered by medical definitions to be at "normal" or "higher" body weights, despite being at a body weight that is too low for their individual physiological needs. This distinction has resulted in many individuals with AAN being underdiagnosed or misdiagnosed. Underdiagnosis for individuals with AAN is particularly concerning, as these illnesses share the same medical complications and psychological impacts (Walsh et al. 2023), and yet those with AAN often do not receive the care or treatment they need.

The Transdiagnostic Cognitive Behavior Theory of Eating Disorders

The current classification system for BED, BN, AN, and their related disorders is problematic in two main ways:

1. It does not match clinical reality. It is common for one's eating disorder symptoms to "migrate" or move around eating disorder categories (Fairburn, 2008). Many patients present to our clinics having met several eating disorder diagnoses in their lifetime. For example, a patient may present with BED which started out as AN. It would be misguided to think that they were recovered from AN and had now developed a new eating disorder, BED. A more accurate view may be that they have had one continuous eating disorder and the features have changed over time.
2. It encourages the view that there are several distinct disorders that require individually targeted treatments. This poses a challenge to patients accessing evidence-based treatments, as treatments would need to be distinct for each disorder, with separate training and expertise.

Rather than focusing on their diagnostic differences, Enhanced CBT (CBT-E) offers a potential solution by focusing on the common characteristics or "core" psychopathology across these disorders. This core psychopathology is driven by a dysfunctional scheme of self-evaluation based on an over-evaluation of shape, weight, and their control. In turn, this dysfunctional scheme maintains all the eating disorder symptoms. These behaviors can include weight-control behaviors (e.g., dieting, self-induced vomiting, driven exercise) and shape and weight-related behaviors and thoughts (e.g., body shape and weight avoidance,

Table 2.1 Eating Disorder Behaviors and Features That Maintain, and are Maintained by, an Over-evaluation of Shape, Weight, and Their Control

Eating habits and weight-control behaviors	Dieting behaviors
	Following diet-related rules
	Objective binge eating
	Subjective binge eating
	Self-induced vomiting, laxative and diuretic abuse
	Diet pill/other appetite-suppressing substance use
	Driven exercise
Shape and weight-related behaviors and features	Weight checking
	Body shape checking
	Reflection checking
	Body comparisons
	Social media body checking
	Body shape and/or weight avoidance
	Experiencing body dissatisfaction spikes

body dissatisfaction), and for some, binge eating in response to weight-control behaviors [see Table 2.1]. In addition, for many individuals, the eating disorder maintains, and is maintained by, the impact and response to life events and emotions. Treating these maintaining processes (what keeps the eating disorder going), shared across multiple diagnostic categories, makes a single – *transdiagnostic* – treatment possible.

Enhanced Cognitive Behavior Therapy for Eating Disorders

CBT-E has a robust evidence base and is considered a frontline treatment for BN, BED, and OSFED (National Institute of Care and Health Excellence, 2017). For AN, CBT-E is one of a few recommended treatments. CBT-E has several benefits:

1. As described, CBT-E is a transdiagnostic treatment specially designed to target the shared underlying eating disorder core psychopathology.
2. It can be applied through the lifespan from adolescents to older populations (Atwood and Friedman, 2020; Bailey-Straebler et al., 2022; Dalle Grave et al., 2023).
3. It can be implemented at a range of levels of care from outpatient through to inpatient settings (Dalle Grave et al., 2013; Fairburn et al., 2015).
4. Training in CBT-E is widely accessible with an asynchronous evidence-based training program (https://www.cbte.co/for-professionals/web-based-training/) (Cooper et al., 2017).
5. It is often well liked by patients and is a short-term intervention that helps to reduce waitlists and increase access.

CBT-E is a highly individualized and focused psychological therapy. It is a structured treatment, guided by the therapist with a clear beginning, middle, and end. CBT-E targets the maintaining mechanisms of the illness and is guided by a patient's personalized formulation. The treatment is spread over four stages. The first stage encourages behavior change and establishing a regular pattern of eating. Stage 2 is a review stage when patients and therapists consider progress in treatment and design the next stage of treatment. Stage 3 focuses on skills related to body image, dieting behaviors, and event- and emotion-related changes in eating. The final stage provides guidance on maintaining progress and preventing relapse. The treatment also includes a follow-up session five months post treatment to support continued change. For patients who do not require weight regain, the treatment is approximately 20 sessions over 20 weeks, and for patients who do require weight regain, it is 40 sessions over 40 weeks. There is also an extended "broad" version of the treatment. The broad version addresses additional maintaining mechanisms external to the eating disorder that may affect a subgroup of patients. The additional mechanisms include clinical perfectionism, core low self-esteem, and interpersonal difficulties.

An Illustration of CBT-E Theory: The Transdiagnostic Formulation

CBT-E is guided by a jointly created formulation. In CBT generally, a formulation, or case conceptualization, is a standard tool. Formulations provide therapists and patients with a strong clinical theory to inform treatment planning, and a blueprint or map of what keeps the disorder going, visually depicting what will be targeted in treatment.

The formulation in Figure 2.1 is an example of a CBT-E transdiagnostic formulation. It is included here to provide a visual overview of the CBT-E theory. This version is meant to highlight clinical concepts and includes technical terms for eating disorder features which would not, however, be used with a patient.

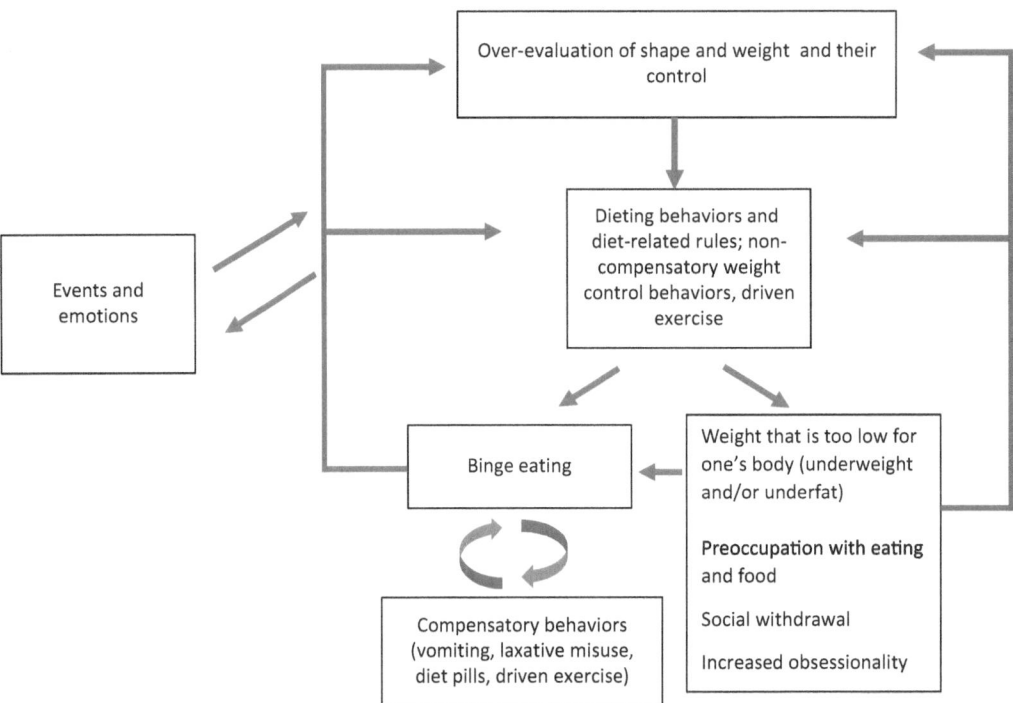

Figure 2.1 Transdiagnostic formulation technical terms.
Adapted from Fairburn, 2008

Although at first glance, the formulation in Figure 2.1 may appear overwhelming, in time it will become familiar. This formulation consists of a number of eating disorder features (the boxes) and the pathways (lines and arrows) that maintain or keep these features going. At the top of the formulation is the core psychopathology (i.e., the over-evaluation of shape, weight, and their control), which drives the eating disorder behaviors. In clinical application, the formulation is personalized to the patients you are working with. Therefore, not every box or arrow will be used for all patients. Understanding the transdiagnostic formulation, and being able to explain it to patients clearly, is essential for delivery of all forms of CBT-E. Appendix B provides detailed information on the formulation, describing the eating disorder features and maintaining pathways typically encountered. It is well worth reviewing this material and taking time to practice both drawing out and explaining a formulation.

A Brief History of CBT-E

In the early 1980s, Christopher Fairburn and colleagues at the Centre for Research on Eating Disorders at the University of Oxford (CREDO) created CBT for BN (CBT-BN). At the time, BN had only recently been recognized as an illness. Throughout the 1980s and 1990s, randomized controlled trials (RCTs) established CBT-BN as a leading outpatient treatment (Agras et al., 2000; Fairburn et al., 1986). In an effort to expand the reach of CBT-BN to both improve results and reach patients with other forms of eating disorders, Christopher Fairburn, Zafra Cooper, and Roz Shafran refined CBT-BN, creating transdiagnostic CBT-E (Fairburn et al., 2003; Cooper & Fairburn, 2011). Numerous RCTs and real-world replication studies have since been conducted providing robust evidence for CBT-E as a leading treatment for eating disorders in adults (e.g., Byrne et al., 2011; Fairburn et al., 2015; Signorini et al., 2018). It is noted that much of the treatment research across all eating disorder treatments, including CBT-E, has been focused on cisgender, white females, and research on diverse groups of patients is needed (Kaidesoja et al., 2023).

Cognitive behavior therapy and eating disorders, published in 2008 and written by clinicians (Christopher Fairburn and colleagues, including Zafra Cooper, Rebecca Murphy, and SB-S), is a practical treatment guide for therapists describing how to implement empirically supported CBT-E. To increase treatment accessibility, CREDO created a more comprehensive CBT-E therapist training consisting of learning modules and illustrations of key interventions with patient/therapist roleplays (Fairburn et al., 2017). Having an accessible treatment guide and training website has greatly increased access to training. At the time of writing this Group CBT-E guide, over 6,000 therapists from nearly 70 countries have completed the online training (R. Murphy personal communication, February 2024).

Riccardo Dalle Grave, Simona Calugi, and colleagues at Villa Garda Hospital, Italy, have further extended CBT-E by adapting it to treat adolescents and patients in HLOC. In 2020, they published a treatment guide specifically for CBT-E with young people: *Cognitive behavior therapy for adolescents with eating disorders* (Dalle Grave and Calugi, 2020).

Group CBT-E is a further extension of the treatment. It benefits from being built on the two treatment guides and real-world experience of implementing the treatment in a group format.

Recommended Reading

Dalle Grave, R., & Calugi, S. (2020). *Cognitive behavior therapy for adolescents with eating disorders.* Guilford Press, New York.

Fairburn, C. G. (2008). *Cognitive behavior therapy and eating disorders.* Guilford Press, New York.

References

Agras, W. S., Walsh, B. T., Fairburn, C. G., Wilson, G. T., & Kraemer, H. C. (2000). A multicenter comparison of cognitive-behavioral therapy and interpersonal psychotherapy for bulimia nervosa. *Archives of General Psychiatry*, 57(5), 459–466.

American Psychiatric Association. (2022). *Diagnostic and statistical manual of mental disorders* (5th ed., text rev.). https://doi.org/10.1176/appi.books.9780890425787

Atwood, M. E., & Friedman, A. (2020). A systematic review of enhanced cognitive behavioral therapy (CBT-E) for eating disorders. *International Journal of Eating Disorders*, 53(3), 311–330.

Bailey-Straebler, S., Redlak-Olcese, A., & Attia, E. (2022). Eating disorder treatment in very old age: A case for using CBT. *International Journal of Geriatric Psychiatry*, 37(1).

*Bailey-Straebler, S., Cooper, Z., Dalle Grave, R., Calugi, S., & Murphy, R. (2022). Development of the CBT-E components checklist: A tool for measuring therapist self-rated adherence to CBT-E. *IJEDO*, 4.

*Bohn, K., Doll, H. A., Cooper, Z., O'Connor, M., Palmer, R. L., & Fairburn, C. G. (2008). The measurement of impairment due to eating disorder psychopathology. *Behaviour Research and Therapy*, 46(10), 1105–1110.

Byrne, S. M., Fursland, A., Allen, K. L., & Watson, H. (2011). The effectiveness of enhanced cognitive behavioural therapy for eating disorders: An open trial. *Behaviour Research and Therapy*, 49(4), 219–226.

Cooper, Z., & Fairburn, C. G. (2011). The evolution of "enhanced" cognitive behavior therapy for eating disorders: Learning from treatment nonresponse. *Cognitive and Behavioral Practice*, 18(3), 394–402.

Cooper, Z., Bailey-Straebler, S., Morgan, K. E., O'Connor, M. E., Caddy, C., Hamadi, L., & Fairburn, C. G. (2017). Using the internet to train therapists: randomized comparison of two scalable methods. *Journal of Medical Internet Research*, 19(10), e355.

*Dalle Grave, R. (2012). Multistep cognitive behavioral therapy for eating disorders: theory, practice, and clinical cases. Jason Aronson, Incorporated.

Dalle Grave, R., & Calugi, S. (2020). *Cognitive behavior therapy for adolescents with eating disorders.* Guilford Press, New York.

Dalle Grave, R., Calugi, S., Conti, M., Doll, H., & Fairburn, C. G. (2013). Inpatient cognitive behaviour therapy for anorexia nervosa: a randomized controlled trial. *Psychotherapy and Psychosomatics*, 82(6), 390–398. doi:10.1159/000350058

*Dalle Grave, R., & el Khazen, C. (2021). *Cognitive behaviour therapy for eating disorders in young people: A parents' guide.* Routledge.

Dalle Grave, R., Sartirana, M., Dalle Grave, A., & Calugi, S. (2023). Effectiveness of enhanced cognitive behaviour therapy for patients aged 14 to 25: A promising treatment for anorexia nervosa in transition-age youth. *European Eating Disorders Review.* doi:10.1002/erv.3019

*Fairburn, C. G. (2008). Eating disorders: The transdiagnostic view and cognitive behavioral theory. In Fairburn C.G. *Cognitive behavior therapy and eating disorders.* Guilford Press, New York, 7–22.

*Fairburn, C. G., & Beglin, S. J. (2008). Eating disorder examination questionnaire (EDE-Q 6.0) 309-316. In Fairburn C.G. *Cognitive behavior therapy and eating disorders.* Guilford Press, New York, 309–316.

Fairburn, C. G., Kirk, J., O'Connor, M., & Cooper, P. J. (1986). A comparison of two psychological treatments for bulimia nervosa. *Behaviour Research and Therapy*, 24(6), 629–643.

Fairburn, C. G., Cooper, Z., & Shafran, R. (2003). Cognitive behaviour therapy for eating disorders: A "transdiagnostic" theory and treatment. *Behaviour Research and Therapy*, 41(5), 509–528.

Fairburn, C. G., Cooper, Z., Shafran, R., Bohn, K., Hawker, D. M., Murphy, R., & Straebler, S. (2008). Enhanced cognitive behavior therapy for eating disorders: the core protocol. In Fairburn C.G. *Cognitive behavior therapy and eating disorders*. Guilford Press, New York, 47–193.

Fairburn, C. G., Bailey-Straebler, S., Basden, S., Doll, H. A., Jones, R., Murphy, R., ... Cooper, Z. (2015). A transdiagnostic comparison of enhanced cognitive behaviour therapy (CBT-E) and interpersonal psychotherapy in the treatment of eating disorders. *Behaviour Research and Therapy*, 70, 64–71. doi:10.1016/j.brat.2015.04.010

Fairburn, C. G., Allen, E., Bailey-Straebler, S., O'Connor, M. E., & Cooper, Z. (2017). Scaling up psychological treatments: a countrywide test of the online training of therapists. *Journal of Medical Internet Research*, 19(6), e214.

Grilo, C. M. (2013). Why no cognitive body image feature such as overvaluation of shape/weight in the binge eating disorder diagnosis? *International Journal of Eating Disorders*, 46(3), 208–211.

Kaidesoja, M., Cooper, Z., & Fordham, B. (2023). Cognitive behavioral therapy for eating disorders: a map of the systematic review evidence base. *International Journal of Eating Disorders*, 56(2), 295–313.

National Institute of Health and Care Excellence. (2017, May 23). *Eating disorders: Recognition and treatment*. https://www.nice.org.uk/guidance/NG69

*Puhl, R. M., Latner, J. D., King, K. M., & Luedicke, J. (2014). Weight bias among professionals treating eating disorders: attitudes about treatment and perceived patient outcomes. *International Journal of Eating Disorders*, 47(1), 65–75.

Signorini, R., Sheffield, J., Rhodes, N., Fleming, C., & Ward, W. (2018). The effectiveness of enhanced cognitive behavioural therapy (CBT-E): A naturalistic study within an out-patient eating disorder service. *Behavioural and Cognitive Psychotherapy*, 46(1), 21–34.

*Waller, G. (2009). Evidence-based treatment and therapist drift. *Behaviour Research and Therapy*, 47(1), 1–9. https://doi.org/10.1016/j.brat.2008.10.004

Walsh, B. T., Hagan, K. E., & Lockwood, C. (2023). A systematic review comparing atypical anorexia nervosa and anorexia nervosa. *International Journal of Eating Disorders*, 56(4), 798–820.

Wang, S. B., Jones, P. J., Dreier, M., Elliott, H., & Grilo, C. M. (2019). Core psychopathology of treatment seeking patients with binge-eating disorder: a network analysis investigation. *Psychological Medicine*, 49(11), 1923–1928.

*References with asterisks appear for the first time in later chapters.

Chapter 3

Pre-treatment Assessment and Contraindications to Starting Outpatient Group CBT-E

Group CBT-E can be implemented sequentially as a complete treatment in outpatient settings or modularly at higher levels of care. There is no need to complete an assessment prior to offering modular sessions of Group CBT-E at HLOC, as this will have been completed as part of the program's comprehensive assessment. Equally, there are no specific contraindications to participating in Group CBT-E at HLOC, and suitability should be guided by individual program guidelines. This chapter focuses on assessment and contraindications for starting *outpatient* Group CBT-E.

Pre-treatment Assessment

Food Insecurity

Food insecurity can play a major role in the development and maintenance of an eating disorder. It is important to assess a patient's ability to regularly access adequate amounts of nutritious food and history of food insecurity.

Neurodivergence

Eating disorders are common among neurodivergent individuals and should be asked about as a part of your screening process. Neurodivergence, including autism, attention-deficit/hyperactivity disorder (ADHD), dyslexia, and other cognitive or developmental differences can influence how individuals perceive and interact with food, body image, social situations, and their environment. Group CBT-E was developed with neurodiversity in mind. The use of handouts to organize materials, following a clear structure, and avoiding confusing metaphors are some of the strategies included to make the therapy more accessible for all. The *Getting to Know Me* handout (Appendix E, included as a part of a Welcome Packet described in Chapter 5) can be especially helpful, setting the foundation for understanding sensory needs and ensuring that the group environment is inclusive.

DOI: 10.4324/9781003450849-3

Motivation and Engagement

In assessing patients for Group CBT-E, careful attention to their desire to engage in treatment is essential. Unlike Individual CBT-E, in Group CBT-E, less time is devoted to engendering motivation to change. Outpatient Group CBT-E is most appropriate for patients who are already in a place of wanting to change. In addition to assessing general motivation to start treatment, specifically consider the patient's interest in engaging in a *group* treatment. Group treatments are not a good fit for all patients. Be sure to assess a patient's history with group-based therapy, their reactions to being offered group-based therapy, and any barriers to fully engaging in the treatment. Be sure to also ask patients their motivation for wanting to start therapy now.

Attendance

In your screening process, assess for barriers to regular attendance and stress the importance of attending all sessions. Consistent attendance is important for the group, but also for the individual in terms of getting the most out of treatment. During the screening, it can be helpful to map out when the sessions will be held, including the end date, and ask about upcoming vacations or events that would prevent complete attendance.

Preferences and Other Considerations

At the end of the screen, ask patients if there is anything else about them that would be helpful for you to know. Asking this question has two aims: 1) to give the patient the opportunity to add anything else about the eating disorder that may not have been elicited during the screening; and 2) to allow the patient to add anything else that is important about themselves to share.

Outpatient Group CBT-E is ideally suited to patients with an eating disorder who:

• have a primary diagnosis of BED, BN, and their subthreshold versions
• do not require substantial weight regain
• are motivated to engage in treatment and
• are comfortable in group settings.

Screening patients for suitability for Group CBT-E requires assessing eating disorder symptom severity based on symptom duration, frequency, intensity, and impact on functioning. These factors interact with one another to inform the appropriateness of Group CBT-E and therefore cannot be considered in isolation. For example, a recent onset of eating disorder behaviors, or a short duration of symptoms, may indicate that outpatient treatment is appropriate, but the frequency of the symptoms and impact on functioning will fully determine this. For example, for a patient with a short duration of illness, but high frequency of self-induced vomiting (e.g., three times a day) and symptoms of dizziness, outpatient Group CBT-E is likely inappropriate. Another patient who has been vomiting daily for many years without medical impact may well be appropriate for this group.

Appendix C provides a more thorough sample assessment tool, with specific questions to ask patients. The information below covers some of the general considerations when conducting an assessment.

Eating Disorder-related Behaviors

It is essential to understand which eating disorder symptoms a patient is struggling with and if these symptoms occur within the context of body shape or weight concerns. The main symptoms to assess are food restriction, binge eating, self-induced vomiting, medication misuse (e.g., laxatives, diuretics, diet pills), and driven exercise.

A helpful place to begin is to ask for a 24-hour food and fluid intake recall. Many patients will have what they describe as a "good" day, when they are highly in control of their eating, and a "bad" day, when they experience episodes of out-of-control eating. You will want a recall for both types of day, listening for differences in intake (including delayed eating, undereating, and/or avoiding certain types of foods), what may have led to any out-of-control eating, specifics related to the food that they are consuming (e.g., portions, diet-type foods), and how frequently they experience "good" and "bad" days per week. Be sure to ask about frequency, duration, and intensity of reported binge eating (assess for both subjective – a small or moderate amount of food that is perceived as large – and objective binge eating), compensatory behaviors (e.g., self-induced vomiting, laxative abuse), and driven exercise.

Driven Exercise

Driven exercise can either be compensatory (to counteract calories consumed) or non-compensatory (as a routine weight-control method). Clues to identify driven exercise include: feeling guilty if unable to exercise, exercising through injuries, following a rigid exercise routine, exercising to the exclusion of other enjoyable life activities, and exercising to "earn" food.

Eating Disorder-related Thoughts

In addition to eating disorder symptoms and behaviors, you will assess for eating disorder-related thoughts. Here you are assessing: 1) whether the patient has eating disorder-related thoughts and 2) the frequency or intensity of these thoughts. These thoughts most often consist of negative body image judgments, a fear of gaining weight, and/or a preoccupation with weight, shape, body, or appearance, often to the exclusion of other aspects of life. If the patient reports no body shape or weight concerns but does endorse eating disorder behaviors, such as a loss of control when eating, this could indicate a diagnosis of BED. If, in this situation, the patient does not meet the criteria for an eating disorder, determine if the symptoms are due to another mental health diagnosis (e.g., anxiety, depression) or another eating disorder diagnosis that is not treated in Group CBT-E (e.g., ARFID).

Table 3.1 Symptoms Indicating the Need for a Same Day Visit with a Medical Provider or an Emergency Room Visit

- Dizziness
- Faintness
- Feeling disoriented
- Confusion or memory loss
- Heart palpitations
- Chest pains
- Shortness of breath
- Blood in vomit
- Edema (swelling) of ankles or face
- Acute food or fluid refusal
- Recent rapid weight loss of more than 3lbs/week for the previous several weeks.

Physical Symptoms

Eating disorders are associated with a number of physical symptoms (detailed in Appendix C). Ask patients if they are experiencing any of the following: menstrual irregularities or lack of menstruation (if applicable), fatigue, poor sleep, bone aches and pains, feeling cold much of the time, gastrointestinal distress, muscle pain, constipation, watery stool, acid reflux, dental cavities, issues with energy, weakness, issues with concentration/memory, or hair loss. If any of the symptoms listed in Table 3.1 are endorsed, this indicates the need for a same day medical appointment.

Height and Weight

Understanding a patient's weight history (and their current height) can be helpful in determining if outpatient group treatment is an appropriate fit. In evaluating this data, consider current weight relative to a patient's individual weight trend history, and height.

Many patients will be maintaining a weight that is *somewhat* lower than their body needs (underweight) and/or are *somewhat* underfat (body fat percentage that is too low). This is common in individuals with eating disorders and is often a factor maintaining the illness. Group CBT-E can be suitable for these patients. It is essential to emphasize to patients that some weight regain/increased fat intake is often required to fully overcome the eating disorder (described further on *Underweight/Underfat* handout).

Weight Suppression

You may notice that we use the phrase *maintaining a weight lower than one's body needs* or *being underfat*. In some literature, weight suppression is used to describe this state. However, more standardly, weight suppression is defined as the difference between one's highest weight and one's current weight, which we believe does not accurately reflect each instance of maintaining a weight lower that one's body needs or an underfat state.

Patients who have lost *significant* amounts of weight or are maintaining a weight too low for their body are not appropriate for the outpatient version of Group CBT-E as it does not cover weight regain. To determine if a patient is at a weight too low for their body, consider the following:

- for adults: weight history timeline (highest adult weight outside of pregnancies; lowest adult weight)
- for adolescents/transition aged youth: previous and current growth charts (if available)
- rapid, recent weight loss (>3 lbs/week for several weeks)
- presence of physical symptoms listed above
- weight during periods of time without eating disorder symptoms (if applicable)
- current eating patterns and adequacy of overall nutritional intake
- evidence of undereating as a method of weight control: missing meals or snacks; low caloric intake; lack of variety; significant avoidance of dietary fats, carbohydrates, and/ or protein
- consultation with their primary care provider (PCP)
- a nutrition assessment with a dietitian

If patients report that they do not know their weight, or sound hesitant to share their weight history, be sure to balance empathy with providing a rationale for why you need this information to ensure that Group CBT-E is best suited for their particular needs. Initial weights can be obtained by a PCP and shared directly with the intake team/therapist if the patient prefers this.

Diagnoses and Medication

Understanding the patient's current and past medical and psychiatric diagnoses, as well as any current medication regimen, is an important component of screening for appropriateness. Group CBT-E may not be an appropriate intervention for patients with specific comorbidities (see section below, 'Counterindications to Group CBT-E') and these need to be assessed and alternative treatment plans identified.

Self-Report Measures

Self-report outcome measures provide additional information on current symptoms. The Eating Disorder Examination Questionnaire (EDE-Q; Fairburn & Beglin, 2008) and the Clinical Impairment Assessment (CIA; Bohn et al., 2008) are standardly used measures in CBT-E. The EDE-Q and CIA are self-report measures focusing on the previous 28 days. The EDE-Q is a measure of eating disorder symptomatology and evaluates eating disorder behaviors and thoughts related to the disorder. The CIA is a measure of how the eating disorder impacts quality of life, assessing the secondary psychosocial impacts of the disorder. Both of these measures can be administered as part of an initial patient pre-assessment and are used at specific time points during treatment. They are both freely available at: www.cbte.co

Information to Share During an Assessment

Group CBT-E Education

Treatment suitability relies on the patient receiving a brief description of the treatment to allow them to make an informed choice about participating in the therapy. The description should include the focus of the treatment (e.g., what is keeping the eating disorder going now, not what caused it to start), that treatment is active and centers around making change, and that handouts are used to convey important treatment information with follow-up between session work (see Chapter 5 for more details). Finally, patients should be aware that the treatment consists of 14 weekly groups with a clear beginning and end. In our experience, few patients and providers are familiar with short-term psychological treatments like CBT-E. It is therefore essential to explain the treatment and treatment expectations to patients before they commit to joining the group. The focus and style of Group CBT-E may not be compatible with what patients are looking for in their care.

Consent to Speak with Other Providers

We request consent to speak with other members of the patient's outpatient medical and psychological treatment team (e.g., adolescent medicine providers, dietitians, PCPs, psychiatrists, psychiatric nurse practitioners, and therapists). We recommend sharing the *Guide for Outpatient Providers* (found in Appendix E) at the start of the patient's course of treatment with all outpatient providers.

Information to Share with Support People

For patients who are under the age of 18, parents/guardians will be involved in some aspects of the screening to provide their concerns and observations. For adults, support people may be a part of the screening process. With the patient's consent, we involve these support people in conversations about the structure, nature, and expectations of CBT-E, and the potential involvement of support people as a part of between-session work.

Contraindications to Group CBT-E

There are times when Group CBT-E is not the appropriate fit. It goes without saying that patient safety is the highest concern when delivering any form of psychological treatment. Eating disorders are associated with numerous medical consequences, though these are far less common when working in outpatient settings. Eating disorders are also associated with high levels of psychiatric comorbidity, including depression and suicidality. Therefore, screening for both medical symptoms and psychiatric comorbidities is essential.

Medical Safety and Stability

While it is less common for patients suitable for outpatient care to have a medical symptom that makes them ineligible to start Group CBT-E, we rely on PCPs to assess medical stability for outpatient treatment. This typically includes complete routine bloodwork and vital signs check, and sometimes an electrocardiogram (EKG). Unless you are a therapist with the medical training required to review and interpret the results, it is important to confirm with the PCP that the results indicate medical stability prior to starting treatment.

If during the screening (or at any point during treatment) a patient reports any of the symptoms in Table 3.1, they are advised to see their PCP with a same day or "sick visit" appointment. If they sound or appear to be in acute distress, they should go to their local emergency department.

Suicidality and Non-suicidal Self-injurious Behaviors

In the outpatient setting, patients who are actively and acutely suicidal are not appropriate for starting Group CBT-E. Similarly, patients who become suicidal during the group treatment need to have the focus of their treatment shifted to one of safety management. For some patients, low-level, chronic suicidality is not an exclusion criterion. In addition, actively engaging in non-suicidal self-injurious behaviors (e.g., cutting and/or burning skin) may not be a reason to determine Group CBT-E is inappropriate, depending on the severity of the behavior. You need to be aware of your own comfort level and experience with including patients with chronic suicidality or non-suicidal self-injurious behavior in your groups.

Patients who report previous suicidal ideation, chronic suicidality, a history of substance misuse, or a history of engaging in self-harm are at risk of experiencing an increase or return of these concerns while undergoing treatment for their eating disorder. This risk may increase as a result of eliminating eating disorder behaviors that may have been acting as coping mechanisms. These patients require additional assessment to consider how removing the eating disorder may affect them.

Patients who report previous suicidal ideation, chronic suicidality, or current or historical self-harm behaviors may be at risk of increased suicidal thinking or urges to engage in self-harm as a result of attending the group. This is due to the likelihood that the eating disorder behaviors are functioning as self-soothing behaviors, distractions, or a method of self-regulation. By removing the eating disorder behaviors – the treatment goal of Group CBT-E– patients may be vulnerable to returning to these other behaviors. We speak openly with patients and their providers prior to the start of group to allow them to assess their current stability related to safety and consider the impact that removing the eating disorder may have. Throughout Group CBT-E, assess for increases in suicidal thinking or urges to engage in self-harm behaviors.

Patients who experience severely intense emotion dysregulation that causes significant dysfunction and an inability to receive treatment as intended may not benefit fully from Group CBT-E. For these patients, a course of treatment that targets this directly, such as Dialectical

Behavior Therapy (DBT), may be a necessary step before addressing the eating disorder. Another option may be to offer Individual CBT-E, which provides strategies for more comprehensive work in this area.

Psychiatric Comorbidities

Psychiatric comorbidities are common in individuals with eating disorders. Mood disorders, anxiety disorders, previous trauma, post-traumatic stress disorder (PTSD), obsessive compulsive disorder (OCD), and some personality disorders/characteristics frequently co-occur with eating disorders. Determining the best order of treatment is an area currently receiving increased attention. In time, clear guidelines may be developed on how and/or when to combine treatments or use protocols that target underlying shared mechanisms. At the time of writing this book, our view is:

- When possible, the eating disorder should be treated first, the rationale being that treating the eating disorder first, and any related malnourishment or preoccupations with eating, shape, and weight, will allow the individual to more actively engage in treatment focused on other mental health concerns. It should also be noted that often treating the eating disorder first can resolve other mental health symptoms that were initially present. We have seen many patients struggling with symptoms of depression or anxiety at the start of eating disorder treatment who no longer had these symptoms, or the symptoms significantly decreased in severity, by the end of their eating disorder treatment. This may be because they were eating regularly, were more engaged in life as a result of their recovery progress, and/or had learned new skills/strategies that could also be applied to their comorbid symptoms.

- There are times when it is essential to treat the co-existing disorder(s) as primary. Some cases where this is true include occasions where the comorbid disorder interferes fully with eating disorder treatment engagement. For example, some patients have a separate (not caused by the eating disorder) clinical depression. In these cases, depression must be treated prior to starting Group CBT-E.

- Sometimes you will not know which disorder needs targeting first before starting treatment. In these cases, we suggest that you begin Group CBT-E and change the patient's treatment course if they are unable to make progress, possibly related to a comorbidity. At times, patients may benefit from concurrent treatments.

Substance Misuse

Co-existing substance use disorder is a contraindication to starting Group CBT-E and should be targeted prior to starting eating disorder treatment. Occasional use of substances would not prevent someone from joining the group. However, attending group intoxicated is not permissible as it can be harmful to other group members and also greatly interferes with the individual's ability to make use of the treatment.

In a similar way to individuals who engage in non-suicidal self-injurious behavior, those who use substances to regulate their emotions or mood are at higher risk of using more substances as the eating disorder behaviors are removed and ideally replaced with more recovery-aligned coping mechanisms. Patients should be made aware of this increased vulnerability and supported throughout the group with check-ins and encouragement to continue with any substance abuse program they may be involved with.

Not Providing Consent to Speak with Other Providers

Some patients may not have disclosed to other providers about their eating disorder (perhaps related to shame and embarrassment) and therefore do not want you to speak with them. Despite wanting to honor our patients' wishes regarding disclosing information about their eating disorder, we have decided that we cannot safely implement Group CBT-E with patients who do not give us permission to speak with their other providers. This is especially important with regard to medication prescribers, as there are some medications which are harmful to take when one has an eating disorder. Eating disorders can thrive in secrecy and we believe that the most effective way to treat a patient is to ensure that all treatment team members are openly communicating about the treatment plan, patient goals and needs, and provider concerns. We acknowledge this may be a barrier to care for some patients. Without this team approach, however, we cannot provide safe and effective care.

Weight Loss Treatment

Group CBT-E is not a weight loss treatment and is incompatible with concurrent weight loss treatment. It is inadvisable for patients engaged in weight loss treatment, or planning to start weight loss treatment while in group, to start Group CBT-E. Provide education that the goal of Group CBT-E is to focus on resolving eating disorder symptoms, not to lose weight.

Chapter 4

Group CBT-E

Overview and Treatment Structure

Group CBT-E: A Brief Overview

Group CBT-E contains the main elements of the focused format of Individual CBT-E (Fairburn et al., 2008), adapted for group delivery. Sessions can be implemented at all levels of care: higher levels of care (HLOCs; inpatient units, residential treatment centers, partial hospital programs, intensive outpatient programs) and outpatient programs.

To accommodate these different settings, Group CBT-E can be delivered in two ways: sequentially for outpatient treatment or modularly/non-sequentially (sessions delivered in any order as appropriate), as part of a treatment package at HLOCs. The ability to use the guide in this flexible manner allows for access across levels of care. The goals of treatment differ somewhat between these two versions. The sequential version is considered a complete standalone treatment, while the modular version aims to introduce some of the concepts of CBT-E and provides foundational psychoeducation. Multiple factors at HLOCs make sequential delivery impractical, due to varying number of treatment days, different treatment start dates, and/or patients who require weight regain. We have found that offering groups modularly at HLOCs is well liked by both patients and therapists. Group CBT-E session content can be implemented in a similar way in both outpatient settings and HLOCs. At the end of each session chapter, HLOC modification considerations are presented.

> **Group CBT-E Delivery Methods**
>
> Outpatient: **Sequential**
> Higher Level of Care: **Modular**

Treatment Goals

Described by Dalle Grave and Calugi (2020), CBT-E has several main goals:

1. To engage patients in treatment and involve them actively in the process of change.

2. To reduce and/or fully remove all eating disorder psychopathology and related behaviors, including dietary restriction, binge eating, compensatory behaviors, driven exercise, and the over-evaluation of shape and weight.

DOI: 10.4324/9781003450849-4

3. To disable the mechanisms that keep the eating disorder psychopathology and related behaviors active.

4. To ensure lasting change.

Differences Between Group CBT-E and Individual CBT-E

Group CBT-E closely follows Individual CBT-E, and mirrors the treatment goals above with some structural and intervention adaptations. For those with a background in CBT-E, you will notice these differences. Table 4.1 captures the main changes and provides a rationale for doing so. Our goal in making these essential adaptations is to allow increased access to the treatment without diluting the treatment effect.

In addition to these adaptations, some Individual CBT-E-specific terms have been updated. These include "urge surfing," "feeling fat," and "mirror checking." The changes to the language for urge surfing and feeling fat were made, in collaboration with patient input, to "urge tolerating" and "body dissatisfaction spikes." "Mirror checking" has been changed to "reflection checking" to capture the behaviors of checking one's reflection in photographs (e.g., selfies) and video (e.g., virtual meetings) which are now more prevalent than when Individual CBT-E was designed.

There are also two new intervention acronyms introduced in Group CBT-E. The acronyms do not change the underlying principles of the interventions as presented in Individual CBT-E, but are used to efficiently, and memorably, describe tools to support change. These are the RAD Approach and the AIM for Change strategy. Both are initially described in detail in Sessions 4 (Chapter 9) and 8 (Chapter 13). The RAD Approach is a tool to support addressing feelings of fullness and body dissatisfaction spikes and AIM for Change is used to reduce body shape and weight checking, and avoidance.

Overview of Group CBT-E Stages and Session Content: Sequential Version

Outpatient Group CBT-E is a standalone treatment. It consists of 14 sessions divided over four treatment stages. Sessions are designed to be one hour in length and held weekly. Table 4.2 contains a treatment outline for sequential application.

Stage One: Achieving Early Change

- *Duration: 4 sessions*
- *Sessions numbers: 1–4*
- *Corresponding Chapters: Chapters 6–9*
- *Goals*:
    - *Engage in treatment and the idea of change*
    - *Create a personalized formulation*
    - *Establish regular eating*

Table 4.1 Group Adaptations to CBT-E

Areas with Adaptations	Individual Format	Group Format	Rationale
Treatment and Session length	~20 total sessions 45–50-minute sessions	14 total sessions 60-minute sessions	Group CBT-E contains the major treatment interventions of Individual CBT-E, but in a shorter overall timeframe. Group sessions last longer, making the total treatment time comparable to Individual CBT-E. The use of handouts in Group CBT-E allows for more efficient treatment delivery.
Session frequency	Twice weekly for four weeks, then weekly for 10 sessions, then every other week for the final three sessions	Weekly throughout	Patient feedback indicated that patients found they were better able to commit to weekly rather than twice-weekly sessions.
Agenda setting	Collaborative between therapist and patient	Set by therapist	Collaborative agenda setting is not possible in this group format, due to an inability to attend to each patient's individual items.
Treatment led by	Therapist	More jointly led by therapist and patient (aided by handouts)	Patients lead their own therapy, facilitated by the therapist and handouts that are completed individually by patients.
Weekly weighing	Collaborative with patient initiated in Stage 1	Led by patient, initiated in Stage 3 along with other body checking and avoidance behaviors	As designed for Individual CBT-E, collaborative weighing is not possible in a group setting without additional individual time to allow for proper implementation of the intervention. Additionally, we wanted to move the emphasis away from weight as a specific intervention in Stage 1 and conceptualize it similarly to other body checking and avoidance behaviors in Stage 3.
Delivery method	Sequentially	Sequentially or non-sequentially (modularly)	Group CBT-E is ideally implemented sequentially; however, sequential treatments are not always possible or practical, especially at HLOC. In higher levels of care, introducing patients to these helpful topics, that can be incorporated into later stages of treatment, provides for a useful continuum of care.
Joint sessions with support people	0–3 (adults) 8–10 (adolescents)	No individual sessions; regular sharing of treatment materials	Group CBT-E does not utilize individual joint sessions with support people; however, use of support people is greatly emphasized in most sessions as a part of between-session work. Additional guidance on involving support people is provided in Appendix D.
Post-treatment review session	20 weeks after treatment ends	No follow-up	Patient feedback indicated that returning for a follow-up group session was challenging in outpatient care and impractical at higher levels of care.

Table 4.2 Group CBT-E Stages and Sessions – Sequential Version

Stage 1 Achieving Early Change	Session 1: Introductions, Personalized Formulations, and Self-monitoring Session 2: Personalized Formulations and Self-monitoring Review and Regular Eating Session 3: Regular Eating and Alternative Activities Session 4: Regular Eating, Urge Tolerating, and Feelings of Fullness
Stage 2 Reviewing Progress	Session 5: Progress Review
Stage 3 Dismantling the Eating Disorder-maintaining Mechanisms	Session 6: Dieting Behaviors and Diet-Related Rules Session 7: The Over-evaluation of Shape and Weight and Its Consequences Session 8: Body Shape and Weight Checking – Part I Session 9: Body Shape and Weight Checking – Part II Session 10: Body Shape and Weight Avoidance Session 11: Stage three Check-in and Body Dissatisfaction Spikes Session 12: Events, Emotions, and Eating
Stage 4 Ending Well	Session 13: Historical Review of the Eating Disorder Behaviors and Thoughts Session 14: Relapse Prevention and Ending Treatment

The first stage of Group CBT-E is focused on quickly engaging the patient in treatment and collaborating on a CBT-E treatment plan, using techniques such as group introductions and personalized formulation creation. The main focus of this stage is on behavior modification, or how to make behavior changes to achieve a pattern of regular eating. These sessions incorporate psychoeducation, self-monitoring to increase awareness of eating disorder behaviors and the mechanisms that maintain them, and applying specific interventions to strengthen regular eating (e.g., alternative activities, urge tolerating, addressing feelings of fullness).

Stage Two: Reviewing Progress

- *Duration: 1 session*
- *Session number: 5*
- *Corresponding Chapter: Chapter 10*
- *Goals:*
  - *Review progress*
  - *Identify barriers to change*

Stage 2 focuses on reviewing progress in treatment, both the patient's progress, and your own as the Group CBT-E therapist. Any barriers to change are identified and feedback is provided on taking action steps to continue with making changes. This stage is an opportunity to collect updated outcome measures and to have patients review these to explore their response to treatment thus far. Stage 2 also provides an opportunity for patients and the therapist to collaboratively identify any concerns about the patient's continuation in the group treatment and to identify an alternate treatment plan, if needed. Following this session, be sure to assess your progress as a group leader and identify barriers to effective group implementation.

Stage Three: Dismantling the Eating Disorder-maintaining Mechanisms

- *Duration: 7 sessions*
- *Sessions: 6–12*
- *Corresponding Chapters: 11–17*
- *Goals*:
  - *Identify and address the remaining maintaining mechanisms that keep the eating disorder going*

In Stage 3, the focus of the sessions is on addressing the primary mechanisms that maintain the eating disorder. These mechanisms can be thought of as the behaviors, thoughts, emotions, or situations that continue to trigger the eating disorder. Maintaining mechanisms such as dieting behaviors and diet-related rules, the over-evaluation of shape and weight, and event- and emotion-related changes in eating will be the focus of this stage. Addressing each of these mechanisms provides patients with the skills needed to overcome common triggers of eating disorder symptoms both in the short and long term.

In Session 6, patients are introduced to the concepts of dieting behaviors and diet-related rules. Psychoeducation on how these behaviors directly impact and increase eating disorder symptoms, as well as strategies to reduce this impact, are provided. Specific CBT-E skills include psychoeducation on diet culture, behaviors, and rules, as well as introducing exposure to avoided foods.

Sessions 7–11, focus on the over-evaluation of shape and weight to define self-worth, in which patients address behavioral and cognitive aspects of body image. Specific CBT-E skills in these sessions include: increasing areas of life unrelated to shape and weight that have been minimized by the eating disorder; addressing body shape/weight checking and avoidance; and addressing body dissatisfaction spikes.

Session 12 addresses event- and emotion-related changes in eating and how events and emotions impact eating disorder symptoms (and vice versa). Specific CBT-E skills include problem-solving, symptom/urge analysis, and breaking the emotion and eating disorder connection.

Stage Four: Ending Well

- *Duration: 2 sessions*
- *Sessions: 13 and 14*
- *Corresponding Chapters: Chapters 18–19*
- *Goals*:
  - *Consider the historical origins of the eating disorder*
  - *Ensure that changes are maintained*
  - *Reduce the risk of relapse*
  - *Process the ending of group therapy*

The final stage of Group CBT-E focuses on understanding the historical origins of the eating disorder, relapse prevention, and ending treatment. Session 13 explores the origin of the eating disorder behaviors and thoughts, and patients engage in between-session work to symbolically let go of their eating disorder. In Session 14, patients reflect on their learning and progress throughout the group. Specific attention is placed on continuing to use the skills learned in treatment moving forward and recognizing signs that the eating disorder is becoming activated. This stage also addresses feelings about treatment ending and setting up a plan for weekly self-check-ins.

Overview of Group CBT-E at Higher Levels of Care: Modular Version

Like Dalle Grave (2012), when applying Group CBT-E in HLOCs, we advise matching CBT-E stages to the appropriate level of care, based on patient needs. For example, the highest levels of care may focus exclusively on medical stabilization and the behavior changes that are the focus of Stage 1, while lower levels of care may introduce Stage 3 concepts, such as diet-related rules, body image, and the connection between events, emotions, and eating.

For HLOC programs that are not CBT-E based, Table 4.3 is intended to help guide the implementation of Group CBT-E and lists the content that can be offered in more intensive treatments. Keep in mind that this list serves as a sample only. Some particular considerations include:

• As mentioned, at the end of each of the group session chapters, there is specific guidance on HLOC adaptations of the treatment. Included in this guidance are recommendations for instances when group sessions could be broken down into several HLOC group sessions, as presented in Table 4.3.

Table 4.3 Examples of Higher Level of Care Group CBT-E Sessions

Personalized Formulation	Other Areas of Life
Psychoeducation (Dieting, Binge Eating, Underweight/Underfat, Driven Exercise, Medication Misuse)[a]	Body Shape and Weight Checking
Self-monitoring Review[b]	Reflection Checking
Regular Eating[b]	Body Comparisons
Alternative Activities	Social Media Body Checking
Urge Tolerating	Body Shape and Weight Avoidance
Feelings of Fullness	Body Dissatisfaction Spikes
Progress Review[b]	Events, Emotions, and Eating
Dieting Behaviors and Diet-related Rules	Historical Review
Over-evaluation of Shape and Weight	Relapse Prevention

[a] This group may require multiple sessions.
[b] These groups likely require more frequent repetition.

- It can be helpful to repeat certain CBT-E groups during a patient's treatment stay. In particular, the interventions related to self-monitoring, regular eating, and progress review would be beneficial to regularly review throughout treatment and not always as part of a group. This can be done in a variety of different formats in addition to group therapy sessions, including adding these components to individual meetings with therapists, psychiatrists, or dietitians; before or after therapeutic meals; or to community meetings.

- In HLOCs, many patients have eating disorder symptoms that lead to being at weights that are substantially lower than one's body needs and/or are substantially underfat. Group CBT-E can be applied modularly in HLOCs for these patients as a part of a more comprehensive treatment plan. Additional topics are encouraged, such as education about the effects of this weight status, motivation, and working toward weight restoration, and these are well described in Fairburn (2008) and Dalle Grave et al. (2013).

Chapter 5

Group CBT-E
Elements and Therapist Characteristics

This chapter reviews important considerations for group preparation, agenda items that carry through session by session, and therapist style. Understanding these considerations is necessary to adequately prepare for implementing Group CBT-E. Appendix D is a helpful supplement to this chapter and offers additional considerations prior to implementing Group CBT-E.

Preparation for the Start of Group CBT-E

Prior to starting treatment, each patient should receive a Group CBT-E Welcome Packet. This Welcome Packet includes important information for the patient to review or complete ahead of the initial session. We recommend that the following resources are included in the Welcome Packet (the first three are located in Appendix E, the final two can be found at www.cbte.co):

- *17.1 Group CBT-E* handout
- *17.2 Group Session Content* handout
- *17.3 Getting to Know Me* handout
- *EDE-Q*
- *CIA*

Common Elements of Each Group Session

Each group session will generally follow the following agenda:

1. Agenda setting and orientation to session
2. Between-session work self-review
3. Specific CBT-E session content
4. Group wrap-up

1. Agenda Setting and Orientation to Session

Group CBT-E relies on a clearly stated agenda to structure each session, listed at the start of each session chapter. We have found that providing patients with the planned session

DOI: 10.4324/9781003450849-5

content for all groups at the start of the treatment can be useful for those who like to prepare for what is coming. The *Group Session Content* handout can be given to patients at the outset as part of the Welcome Packet. At the start of each session, openly share with the group the agenda for that particular session and visually display agenda items, using a tool such as a whiteboard.

The presentation of an agenda should include four important elements:

1. A positive, encouraging welcome to set the tone for the rest of the session
2. Current session number and treatment stage
3. Number of sessions remaining
4. Clearly listed CBT-E content that will be the focus of the session

2. Between-session Work Self-review

Between-session work, sometimes called "next steps" or "homework" in other therapies, are the skills learned in group, and goals identified, that patients will practice outside of the sessions. The importance of between-session work cannot be overstated. This works allows patients to apply therapeutic skills outside of the sessions in their own environments under the stress of their daily lives. Work between sessions is critical for the treatment to be effective. Introducing the importance of between-session work starts at the beginning of Session 1 when introducing group therapy expectations. Between-session work is additive. Once a patient has worked on a particular goal, it will likely require continued practice and focus throughout all subsequent weeks and may be included in a relapse prevention plan.

At times, a patient may decide to include a support person to augment their between-session work. We recommend that patients use their supports as much as possible in this treatment and, if willing and appropriate, provide an update to their support person after each group, perhaps reviewing handouts and Action Plans with them. Not all patients will have someone they feel could be a support person and they may share feelings of sadness or embarrassment about this. Meet this with empathy, consider with the patient if there may be supports in their lives that they haven't considered (e.g., colleagues, neighbors, friends that they have lost touch with, family they believe are too busy), and, if there is not a support person available, remind the patient that all between-session work is individualized and can be completed independently.

Group CBT-E starts each session, apart from Session 1, with patients completing a brief self-review handout, the *Between-session Work Self-review* handout. Starting in Session 2, there is one handout for each session which is individually tailored to that specific session and expected to be completed at the start of the session. The self-review handouts allow patients to assess how much of the between-session work they have completed, as well as identify areas to take action for the following week. This self-review allows the patients to quickly assess progress and identify barriers to progress, as well as reinforce the importance of between-session work completion and identify clear goals going forward. After completing the handouts independently, patients are offered a brief opportunity to discuss the self-review as a group, before the main group content begins.

3. Specific CBT-E Session Content

Each session will cover specific CBT-E interventions. The interventions or skills are the tools that will support a patient in overcoming their eating disorder. The content is delivered through a combination of therapist facilitation, peer support, and handouts. A main goal of the therapist is to ensure that all patients are provided with the essential tools by the end of treatment. Not only will learning these skills help a patient in the active phase of their eating disorder, but it also is extremely important to preventing relapse and staying well.

4. Group Wrap-up

You will cover a lot of detailed and useful material in each session. It can be hard for patients to remember it all. Having a group wrap-up at the end of each session is necessary. Group wrap-up scripts are included in each session chapter. The wrap-up has two aims:

1. Briefly summarize the main content and skills learned in the session
2. Have patients write down the between-session work

Other Group CBT-E Treatment Elements

Handouts

As discussed in Chapter 1, each group session includes handouts that group members personalize to their specific experience and eating disorder symptoms. Handouts in Group CBT-E make the therapy more patient led by guiding the session, rather than relying primarily on the therapist. These handouts are essential because they allow for individualization within group therapy, ensure that each patient receives key treatment content, provide visual tools that reinforce verbal material, and emphasize that treatment extends beyond group sessions. As such, they are designed to be reviewed and worked on both during the course of treatment and afterward as part of relapse prevention. Many handouts also include an Action Plan. Action Plans allow patients to describe, in specific ways, how they intend to implement a skill or tool. By writing down a defined plan, patients have a clear idea of what to work on, increasing the likelihood of completing the task. By the end of a session, patients may have created multiple Action Plans to reach their goals. Additional blank Action Plans can be found in Appendix E.

Handouts continued throughout treatment are referred to as Standard Weekly Handouts, while others will change with the session and are Session-specific Handouts. At the start of each session, there is a list of all necessary handouts. In the text, the relevant handout is labelled under the corresponding agenda item.

Assessment Measures

Table 5.1 provides suggested times to use assessment measures (described in Chapter 2) when the treatment is delivered sequentially. In Sessions 5 and 14, these measures will be reviewed by the patients in the group to highlight progress and identify areas requiring additional therapeutic focus.

Table 5.1 Measurement Administration Timetable

Measurement	Frequency
EDE-Q	Time point 1: Prior to session 1 Time point 2: Session 4 Time point 3: Session 13
CIA	Time point 1: Prior to session 1 Time point 2: Session 4 Time point 3: Session 13
EPCL	Weekly (optional)

Settings and programs that require, or are interested in, a weekly questionnaire are encouraged to use the Eating Problem Checklist (EPCL; Dalle Grave and Calugi, 2020). The EPCL is a self-report measure that assesses eating disorder symptomatology on a weekly basis and is meant to be used session by session to assess improvement or deterioration. The frequency of administration of the EPCL makes it a helpful choice not only to assess week-by-week changes, but also at HLOCs where treatment length varies.

Therapist Preparation

All sessions require a certain amount of therapist preparation. A preparation checklist is provided in each session which includes items to review in advance and/or guidance on a particular session or intervention.

Group Therapy Process and Patient Participation

As a group therapy, this treatment offers a multitude of unique group-based benefits including:

- Increased social support and connectedness
- Interpersonal learning
- Exposure to new perspectives
- Group belongingness and opportunities to decrease shame related to stigma
- Social skill practice

Group Therapy Process

Each group session will utilize the group process to support patients in better accessing and applying the treatment interventions. Some examples of important group techniques include:

- *Group Discussion*: Discussing information and skills as a group is widely utilized throughout this treatment. The therapist engages the group in discussion topics that may include psychoeducation, responses to a between-session work activity, or aspects of a topic that the therapist would like the group to reflect on. For example, when discussing body checking (Session 8), the therapist engages the group in a discussion about what they learned from a body checking self-monitoring activity. This allows patients to learn from one another and potentially decrease shame related to these sometimes embarrassing behaviors.

The process of discussing interventions as a group helps patients to learn from one another, consider others' learning and perspectives, and, at times, shift perspectives through accepting a fellow group member's support. This support sometimes means having one group member compassionately challenge another's assumption or viewpoint; while at other times, it may mean one group member sharing how they relate to another based on personal experience. Patients may hear from another group member something that they relate to that they otherwise would not have thought to consider. An example of this style of intervention is the creation of the food rules list (Session 6). In this session, patients have the opportunity to share aloud food rules that they hold. Oftentimes hearing others' food rules can remind patients of their own rules, which allows for the ability to make an Action Plan to thoughtfully challenge such rules.

- *Use of Whiteboards*: In combination with group discussion, whiteboards are a great way to keep patients engaged with a variety of learning styles. Throughout the treatment guide, there will be references to using a whiteboard (or another similar tool) to share information visually. Included in the session text are many whiteboard examples. The examples show what collaboratively created lists generated in group may look like. Having an easily accessible tool to record material that is discussed in group is very useful. Not only does displaying this material on a whiteboard help with visual learning, but it also allows for the material to be more easily transcribed by the patients onto their own handouts.

- *In-Session Ratings*: To aid with collecting a lot of group feedback at once and to keep patients engaged, we recommend setting up a clear and consistent rating system for the patients to use to provide quick answers. For example, we find that asking patients to give a thumb rating works well (thumb up=yes, thumb down=no, thumb side=sometimes/maybe/I don't know). Have fun coming up with an idea – consider emojis, green/yellow/red cards, or raising hands. This is an engaging and efficient way to collect information and have patients provide information to each other. It also provides a non-verbal way to participate and share emotions and progress, which may be more comfortable for some group members. Once a rating is collected, depending on the responses and the agenda, you may have additional follow-up discussion, or you may be well set up with the information that you need and can quickly move to the next agenda item to stay within the time limits of the session.

- *Patient Examples*: Certain interventions or skills are best implemented when one group member shares their individual experience as an example and then each member applies this to their own experience, by completing the related handout. For example, drawing a personalized formulation (Session 1) starts with a group member sharing their experience. The volunteer's formulation is drawn on a whiteboard. Then, other group members use their accompanying handout to create their own personalized formulation. This process can be useful to help to decrease shame and guilt, normalize symptoms experienced, and offer validation.

- *Shifting Group Responsibility Over Time*: A skilled group therapist will not only challenge patients, as they are ready, more and more over time in relation to the session content and between-session work, but also in relation to the group process. This means that as the group progresses and group members become more comfortable in the group and with each other, you will encourage patients to challenge themselves more with group-based behavior. This will look different for each patient, but could include participating more, participating less, completing homework less perfectly, sharing more about one's own experience as opposed to giving advice, or balancing out sharing both successes and struggles. From a group perspective, over time, patients should become more responsible for their own group, which includes supporting one another more by helping to identify ways in others that the eating disorder may be impacting them, and challenging each other to do the hard work to make change.

- *Praise*: Praise is an important therapeutic skill to be implemented throughout Group CBT-E. Initially, praise will likely be modeled by you, and hopefully it will then be initiated by group members to support one another. Look for as many opportunities to offer praise as possible – completing between-session work, engaging in a discussion, identifying Action Plans, supporting a peer, making a recovery-oriented statement, engaging in a particularly difficult between-session challenge, etc.

- *Staying on Time and Following the Agenda*: Following the agenda ensures that each patient will receive the necessary tools to overcome their eating disorder. Keeping to the suggested times included in each session will allow for adequate coverage of each agenda item. It is common for therapists to struggle to keep to time, especially when they first start implementing a new therapy. Setting alarms to gently remind you when you are coming to the end of a section can be a useful tool.

Patient Participation

Patient engagement and participation in therapy is a key element in any psychological treatment. As it pertains to group, patients report that verbally participating in group helps to get the most out of their treatment. Generally, individuals have different levels of comfort in speaking and sharing. These differences can sometimes be more pronounced in a group. As a group leader, be attuned to the particular needs of the patients in the group. Be sure that all patients have equal access to sharing in a way that is most comfortable for them. As discussed above, it is important to apply group process interventions to encourage patients to support one another to help to problem solve, consider alternative perspectives, brainstorm, validate experiences, and therapeutically confront eating disorder thoughts, feelings, and behaviors. This can be particularly therapeutic, as patients often report that receiving this type of support from others that have also struggled with eating disorder symptoms is more relatable. It is very common for patients to report that receiving support directly from a peer who can relate to the difficulties of recovery has a unique benefit, compared to receiving the same support from a professional.

Patient Engagement

Do some patients need...

- Extra encouragement to participate by being called on directly?
- Clear support to allow others to speak or redirection on certain topics?
- To write down responses instead of sharing verbally?
- To challenge themselves to speak despite anxiety?

The Group CBT-E Therapist

Training

General knowledge of eating disorders and comfort with eating disorder treatment is necessary, particularly for therapists delivering this treatment in the outpatient setting where the group leader holds clinical responsibility for patients. Previous experience running group therapies is beneficial, though not a requirement. Many new therapists and trainees have described the structure and the use of handouts as helpful in building their confidence implementing the group.

A foundational knowledge or training in Individual CBT-E is advantageous to learning Group CBT-E. Below are a couple of training resources.

- *Web-based training*: Created by CREDO, online training is available for Individual CBT-E. The training is roughly the equivalent of a two-day workshop. It provides an introduction to CBT-E interventions and a library of acted patient role-plays showcasing skill implementation. Evaluations of this asynchronous and accessible training have shown it to be useful in increasing therapist knowledge of CBT-E treatment interventions. At the time of writing, the training continues to be available at low or no cost (www.cbte.co).

- *Treatment guide*: Individual CBT-E is comprehensively detailed in the treatment guide by Fairburn and colleagues: *Cognitive Behavior Therapy and Eating Disorders* (Fairburn, 2008). Group CBT-E is closely modeled on this guide.

- *Group CBT-E Components Checklist*: In Appendix E, you will find a group version of the CBT-E Components Checklist. The checklist is a therapist self-rated adherence scale covering all treatment interventions. This tool can be useful in both learning and delivering CBT-E.

When possible, we encourage ongoing supervision for therapists implementing Group CBT-E. We acknowledge that finding expert supervision is not always feasible and is often costly. Frequent reviews with oneself, as well as organizing peer supervision groups, can be useful alternatives.

Therapist Approach, Style, and the Importance of Instilling Hope

An openness or desire to implement CBT-E is essential. This is not to say that therapists from a variety of therapeutic modalities cannot learn the treatment and implement it well. We have found, however, that some therapists who oppose the use of short-term therapies or whose therapeutic style does not fit with CBT have a harder time implementing the therapy with fidelity (i.e., adherence to the treatment principles), which can impact outcomes.

Some important recommendations related to therapist style include:

- The therapist is genuine, empathic, and warm.

- The therapist is an active, directive participant in the treatment and acts as a guide in helping to support a patient with their treatment goals.

- The patient and therapist form a team – the patient is the expert on their own eating disorder and the therapist is the expert in Group CBT-E and eating disorder knowledge. The therapist is transparent in this approach.

- Ideally, patients are educated consumers of their treatment. Educating them about what to expect and its clinical rationale is important for patient awareness, motivation, hopefulness about the efficacy of treatment, and understanding of how treatment components fit together (i.e., the plan for treatment).

- Working collaboratively, the therapist supports patients in developing a scientific attitude toward learning and experimenting with change. It is highly important that the therapist instills hope that change is possible. Patients can, and do, reach long and lasting eating disorder recovery. Many of our patients hold the view (a shared view held by many, including mental health providers) that eating disorders are intractable illnesses that are chronic in nature. For the great majority of patients who receive well-implemented, recommended treatments, recovery is possible. As the Group CBT-E therapist, it is essential to share this hopeful view and hold the belief that recovery is possible.

Weight Bias

As with all clinical work, it is critical that you explore your biases as a therapist and understand how they may be impacting your treatment and care of patients. This awareness informs any potential changes that may need to be made to assure that you are providing inclusive and equitable care.

Weight bias is one form of bias that may be particularly relevant when working with individuals with eating disorders. Weight bias is a set of negative beliefs, expectations, behaviors, assumptions, stereotypes, judgments, and discriminatory acts aimed at individuals solely because of their weight. It leads to stigmatization. Weight bias is pervasive in our diet-positive culture, and therapists, including eating disorder specialists, are not immune to this bias (Puhl et al., 2014). It is important to consider our own biases, knowing that some biases are implicit, meaning that they are unconscious, and we are not aware of them. Be open to the impact they have on your ability to treat patients effectively and justly. As an eating disorder therapist, it is imperative that you can approach all patients with openness and acceptance without discrimination related to any aspect of themselves, including their weight.

Ideally, Group CBT-E therapists hold a neutral view about bodies and food which comes across in the language used in group. Moral values and judgments should not be placed on body sizes and food choices, despite our culture's diet-positive messages about this. For example, at an outpatient level of care, as a result of Group CBT-E and reducing eating disorder behaviors, patients may gain weight, may lose weight, or may have no change in weight. All of these outcomes are typical and acceptable and should be met with neutrality by the therapist.

Therapist Drift

Therapist drift is when a therapist is no longer implementing the therapy as initially designed or researched (Waller, 2009). It leads to therapies that are not adherent to the treatment protocol, rendering them less evidence based and likely less effective. Therapist drift is common. Despite best efforts to follow a clinical protocol closely, it is human nature to drift at times. There are a number of reasons why drift can occur, including:

- Forgetting certain aspects of the protocol.
- Not agreeing with particular interventions.
- Anxiety that an intervention will cause the patient anxiety.
- Concern that a certain intervention is harmful for patients.
- Not understanding the rationale for interventions.
- Being disinterested in certain aspects of a protocol.
- Thinking that another intervention may be more useful.

To reduce/protect against drift, use the *Group CBT-E Components Checklist* (Appendix E) to assess your own adherence to the treatment on a session-by-session basis. Remember, editing or adding to the protocol takes you away from applying evidence-informed interventions and may lead you astray and delay your patients' care.

Minimizing Dropouts

Dropouts are a part of mental health treatment, and some number of dropouts should be expected. That said, as therapists, we need to put into place our best strategies when noticing warning signs for dropping out. Dropping out of treatment puts patients at greater risk of no longer obtaining mental health treatment in the future, and of their disorder worsening. Increased risk of dropout is associated with:

- Therapist concerns about participation and/or appropriateness of the treatment for the patient.
- Support people who are critical or skeptical of the treatment.
- Practical barriers that get in the way of fully engaging with the treatment (e.g., scheduling concerns, costs).
- The patient missing therapy sessions or being frequently late.
- The therapist missing sessions or being late to sessions.

In these situations, we recommend addressing these issues as swiftly as possible. This discussion is best done in the group format itself; however, due to time constraints, that is not always possible and may require a brief, individual check-in following the group. We recommend engaging in a conversation such as:

I am noticing that you have been late twice in a row to group and that you haven't shared much in group yet. I am wondering about how you are feeling about the group and your level of commitment to the sessions? Are there aspects of the group that you are feeling disengaged from, that you disagree with, or that are prohibiting you in any way from fully immersing yourself in the treatment?

We recommend briefly exploring these with the patient and coming up with a plan to address such barriers. If the patient has external treatment providers, consider collaborating with them regarding the patient's misgivings and sharing the plan identified.

Likewise, as a therapist, it is important to start the group on time and come prepared each session. Therapists who are not engaged in the treatment will struggle to implement the group well. Related to this, when possible, do not start the group if you have extended planned time off approaching. Just as we ask patients to not take breaks during treatment, it is important that therapists also commit to being present throughout the treatment. Where breaks are not avoidable, arrange for a covering therapist if possible.

Concerns about Group Contagion

A common concern when offering group-based eating disorder treatment is the fear of patients triggering each other or learning new eating disorder behaviors from one another. An example of this fear would be that if one patient is discussing that they engage in self-induced vomiting, another patient, who had not considered this behavior, would begin to use this behavior after learning about it. There is limited research on this so called "peer contagion." While this is a concern, peer contagion is not something we have significantly encountered during group. In a time of endless social media, any peer contagion from the group will be minimal compared to what one has access to online. Our guidance is to be aware of the possibility, openly talk about the impact of hearing someone else's symptoms, and ask the patient their experience of having this particular eating disorder behavior. Often, if a patient expresses an interest in trying a new eating disorder behavior, the patient already using that behavior will discourage it. A patient response may be something like: *"Oh gosh, no, you definitely do not want to start using laxatives! I wish that I never started. They make me feel sick and I always worry where the nearest bathroom is when I am out."*

Multidisciplinary Collaboration

As a Group CBT-E therapist, we highly encourage collaborating with all of the patient's established treatment team members at the start of the patient's treatment, with continued follow-up as needed. We suggest using the *Guide for Outpatient Providers* (Appendix E) to help with communication.

Working with Other Therapists

As an outpatient intervention, presented sequentially, Group CBT-E is designed to be a standalone treatment. That said, some patients will come to Group CBT-E with an established therapist and may not be interested in stopping that treatment to start Group CBT-E. Other patients may be in treatment with another provider for a separate mental health concern. In both these situations, we recommend working collaboratively with the established provider to clearly describe Group CBT-E goals and interventions, as well as anticipate with the provider any areas where treatment goals could potentially differ. Addressing these differences directly and creating a plan is strongly recommended. It is important that patients receive consistent messages from all providers. Many times, patients may need to take a pause from other treatments to focus on Group CBT-E.

Working with Dietitians

Dietitians are an integral part of a multidisciplinary eating disorder team at HLOCs. In outpatient treatment, the role of the dietitian is less clearly specified. Individual CBT-E does not include specific nutrition advice and finds that many patients do not require such guidance to successfully overcome their eating disorder. As such, Group CBT-E does not include sessions with a dietitian. However, there are certain circumstances when a nutritional assessment or follow-up nutritional therapy with an eating disorder-informed dietitian is highly recommended. A nutritional assessment is extremely useful in identifying when a patient is maintaining a weight lower than their body needs, are underfat, and/or are not eating in a fully balanced way (e.g., undereating certain nutrients or food categories such as carbohydrates or fats). Additionally, patients requiring specific nutritional advice are also advised to meet with a dietitian. This includes patients with certain health conditions (e.g., diabetes mellitus, celiac disease, food allergies, osteopenia/porosis); patients who have undergone any form of bariatric surgery; and patients with low levels of nutritional knowledge. When indicated, sessions with an eating disorder-informed dietitian can be concurrent with the group. Where possible, working with a dietitian who is well aligned with CBT-E helps to create more unified guidance and is less confusing to patients. It is noted that many patients do not have access to dietitians (let alone eating disorder-informed dietitians) due to insurance coverage barriers and this should be taken into consideration when making referrals. Additionally, while not permissible in all geographical regions, in locations where dietitians are licensed to lead psychological group therapies, the entirety of Group CBT-E can be delivered by a dietitian trained in CBT-E.

Group CBT-E Sessions

Achieving Early Change

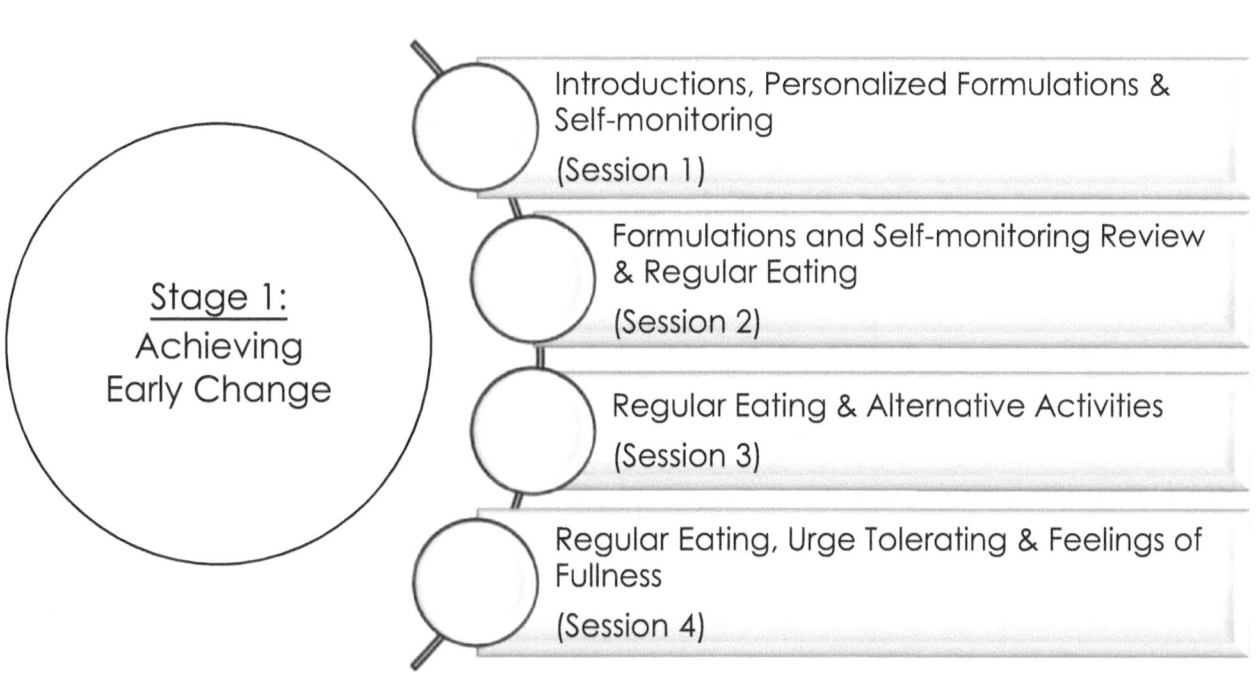

Stage 1:
Achieving
Early Change

Introductions, Personalized Formulations &
Self-monitoring

(Session 1)

Formulations and Self-monitoring Review
& Regular Eating

(Session 2)

Regular Eating & Alternative Activities

(Session 3)

Regular Eating, Urge Tolerating & Feelings of
Fullness

(Session 4)

Chapter 6

Group Session 1
Introductions, Personalized Formulations and Self-monitoring

Stage 1 of Group CBT-E comprises Sessions 1–4 of the treatment. The main focus of these sessions is on achieving early behavior change, in particular the adoption of a regular pattern of eating. Being able to make such changes early in treatment is a robust predictor of positive treatment outcome, thus making it essential that treatment starts well from the very first session. Starting treatment well involves creating a space where patients feel welcome and hopeful about making changes to their eating disorder and providing them with the necessary skills to do so.

Stage 1 emphasizes behavior change which, for many reasons, is important to prioritize from the start. First, decreasing/eliminating certain eating disorder behaviors (e.g., binge eating, self-induced vomiting) is highly reinforcing for patients. Decreasing these unwanted behaviors engages patients in treatment as it indicates that treatment is "working." Second, early establishment of regular patterns of eating aids in repairing some of the physical consequences of the disorder. These physical consequences negatively impact the patient's health and can harm a patient's insight, judgment, concentration, attention, and cognitive flexibility. Being able to reverse these symptoms quickly allows patients a better chance at fully engaging with the CBT-E treatment provided. Third, when behavior change is made consistently, some associated cognitive processes will automatically change to accommodate for this (e.g., when someone changes a behavior repeatedly, the thoughts that were leading to that behavior can eventually change along with the behavior). Overall, behavior change seems to have the greatest impact early on for a patient with an eating disorder in addressing not only behavioral symptoms, but also physical impairment, cognition, and motivation.

Overview

Starting in this first session, patient engagement is highly important. This is often achieved through a combination of a warm welcome, shared patient introductions, and presenting yourself as a safe and compassionate therapist with important knowledge about eating disorders and the treatment. In addition to engaging patients in treatment, Session 1 has two additional main aims:

1. To create a personalized eating disorder formulation
2. To introduce real time self-monitoring

DOI: 10.4324/9781003450849-8

As in all Group CBT-E sessions, the group will end with the group wrap-up. For guidance related to the group wrap-up, an essential component of every session, see Chapter 5.

Therapist Preparation

☐ Ensure in advance that each patient meets criteria for group participation and that Group CBT-E is an appropriate and safe treatment approach (reviewed in Chapter 3).
☐ Check that each patient has received their Welcome Packet, including the *Group CBT-E* handout which will be reviewed in this session.
☐ Review each patient's clinical presentation and their pretreatment EDE-Q and CIA.
☐ Review this chapter in advance.
☐ Review accompanying handouts and have copies available for patients.
☐ Review Appendix B on formulation creation.

Handouts

- Session-specific Handouts
  - *17.1 Group CBT-E (Appendix E)*
  - *1.1 My Formulation*
  - *1.2 My Formulation Information Tool*
  - *1.3 Self-monitoring Form*
  - *1.4 Self-monitoring Example*
  - *1.5 Self-monitoring Instructions*
  - *1.6 Between-session Work Log*

Group Session Agenda

1. Setting the agenda and orienting to the session (2 minutes)
2. Introducing the group (10 minutes)
   a. Reviewing CBT-E education and introducing group expectations
   b. Patient introductions
3. Creating personalized formulations (30 minutes)
4. Introducing real-time self-monitoring (15 minutes)
5. Group wrap-up (3 minutes)

1. Setting the Agenda and Orienting to the Session

As discussed in Chapter 5, start all group therapy sessions by orienting the patient to the group and sharing an agenda.

Hello and welcome to Group Enhanced Cognitive Behavior Therapy for eating disorders, Group CBT-E for short. I'm really pleased to welcome you to this group. I'd like to acknowledge the courage that it must have taken to show up today to embark on this challenging, yet hopefully very rewarding, experience. I know that many of you may feel nervous as this is likely very new for you, and I am hoping that we can work together as a team to best support the changes that you want to see with your eating problem. For today, and all sessions moving forward, I will start the session by sharing what our agenda is for the group session and writing it on our whiteboard. Each session we will work our way through the agenda and use it to structure our sessions.

Therapist Insight

There is a lot of material to get through in each session. Be careful to stick closely to the agenda and to check in with yourself about how you are prioritizing time. Remember that sometimes clinical material that may be interesting for you or a patient to discuss is not always the most important therapy component to prioritize. The priority is to ensure that each patient is given the necessary tools to overcome the eating disorder.

Today is Session 1 of Stage 1. After today, we have 13 sessions left. Today we are going to start by introducing the group and ourselves. After that, I am going to help guide all of you in creating something we call personalized formulations, which are a way to map out what your eating disorder looks like to better understand your disorder and how we will plan treatment. Then I will describe a tool that we will use throughout treatment called self-monitoring. I will show you how to use this tool to help better monitor your behaviors, thoughts, feelings, and situations. Finally, we will end this session, and all of our sessions, by wrapping up the group. I will summarize for you (and have you write down) between-session work to focus on over the course of the upcoming week.

2. Introducing the Group

Handout: *Group CBT-E*

a. Reviewing CBT-E Education and Group Expectations

Prior to the start of group, you will have given group members the *Group CBT-E* handout which introduces the treatment and sets expectations for group guidelines. Determine if group members have read the handout and answer any questions that may arise. Briefly review the group expectations portion of the handout together to ensure understanding.

Before we have the chance to introduce ourselves, as part of your Welcome Packet, each of you received information about Group CBT-E and group guidelines, some of which helps to guide how we communicate in group. I'd like to briefly check in to see if you were able to complete this reading and answer any questions you may have. In particular, I would like to review the group expectations. [Have these prepared on a whiteboard (or similar tool) and ask patients to take turns reading items aloud, or any other method you prefer.]

b. Patient Introductions

Next, ask patients to introduce themselves. This is helpful for group rapport, to expose group members to the act of participating right at the start of the program, and to foster a group belonging process.

> *Let's go around and do some brief introductions to start getting to know one another. I will ask you to share your name, pronouns, a brief statement about why you have chosen to join group, and anything important that you feel we should know about you to best support you in group.*

A patient may introduce themselves by saying,

> *My name is Mariella, they/them/theirs. I am here to finally, after 10 years, get my eating disorder under control. Sometimes I struggle to speak in groups, especially if it is noisy.*

3. Creating Personalized Formulations

Handouts: *My Formulation; My Formulation Information Tool*

The first treatment intervention of Group CBT-E is to guide patients through the process of creating their personalized eating disorder formulation. The formulation serves as a visual representation of the patient's eating disorder, highlighting specific symptoms, the maintaining mechanisms of the illness, and the areas that will be targeted in treatment. Formulation creation gives patients the opportunity to think about their specific eating disorder behaviors and how engaging in these behaviors maintains or keeps the eating disorder going through a variety of vicious circles. It is also intended to offer hope that overcoming the eating disorder is possible by disrupting these behaviors and maintaining mechanisms.

The formulation has three main purposes (Fairburn, 2008):

Therapist Insight

Patients often find creating their formulation to be highly engaging and validating. A common response to viewing the completed formulation is: "This completely describes my eating disorder!" If the formulation does not resonate with a patient, check in that they have included relevant information to describe their individual symptoms. For some, creating the formulation can be difficult as this is often a new way to consider very vulnerable information. Remind group members that group is a safe space to share. Encourage the group to ask questions, openly share confusion, and utilize your support to help organize the formulation.

1. To allow the patient an opportunity to begin to distance themselves from the eating disorder.
2. To increase treatment engagement and provide validation.
3. To visually identify the main targets of CBT-E, creating a blueprint for treatment.

There are several tools in this guide to help teach you about the process of creating personalized formulations:

• Appendix B includes an in-depth explanation of CBT-E formulations and provides other examples of eating disorder behavioral presentations and how they would be reflected in a formulation.
• Table 6.1 offers practical tips for creating formulations.
• The *My Formulation Information Tool* handout offers numerous examples of what thoughts, behaviors, and emotions may be included on a formulation and where these might be included.

The formulation is completed in steps. Creating a formulation can be confusing at first for patients. To reduce confusion, we recommend engaging a group volunteer to collaboratively create their formulation on a whiteboard step by step to serve as an example. Following each step completed by the volunteer, ask group members to complete the same step on their *My Formulation* handout. Keep in mind that all formulations are individual to the patient and therefore will not have all of the same boxes or arrows. If a box or arrow does not apply for a patient, ask them to cross it off or indicate in some way that they are not sure (e.g., using dashed lines or different colors).

Before going through the formulation steps, review the layout of the *My Formulation* handout with the group:

On your My Formulation handout, you will see a bunch of boxes and arrows. In the boxes, we will put the eating disorder behaviors, thoughts, and emotions that make up your eating disorder. The arrows help us to see how the boxes interact with each other and keep the eating disorder going. Everyone's content will be individual to them and not everyone will have all of the boxes filled in. If you do not have something to add for a certain box, it can be crossed out.

Table 6.1 Formulation Tips

1. Be sure that patients use their own words and avoid suggesting technical terms and clinical jargon.
2. Encourage patients to add personalized details for each box. For example, if someone were to add "go on a diet," find out what that means for them. Does it mean eating a certain calorie amount? Does it mean skipping certain meals or snacks? Does it involve avoiding groups of foods and if so, which ones specifically?
3. Encourage patients to personalize maintaining mechanisms (arrows) to fit their view of the eating disorder. Using dashed lines can be helpful to indicate that a mechanism may be at work, but the patient is not sure yet.
4. Encourage curiosity and limit perfection. It is expected that formulations will be updated throughout treatment and are a working document.
5. Avoid making the formulation overly complicated as it can take away from the patient easily recognizing the primary treatment targets and how these maintain the illness.

Step 1: Box A

Box A contains all of the dieting and exercise rules one follows, or attempts to follow, in an effort to change their weight.

Dieting behaviors and having diet-related rules are central to most eating disorders and are a good place to begin when using a standardized approach to formulation creation across all patients in the group. In this box list any dieting behaviors or diet-related rules that the patient follows or attempts to follow. This includes driven exercise when used as a non-compensatory weight control method. The more extreme or rigid the behavior or rule is, the more likely it is to cause further eating disorder behaviors or thoughts. Encourage each patient to be as specific as possible. Examples of dieting and diet-related rules are included on the *My Formulation Information Tool.*

Thank you for volunteering. We are going to draw formulations one step at a time. First, we will draw out [patient's name]'s formulation step on the whiteboard, and then I will ask you to complete the same box on your My Formulation handout. The first box to complete is Box A. In this box write in all of the ways you engage in dieting, attempts to follow diet-related rules, or examples of any driven exercise. Be as specific as possible. Some of the ways you diet, or attempt to diet, may not even be obvious to you. Please use the samples in the My Formulation Information Tool which provides some ideas. If you think something you do may be a dieting behavior, but you are not sure, add it in for now and we can always reconsider keeping it. Be sure to use your own words. If a sample suggestion is not how you would describe it, change the wording to match your experience. [It can be helpful to encourage patients to use erasable methods of writing so that changes can be made while thinking together.]

Step 2: Boxes B and C

Boxes B and C identify two possible consequences of dieting – binge eating and maintaining a weight that is too low/underfat for one's body.

The next boxes I would like you to fill in are the boxes just below dieting behaviors, boxes B and C. These are some of the typical consequences of dieting and having diet-related rules. Not everyone will have information for both of these boxes, and some of you may not have content for either box. That is completely fine. Remember the formulation is personalized to your eating disorder. Cross out the boxes that do not pertain to you.

Box B – Binge eating is a very common outcome of dieting/attempting to diet when you have an eating disorder. This area here [point to the area that leads from dieting to binge eating] *highlights this relationship. This occurs for three reasons. First, undereating places great physiological pressure on our bodies to make up for the missing calories – binge eating is an effective way to replenish an energy deficit quickly. Second, dieting and not eating foods that we may otherwise enjoy causes feelings of emotional or psychological deprivation. Feeling deprived in this way can lead to extreme preoccupation with food or particular foods, making it more likely that a binge will occur when these foods are encountered. Lastly, dieting is often associated with many eating rules that are difficult, if not impossible, to follow all of the time. A common reaction to "breaking" a food rule is thinking that one has failed. Thinking one is a failure in this regard can cause further binge eating, either as a result of "giving up" or in an attempt to soothe away the resulting negative feelings.*

Box C – For some, dieting leads your body to be undernourished. You may be a weight that is too low for your body or you may be underfat for your body to function optimally without further eating disorder thinking. Maintaining a too low weight or being underfat is associated with a number of consequences such as feeling irritable, isolating from friends, and thinking about food a lot (sometimes even dreaming about food). Be sure to add in any consequences of being undernourished that you are currently experiencing.

Underfat is the term we use to describe when an individual's body fat percentage is likely too low. We do not encourage the use of body fat measurement; however, many patients get this information via "smart" scales, and other methods. Clues to suggest being underfat include an intake that is low in calories and/or lacking in dietary fats, a preoccupation with leanness or "ripped" muscle tone, and/or driven exercise. Assessment with a registered dietitian can be invaluable in determining if someone is underfat.

Bring the group's attention to the arrows highlighting that both binge eating and maintaining a weight too low for one's body leads to further dieting behaviors and/or binge eating.

Binge eating:

Can you relate to the reaction of planning to "diet harder or even more" the next day after a binge? The arrow going from binge eating back up to the dieting box shows this relationship.

Maintaining a weight too low for one's body:

Look at the arrows on your formulation from Box C back to dieting and to binge eating. Were you aware that maintaining a weight that is too low for your body puts pressure on you to binge eat? And that it encourages further dieting behaviors?

Step 3: Box D

Box D contains any compensatory behaviors following binge eating used in an effort to minimize the impact of binge eating on one's shape, weight, or feelings of control.

Some of you shared on the assessment measures that a part of your eating disorder involves compensating for binge eating to make up for, or reduce the impact of, the calories eaten. In the box below binge eating, please add in any behaviors that you use to attempt to "undo" the binge eating. Again, the My Formulation Information Tool handout lists some common compensatory behaviors.

Emphasize how compensatory behaviors after a binge can lead to more binge eating. Below is an example of how to address this in relation to self-induced vomiting, but it could similarly be applied to any compensatory behavior.

> *For those that shared they make themselves vomit after every binge eating episode to prevent weight changes- what would happen if you knew that you were not going to be able to throw up? Say there was no access to privacy? Would you still binge eat?*

A common response to the question above is, *"Oh, if I know I will not be able to throw up that almost always stops me from binge eating in the first place."* While this is not every patient's view, share with the group that it is common that when a compensatory behavior is unavailable, binge eating is less likely to occur. This means that a compensatory behavior actually maintains binge eating, as without the opportunity to engage in a compensatory behavior, the binge eating is less likely to occur. Knowing this helps to highlight how binge eating and compensatory behaviors get locked into a vicious circle as shown by the arrows on the handout.

In other situations, a patient may share that there are times when they are engaging in behaviors in Box D, but not to compensate for caloric intake. In these cases, make sure that the arrows on their formulation reflect what seems to trigger this behavior for them (e.g., stressful events, low mood, core psychopathology) and then what the behaviors lead to (e.g., low mood, core psychopathology, binge eating).

Step 4: Box E

Box E contains any emotions and/or events that impact symptoms or are impacted by the eating disorder. Many patients use eating disorder behaviors to regulate their emotions, and changes in emotions can greatly impact eating or eating disorder symptoms. For example, one patient may binge eat in response to stress, another will use control over their eating or driven exercise to reduce stress, someone else may take laxatives to cope, and some will use a combination of symptoms, depending on the situation. Recognizing the impact of emotions on eating disorder symptoms, and vice versa, is often an aspect of the eating disorder that resonates with many patients.

> *Next, we will identify how emotions and stressful events may impact your eating disorder and the behaviors listed so far. What emotions or events do you think are important to include here? What is the relationship? Do you agree with the arrows suggesting that, for example, low mood and increased stress can lead to more eating disorder behaviors, and that eating disorders can lead to low mood/stressful events?*

Step 5: Box F

Box F is the last box to fill in and contains the core psychopathology of the eating disorder that drives the rest of the behaviors. The cognitions listed in this box capture the preoccupation with shape and weight in the patient's own words.

Now, we will fill out the box at the top. In this box goes all of the thoughts you have about your shape and weight that have led you to diet, have diet-related rules, and/or engage in driven exercise. You may believe this to be obvious, but I'd like to know in your own words, why you engage in all of the behaviors you listed in Box A?

Emphasize to patients how the thoughts in Box F often represent the main driver that keeps the eating disorder going:

It makes sense that if you have the thoughts you listed in Box F, for example that you "detest your shape," that you would want to do something about this. Diet culture, which

Therapist Insight

Look for opportunities to normalize behaviors and show understanding. The link between negative thoughts about one's body or a desire to change one's shape and weight is an opportunity to highlight the pressure diet culture places on everyone to look a certain way. Diet culture also encourages the thinking that one has full control over one's shape and weight. While eating disorders affect only a subgroup of individuals, dieting to influence one's shape and weight is extremely common in our society.

we will speak about more in Session 6, tells you that dieting is the solution to obtaining the body you desire. However, as we can see from the arrows, this leads to a whole host of unwanted consequences, including binge eating, maintaining a weight too low for your body, negative mood, and ultimately more focus on your body and so on. In an effort to feel better, you actually feel far worse about yourself and your body. These different maintaining cycles are very strong and difficult to break out of, but it can be done.

Briefly discuss the various arrows and cyclical patterns and ask patients to identify which ones they recognize in their eating disorder. Make sure to emphasize that in an effort to feel better about one's body, engaging in dieting (with its subsequent consequences), actually leads to more negative focus on one's body.

Offer time for other group members to share their formulation aloud and receive feedback from others, process how their formulation impacts them personally, and/or discuss how they would like to see change.

Step 6: Use the Completed Formulation to Provide Hope That It Is Possible to Break Out of the Eating Disorder by Targeting Each Aspect of the Formulation

The discussion serves to motivate patients to consider making changes.

Your formulations serve as a map showing everything we will address in Group CBT-E. In group we will work to remove all of the elements (lines and boxes) of your formulation. Treatment starts by addressing many of the aspects of your formulation that are behavioral, for example modifying your eating patterns. By reducing some of these behaviors, it is likely that some thoughts, emotions, and other behaviors related to the eating disorder will improve. The connections between these factors (i.e., the relationship arrows) will begin to weaken, addressing a significant portion of the model. Once the eating behaviors are directly treated and a regular pattern of eating is established, the focus will shift to addressing other thoughts, emotions, and behaviors that contribute to maintaining the disorder, such as the over-evaluation of shape and weight, and events and emotions. By addressing everything on your formulation you have every chance of reaching a long and lasting recovery.

4. Introducing Real-time Self-monitoring

Handouts: *Self-monitoring Form; Self-monitoring Example; Self-monitoring Instructions*

The second intervention of the session is to introduce real-time self-monitoring. Real-time self-monitoring is recording each day *in the moment* all eating episodes and eating disorder behaviors (e.g., binge eating, self-induced vomiting), along with associated thoughts, emotions, and events. Treatment is unlikely to be successful without the completion of self-monitoring as it is central to treatment and will be utilized throughout the group program. To set patients up for success in completing self-monitoring forms, first share the rationale for the importance of self-monitoring.

Real-time self-monitoring has three primary functions:

1. *To increase awareness of eating patterns.* The goal is to become more aware of the eating disorder behaviors an individuals in engaging in and, how these symptoms may relate to thoughts and feelings, and all of the associated details related to their eating problem.

2. *To help make changes to eating.* When patients are aware of what is going on in the very moment that it is occurring, they are more able to make changes in the moment. Patients will learn that previous behavior that seemed automatic or habit may become more manageable.

3. *To provide day-by-day information about the eating disorder that would otherwise be missed.* It would be challenging to expect patients to recall what they ate, thought, felt, etc. in a weekly review without this information being stored somewhere. The weekly review of self-monitoring records is a key component of Group CBT-E.

Once patients have a good rationale for the purpose of self-monitoring, the next step is to review a sample self-monitoring form together. Using the *Self-monitoring Example* handout, slowly review the instructions on how to complete the monitoring form (see *Self-monitoring Instructions* handout).

Self-monitoring requires time and energy from the patient. As designed, monitoring in this way heightens a person's awareness of what they are eating, which can lead to feelings of

Therapist Insight

Sometimes it can be helpful to share a non-eating related example. If someone is wanting to quit vaping, but they do not realize they are vaping until mid-vape, it makes their goal of stopping this behavior more difficult. If, however, this individual is asked to write down every time they vape (and their associated thoughts, feelings, and the situation) then their increased awareness and focus on this behavior may decrease the frequency of some of the automatic aspects of the behavior and/or help them to better understand the associated factors related to their vaping.

guilt, shame, anxiety, and/or embarrassment. Take time to explore the group's reactions to the idea of self-monitoring and explore anticipated barriers to completing the records. Ask group members to identify any concerns or barriers they may have and address these using the information provided below. Generating a list of concerns on the whiteboard can be an engaging way to encourage group members to share their views. Make sure to address potential feelings of guilt and shame as it relates to seeing their own records, as well as perhaps choosing to share pieces of their forms with the group in future sessions. Some common concerns, adapted from Fairburn (2008), include:

- *"Why do I have to do it in real time?"* Real-time recording allows not only for accurate reflection, but also for insight in the moment. With such insight and awareness, sometimes a patient is able to make different choices related to their eating. Without that reflection in the moment, a new choice cannot be made as one cannot change something that has already taken place.

> **Therapist Insight**
>
> Be sure to stress that records are ideally completed in real time, as the behaviors (e.g., episodes of eating) and thoughts are occurring. This critical step often requires re-emphasizing.

- *"Can I use my phone to record?"* It can be helpful to provide education about how the more obtrusive a self-monitoring system is, the better the effect of the practice. This is because the more that the monitoring draws attention to the act of monitoring, the more likely the individual is to shift attention to the behavior. As such, it is recommended that patients complete self-monitoring on paper. If this seems undoable, then using other options (e.g., electronic methods of self-monitoring) can be explored. The monitoring forms will need to be reliably available to the patient during group.

- *"I can't carry these around with me."* We often hear this as it relates to individuals' place of work or school, in that there is no option to record these confidentially and privately. We recommend using the support of the group in this situation to problem solve how to prioritize this practice. For example, we have seen patients include self-monitoring forms in their planners or create a self-monitoring journal which allows for some privacy.

- *"I've already done this before and it didn't work."* This is often shared by patients and even when it is not, we proactively bring this concern up in the group. A helpful response will include that unless such self-monitoring occurred while in structured CBT-E, the patients have very likely not participated in self-monitoring in the same way that is being asked of them now. Often patients have engaged in recording their food for dieting purposes and/or to count calories, which is the antithesis of this practice. Self-monitoring, under the care of a professional, with the structure described, is likely a different approach with new objectives to support recovery using CBT skills. If patients have used self-monitoring in the way described, it can be useful to encourage them to try again as they are likely in a different headspace with their eating disorder and things may work differently this time.

- *"I don't want to do this because it will cause me to think more about food and I came to this group to think less about food."* It is important to provide genuine empathy in this situation and let patients know that this is true – the monitoring forms will likely cause an increased focus on food and eating disorder behaviors, at least initially. This is the therapeutic intent. To work on their eating problem, the patient must first focus more on that problem to better understand the nature and patterns of the problem and how to make change. Most patients find that self-monitoring is more cumbersome and can increase anxiety for the first couple of weeks. With time the practice becomes more of a habit and less anxiety-provoking. Many patients that are initially hesitant about self-monitoring find it to be incredibly useful during the treatment. Some of these patients find it difficult to consider stopping self-monitoring once treatment ends.

> Treatment is unlikely to be successful without the completion of self-monitoring.

5. Group Wrap-Up

Session Summary

In today's session, we started by introducing ourselves to each other. Again, it is so lovely to meet you all and to be here to help support you on working on your eating disorder. We created personalized formulations to have a better sense of what your eating disorder looks like and how treatment will be used to address your specific needs. I introduced self-monitoring, a principal tool that will be used throughout Group CBT-E to learn about your eating patterns, to make changes to your eating behaviors, and to act as a record to review in group.

Between-session Work

At the conclusion of each session, ask group members to record the between-session work on their *Between-session Work Log* handout. The between-session work for Session 1 is:

- *My Formulation*. Take 15 minutes this week to review your personalized formulation and make additions and edits as needed. Share it with a safe support person, if available.
- *Self-monitoring Form*. Begin real-time self-monitoring immediately following the group session.

The following is an example of how to present between-session work at the conclusion of a session:

Between now and our group next week, there are two items of between-session work – reviewing your personalized formulation and starting your self-monitoring forms. Please take some time, about 15 minutes, to review your personalized formulation and make any edits or additions. Share it with a safe support person if you have someone available. Also, please start completing self-monitoring forms daily, in real time, starting today. Use the Self-monitoring Form, Self-monitoring Example, and Self-monitoring Instructions handouts to help with this. Please take a moment to record all of this on your Between-session Work Log handout before leaving today. Looking forward to seeing you all next week.

Higher Level of Care Adaptations: Modular Implementation

When this session is used modularly, the following adaptations are suggested.

- *Introductions*: Introductions are likely unnecessary as most patients will know each other already in the program and have a sense of the program's expectations and group guidelines. If not, make sure these introductions take place. In either situation, a standard warm welcome to all is encouraged in this session and all sessions.

- *Personalized formulations*: We have used this single agenda item as an entire group at higher levels of care (HLOCs). Patients seem to relate well to the information and find it useful in understanding their eating disorder. At HLOCs, a number of patients are likely to experience starvation symptoms and other medical consequences as a result of recent extreme weight loss, maintaining a weight significantly lower than one's body needs, or engaging in compensatory behaviors. Be sure to spend adequate time providing education about these consequences and how most of them can be reversed with adequate nutritional intake. These more extreme consequences are listed on the *My Formulation Tool Information* handout under Box C.

    Additionally, these symptoms of starvation can negatively impact a patient's cognitive functioning, including concentration, attention, insight, and judgment. As such, some patients newly admitted to the highest levels of care may struggle to understand or focus on this, or other, interventions until they have started the refeeding process. Patients who are struggling with poor insight or judgment may not be able to recognize or acknowledge eating disorder symptoms as they are presented in the formulation. In both cases, meet these patients with validation and know that the most important treatment focus for these individuals initially is renourishment. If they do not respond to this intervention or other interventions at first, they may be able to better interact with these later in treatment as the symptoms of starvation are reversed.

- *Self-monitoring*: Consider the usefulness of this intervention depending on your service. In some inpatient and residential settings, any form of recording could be impractical given possible cognitive limitations of the patients or rules about carrying papers around. While in other settings, recording what one eats may provide less meaningful data as food choices may be decided by the program and individual nutritional needs. In these settings, it may be worthwhile to have patients record only their thoughts and feelings (including eating disorder symptom urges) about what they are eating and/or are required to eat. This information can then be processed in a group setting.

    Monitoring tends to work quite well in partial hospital and intensive outpatient settings and can be implemented as suggested. Along with the benefits to the patient, this monitoring is often a critical and required tool in these programs for the treatment team to have a sense of the patient's food intake and eating disorder symptoms while away from the program. These data are necessary to inform progress, and treatment and discharge planning.

Group Session 1

Handout 1.1 *My Formulation*

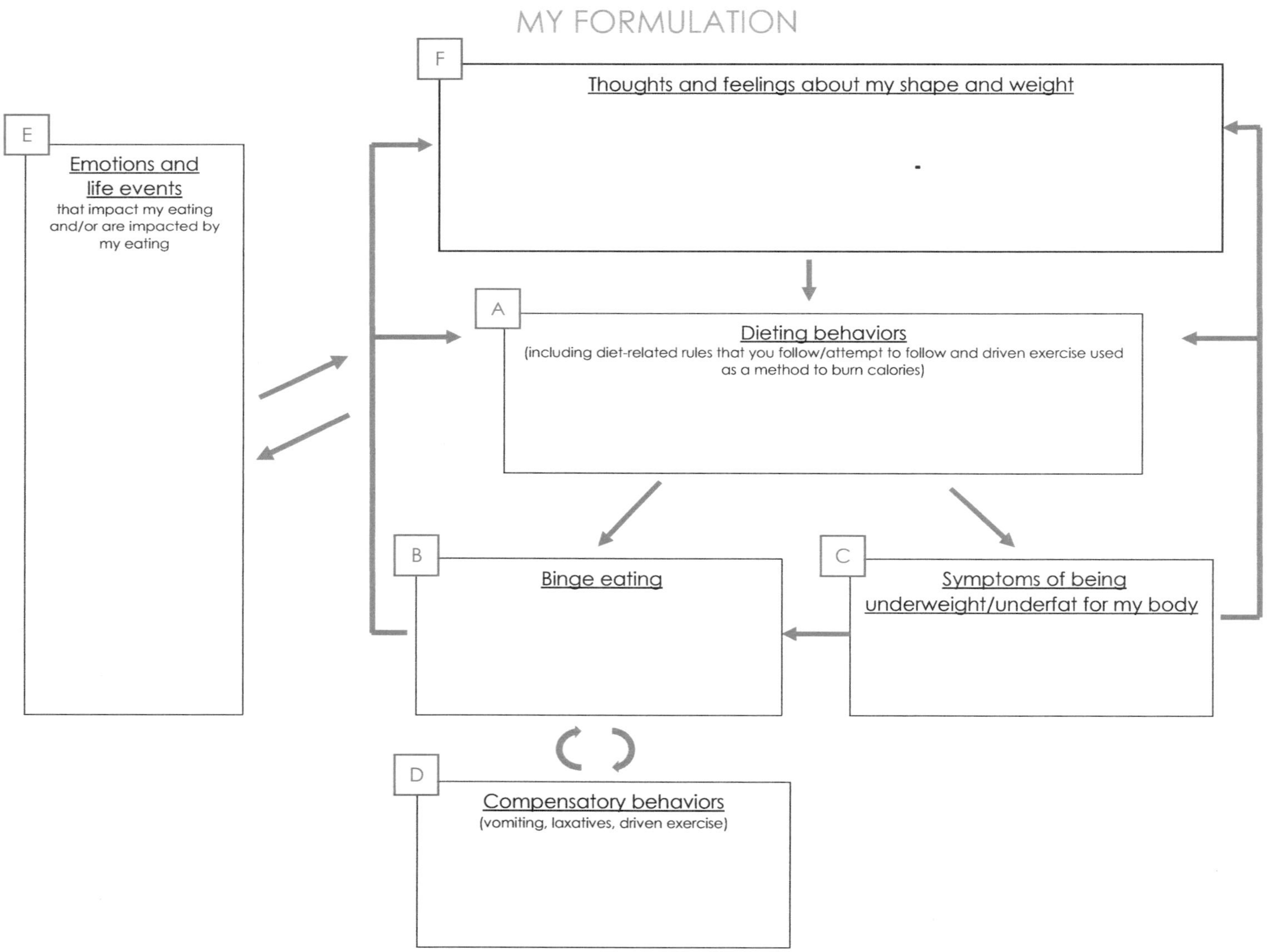

MY FORMULATION

F — Thoughts and feelings about my shape and weight

A — Dieting behaviors
(including diet-related rules that you follow/attempt to follow and driven exercise used as a method to burn calories)

C — Symptoms of being underweight/underfat for my body

B — Binge eating

D — Compensatory behaviors
(vomiting, laxatives, driven exercise)

E — Emotions and life events
that impact my eating and/or are impacted by my eating

Handout 1.2 *My Formulation Information Tool*

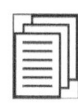

MY FORMULATION INFORMATION TOOL

This tool provides examples of the kinds of information to include on your *My Formulation* handout.

A

Dieting behaviors

(including diet-related rules that you follow/attempt to follow and driven exercise used as a method to burn calories)

- Counting calories and only allow myself x amount each day
- Only eating lean proteins
- Trying not to have bread with my dinner when out to eat
- Exercising before I allow myself to eat
- Only eating when I'm at home
- Only having one meal per day
- Chewing and spitting food
- Avoiding all "bad" fats – fried foods, cheap oils, butter, ice cream
- Avoiding starchy vegetables
- Avoiding most carbohydrates – especially white pasta and rice
- Lifting every day, even when I am tired or injured
- Only having two meals on weekdays
- Drinking a lot of coffee
- Taking diet pills

B

Binge eating

- Eating everything in my cupboard when alone
- Eating completely out of control, can't stop
- Eating out of control on the weekends (my "cheat" days)

C

Symptoms of being underweight/underfat for my body

- Increased obsessiveness
- Feeling full even when my partner says I've barely eaten
- Irritability
- Thinking about food a lot
- Feeling cold all of the time
- Can't sleep – I dream about food when I do!
- Constipated
- No periods

D

Compensatory behaviors

- Making myself throw up
- Using laxatives
- Pushing myself really hard at the gym
- Pumping extra breastmilk
- Using diuretics
- Misusing insulin

E

Emotions and life events

that impact my eating and/or are impacted by my eating

- Feeling depressed
- Feeling anxious
- Preparing for my son's wedding
- Loneliness
- Going on vacation with others
- Feeling angry
- Loneliness
- Trying to get pregnant
- Work/ school stress
- Coping with difficulties with my family

F

Thoughts and feelings about my shape and weight

- I hate my body.
- I am so disgusting.
- My jawline is barely noticeable and just looks bad.
- I can't stand the way that I look.
- I just want to be smaller.
- My waist/thighs are too big.
- I am not good enough in this body.
- I have zero muscle definition and look like a blob.

Handout 1.3 *Self-monitoring Form*

Name: _____

SELF-MONITORING FORM

Date: _____   Day of the Week: _____

Time	Food and Drink	Place	*	v/l/d	e	Context and comments

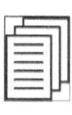

Handout 1.4 *Self-monitoring Example*

SELF-MONITORING EXAMPLE

Name: __Ezi__   Date: __11/02__   Day of the Week: __Wednesday__

Time	Food and Drink	Place	*	v/l/d	e	Context and comments
7:00 AM	Coffee with milk	Kitchen			e	Yesterday was so bad, I am ready to start this day off on the right foot. I went jogging (3 miles) before my coffee.
11:00 AM	Granola bar	Desk				I am so bored at my job and this granola bar feels like something to look forward to. I have a pounding headache.
12:30 PM	Small salad with cottage cheese	Desk				So far, so good. I really like this salad and feel like it is a good choice.
7:00 PM	Chicken, rice, broccoli	Living Room				This is a typical dinner. I guess I like it. Still hungry though. What is wrong with me?
7:30 PM	Bowl of ice cream	Living Room	*			Ugh. Why am I eating more? I feel like I can't stop. Once I am done with one thing, I feel like I am thinking about the next and have no control. What's wrong with me? I am embarrassed to be writing this.
	Half a bag of Doritos		*			
	Another 2 plates of dinner		*			
	Another bowl of ice cream		*			
10:00 PM	Banan a with peanut butter	Living Room				Why did I eat again? I know that I wasn't hungry – I just can't stop. Gross. I will get up early to jog again.

SELF-MONITORING INSTRUCTIONS

Real-time self-monitoring is an **essential** tool used throughout Group CBT-E. It is a critical component of Group CBT-E!

There are 3 main functions of self-monitoring:

1. **To slow down and become more aware** of your behaviors (i.e., eating, eating disorder symptoms), thoughts, feelings, and all of the associated details related to your eating problem (i.e., arguments, stress), in real time.

2. **To highlight areas for change**. Sometimes these changes can occur in the moment you are writing in your record and other times these changes can occur later after reviewing your eating patterns.

3. **To have a record of your eating patterns** that you can use as an evaluation tool during the week and in group.

At first, self-monitoring may seem challenging and scary (or boring and time consuming). Monitoring can also increase your focus on eating, leading to distress, which is precisely what you'd like to focus less on. Remember, the intention of self-monitoring is to focus *more* on your behaviors, in the short term, to increase your awareness and understanding of these behaviors which will lead to you being able to change them. It can feel distressing and inconvenient initially, but becomes second nature after the first 2 weeks or so.

All recording should be done in **real time**, when the eating or behaviors are occurring. It is very difficult to remember the details surrounding an eating event later on and impossible to make change to that event after the fact.

Follow these guidelines to help in completing the forms:

Item	Guideline
Time	Record the time of all eating, drinking, and other behaviors.
Food and Drink	• Record **all** food and drink. • It is important to put a general description and size of a meal; however, calories should not be recorded and food should not be measured or counted. • Identify eating episodes that you see as meals in **brackets**. • Sometimes it can be difficult to write foods down, especially if they were part of a binge. If you feel that you have eaten excessively, it is important to include all foods that were a part of this eating episode. Don't let the eating disorder encourage you to keep things hidden.
Place	Write the place (including room) where you have eaten.
*	Place an asterisks if you think that you have eaten excessively and/or times when you felt a loss of control when eating.
v/l/d	• v = self-induced vomiting • l = laxative use • d = diuretic use
e	Record all exercise. If you know it is compensatory in nature, add this too.
Context and comments	• Record all thoughts, feelings, and events that may have influenced your eating (e.g., getting into an argument with your friend and then binge eating). • Try to write a brief comment each time you eat. • You may want to include information about other thoughts, feelings, and events, even if they didn't seem to impact your eating. • Include details about any exercise.

Handout 1.6 *Between-session Work Log*

BETWEEN-SESSION WORK LOG

This is a place to keep track of all of your between-session work. At the end of each group, together with your therapist, you will decide what to put in each box. Be sure to bring this log to every session.

Session 1		Session 8	
Session 2		Session 9	
Session 3		Session 10	
Session 4		Session 11	
Session 5		Session 12	
Session 6		Session 13	
Session 7		Session 14	

Chapter 7

Group Session 2

Personalized Formulation and Self-monitoring
Review and Regular Eating

Overview

Session 2 focuses on:

- Reviewing the patients' thoughts and reflections about their personalized formulation
- Exploring patients' first attempts at self-monitoring
- Introducing regular eating, a major component of treatment

Additionally, this session begins by introducing, for the first time, a between-session work self-review and the accompanying handout. The review handout guides the patients through an assessment of their between-session work. In this session, the self-review focuses on their formulations and the start of their self-monitoring. The self-review also supports patients in making clear Action Plans to continue to progress in these areas. Following the self-review, a detailed joint in-session review of self-monitoring forms is conducted. This review allows patients to begin recognizing and understanding their behavior patterns related to eating. The last part of this session introduces the main components of regular eating.

Therapist Preparation

☐ Review this chapter in advance.
☐ Review accompanying handouts and have copies available for patients.

Handouts

- Standard Weekly Handouts
    - *1.1 My Formulation*
    - *1.3 Self-monitoring*
    - *1.6 Between-session Work Log*
    - *2.1 Between-session Work Self-review – Session 2*

DOI: 10.4324/9781003450849-9

- Session-specific Handouts
  - *2.2 Self-monitoring Review*
  - *2.3 Regular Eating*
  - *2.4 Planning Ahead*

- Optional information handouts
  - *2.5 Dieting*
  - *2.6 Binge Eating*
  - *2.7 Underweight/Underfat*
  - *2.8 Self-induced Vomiting and Medication Misuse*
  - *2.9 Driven Exercise*

Group Session Agenda

1. Setting the agenda and orienting to the session (2 minutes)
2. Between-session work self-review (10 minutes)
3. Reviewing the personalized formulations (10 minutes)
4. Reviewing the self-monitoring process (20 minutes)
5. Introducing regular eating (15 minutes)
6. Group wrap-up (3 minutes)

1. Setting the Agenda and Orienting to the Session

Begin with a positive, encouraging welcome; share that this is Session 2, Stage 1 with 12 sessions remaining. Clearly list the session agenda.

2. Between-session Work Self-review

Handout: *Between-session Work Self-review – Session 2*

As this is the first time patients will be introduced to the concept of the between-session work self-review, and this review also provides time for generally checking in on feelings about having started treatment, more time is allotted for this on the agenda in this session. For more information about the between-session work self-review, see Chapter 5. In this session, both reviewing the personalized formulation and using the self-monitoring handout will be explored in depth as separate agenda items. The *Between-session Work Self-review – Session 2* handout does not have a box for follow-up Action Plans, something you will see in subsequent sessions. Be sure to introduce the self-review to patients and emphasize its importance:

Today, and in all of the group sessions moving forward, you will start by completing a between-session work self-review handout. These reviews allow you to check in with yourself about how much of the between-session work you completed. Completing between-session work, and identifying obstacles to completing it, are some of the best ways for you to reach your recovery goals and overcome the eating disorder. As you can see on the Between-session Work

Self-Review – Session 2 handout, this review asks specific questions about the content from last session – your personalized formulation and the self-monitoring forms. You will also see in this review a space to write down your initial thoughts and feelings about the first week of treatment. It would be helpful to know how you are feeling and what you are thinking at this point. Please take a few minutes to complete the handout and then we will go around the group and share general impressions and also how you feel you did in getting started with the first two skills, which we will talk much more about throughout this session.

3. Reviewing the Personalized Formulations

Handouts: *My Formulation; Optional information handouts: Dieting; Binge Eating; Underweight/Underfat; Self-induced Vomiting and Medication Misuse*; and *Driven Exercise*

Following the between-session work self-review, engage the patients in reviewing their personalized formulations created in the previous session. These formulations will be reviewed not only in this session, but throughout the treatment, as they are often referred to, added to, and amended. Encourage patients to bring them (a picture on their phone works well for portability) to each session.

For this review, ask patients to take out their *My Formulation* handout and share any further thoughts they had or questions about their formulation. Perhaps they added some additional information, crossed off a box, or added a maintaining arrow. Check in to see if they shared the formulation with a support person and how that went. The following questions can be used to guide this discussion:

- *Did you have other thoughts about the formulation when you reviewed it?*
- *Did you change or amend your formulation?*
  - *Were there any boxes that you added information to or content you decided to remove?*
  - *How about the arrows? Did you add any new ones or take any away?*
  - *Did you have any new reactions/thoughts related to the formulation? Any additional thoughts about how seeing your eating disorder presented this way may impact your motivation for treatment?*
  - *If you did not review it, are there ways we can understand what got in your way and support you in reviewing it this week?*
- *Did you share your formulation with your support person?*
  - *If you did share it, was this challenging to do? Or helpful in some ways?*
  - *If you were not able to share it, why not? Is this something you would like to do for next week?*
  - *If you wanted to share it, but encountered an obstacle, are there ways the group can help you think through ways around the obstacle?*
  - *If you did share it, what kinds of questions did your support(s) have?*
  - *Was anything added/edited after looking at it with a support?*

Providing Psychoeducational Handouts Related to Specific Symptoms on Personalized Formulations

At the end of the formulation review, ask patients to consider which of the following symptoms they have included on their formulation: dieting (Box A on the formulation); binge eating (Box B); underweight/underfat (Box C); self-induced vomiting and medication misuse (Box A and/or D); and driven exercise (Box A and/or D). When present, these symptoms are a critical component of a patient's eating disorder and maintain the cyclical processes reflected in the personalized formulations. These symptoms need to be addressed to overcome the eating disorder. To support patients in making changes to these behaviors, Group CBT-E includes specific information handouts on these topics: *Dieting; Binge Eating; Underweight/Underfat; Self-induced Vomiting and Medication Misuse*; and *Driven Exercise*. Provide the appropriate handouts to patients based on their individualized eating disorder symptoms. Not all handouts will be given to each patient, just those that are relevant. These handouts include psychoeducation about the symptoms themselves and ask patients to consider reasons to change, as well as to create Action Plan(s) to start making such change. For between-session work, ask patients to review and complete the relevant handouts, including creating at least one Action Plan for each symptom that is relevant.

4. Reviewing Self-monitoring

Handout: *Self-monitoring Review*

The next agenda item is to review the process of each patient's self-monitoring. To start, engage the group in a conversation about the self-monitoring process using the *Self-monitoring Review* handout.

> *Let's now take some time to look at the self-monitoring work that you did this week. We'll start by thinking about how the process of self-monitoring went for you. Please complete the checklist included on the Self-monitoring Review handout and let's think together about surprises, barriers to completion, difficulties related to self-monitoring, and any benefits.*

Therapist Insight

Praise is a very important component of many group discussions throughout Group CBT-E. Remember how difficult new skills are for patients to acquire and any efforts toward implementing such skills should be praised using a warm, genuine, and encouraging tone.

During this discussion, praise patients for all efforts that they have put into self-monitoring. Self-monitoring is a difficult task. It takes up time and for many patients, it is emotionally distressing to see what they are eating and what eating disorder behaviors they may be engaging in. If any group members did not start self-monitoring, or complete self-monitoring consistently, engage the group in identifying a list of barriers to completing the task as intended (using the commonly identified barriers listed in Session 1), and consider recording these on a whiteboard. Then, support patients in identifying specific Action Plans to help with starting/restarting/continuing with self-monitoring. Re-emphasize the importance of completing the task as intended and the necessity of this intervention for working toward behavior change goals.

It is great to see the effort that many of you put into prioritizing self-monitoring this week. I know that it is a time-consuming task that can sometimes increase discomfort. Well done on completing this important treatment component despite this! For some of you, it was more difficult to get started with, or fully complete, self-monitoring. Given what a challenging task completing the monitoring can be, this is understandable. Since monitoring is such a critical part of this treatment – we really cannot do Group CBT-E without it – I'd like to brainstorm some of the barriers you encountered to completing the task. Let's aim to come up with at least one Action Plan to help support you to overcome barriers that got in your way. For those of you that were able to complete self-monitoring this week, please join in with tips and support related to what was helpful for you. Also, if you found self-monitoring to be helpful for you so far, please let us know how you found this tool to be useful.

5. Introducing Regular Eating

Handouts: *Regular Eating; Planning Ahead*

The next agenda item is to introduce regular eating. Regular eating is one of the principal treatment interventions in CBT-E. Regular eating is an organized eating structure and plan that is prescribed to patients to minimize the likelihood of eating disorder symptoms. Regular eating aims to provide nourishment throughout the day to keep the body satiated and in a state of homeostasis; offer adequate caloric energy; reduce urges to binge and restrict; increase a sense of structure and control; and attempt to repair potential metabolic slowing. For example, for patients who are stuck in a cycle of restricting and binge eating (with or without compensatory behavior), regular nourishment throughout the day often leads to significantly decreased urges to binge eat as the body is better nourished and there is less physiological pressure to overeat.

Regular eating consists of two steps. Step 1 establishes eating at regular intervals, that is, eating every few hours. Step 2 considers the content of the food and if it is an appropriate amount in terms of calories and balance (e.g., containing fats, proteins, and carbohydrates, including fruits and vegetables.). Not all patients will need to work on Step 2 as they are not undereating and are already eating in a balanced way. For patients who do require modifying the content of their food, some of these issues will be addressed in Session 6 (dieting behaviors and diet-related rules). It is still helpful to highlight that for some patients to fully establish regular eating, additional consideration about the amount of food they are consuming will be necessary. For now, the priority is to encourage patients to feed their bodies at regular intervals.

Using both the *Regular Eating* and *Planning Ahead* handouts, review with patients what regular eating looks like, why regular eating is recommended, tips for how best to accomplish this pattern of eating, and how to apply planning ahead as a tool to help support regular eating patterns. Take adequate time to discuss each guideline carefully and leave time for questions. Emphasize the following components of regular eating:

Regular eating is:

- Feeding your body at regular intervals throughout the day – usually 3 meals and 2–3 snacks.
- Trying to eat roughly every 3 hours and not going over 4 hours.
- Making a commitment to not skip meals or snacks.
- Trying to stick to the pattern and eat at the eating times and not in between. This means having periods of time for eating and for not eating.
- Knowing in advance of eating **when** you will eat next.
- Having an idea of **what** you will eat. A rough idea is enough information – you do not need to be precise (e.g., planning a bowl of cereal versus a specific amount of two cups of cereal).
- Choosing foods, for now, that you are comfortable with and are less likely to cause you to have urges to engage in eating disorder behaviors (e.g., self-induced vomiting, food restriction).
- Prioritizing regular eating in your day.

Stress to the group that regular eating is one of the most important ways to move towards their recovery goals.

You may introduce the concept of regular eating by stating:

Let's spend some time thinking about how we can feed our bodies in a way that helps to reduce eating disorder symptoms. In group, we will call this regular eating. Regular eating is a style of eating where you feed your body every few hours at planned intervals. Looking back at your formulations, regularly eating will help to break down particular maintaining cycles, for example the cycle caused by dieting that can lead to binge eating. Regular eating includes eating 3 meals a day and 2–3 snacks without gaps of 4 hours or more between eating episodes. Planning in advance <u>when</u> you will eat is very important. To help you get started, let's look at the Regular Eating and Planning Ahead handouts.

After patients have made a tentative eating plan in the *Planning Ahead* handout, ask them to attempt to establish a regular pattern of eating as a part of between-session work this week. Emphasize that regular eating is a skill that starts in Session 1 and is practiced each week throughout treatment and beyond.

The ability of a patient to implement regular eating well depends on a variety of factors: their motivation level, how different their current eating is from regular eating, fears about what regular eating may do to their shape/weight, and availability of food. As such, share with patients that making changes to their eating is difficult, but worth it. Take a motivational, optimistic, and encouraging approach to regular eating.

Regular eating is one of the primary skills that we will be working on in this group. It will be a major focus of the rest of Stage 1 of CBT-E (the next 2 sessions) and will be a critical skill to practice throughout the entire group and beyond. In Stage 1, we are going to focus on skills that will help to better support regular eating goals. We will work together to learn from times where you struggled with regular eating to identify plans for how best to support yourselves with these goals. Of course, it is not expected that you will return to group next week with

100% regular eating behaviors, but attempting each day to follow the pattern, as best as you can, is beneficial. The sooner you can find stability with your eating in this way, the more you will benefit from treatment overall. That said, this is likely going to be a challenging skill for many of you, so please keep an open mind when you experience difficulties – that is all a part of the process. The group is here to help and support you.

6. Group Wrap-up

Session Summary

In today's session, we took a close look at your personalized formulations, and you shared your reflections and the modifications that you made. We then reviewed your self-monitoring forms and assessed how the process of self-monitoring is going for you. We finished the group by introducing a very important tool to overcome your eating disorder: regular eating.

Between-session Work

Remember to encourage patients to write the between-session work on their *Between-session Work Log* handout. The between-session work for Session 2 is:

- Continue work from Session 1:
  - *Self-monitoring* – to be completed daily, in the moment.

- New work from Session 2:
  - *Regular Eating* and *Planning Ahead* – Begin implementing a regular pattern of eating, focusing initially on the times of eating.
  - Additional information handouts – Review relevant handouts: *Dieting, Binge Eating, Underweight/Underfat, Self-induced Vomiting and Medication Misuse,* and/or *Driven Exercise.* Complete at least one Action Plan as described in each handout.

Higher Level of Care Adaptations: Modular Implementation

When this session is used modularly, the following adaptations are suggested.

Formulation review: In settings where most of the same patients return for this group having completed Session 1, reviewing the formulations as described works well. For new patients, for this session and all sessions, it can be helpful to ask current group members to briefly review the previous session's work. This serves as a way to reinforce the learning for current group members and share missed information with new patients. Encourage new patients to actively listen to the group content and ask questions.

Optional information handouts: Reviewing the optional information handouts can serve as an entire psychoeducation group, or groups, at HLOCs. Material can be read aloud, and the information processed collaboratively as a group. Patients can share their experience of engaging in certain behaviors and why they want to stop engaging in these behaviors and/or feel scared about stopping. They can start to make plans for how they will cope with stopping these behaviors while they are in HLOC. These psychoeducation groups could be facilitated by members of the treatment team other than a therapist, depending on scope of practice and expertise. When necessary, consider using creativity when presenting this information, while still committing to all the educational components. Sometimes HLOC patients may see material repeatedly and group leaders will find creative ways to introduce the material in a manner that captures the group's attention (e.g., creating psychoeducation posters; breaking into pairs to discuss the concepts and then returning to present to the group; asking an established patient to help facilitate the group psychoeducation discussion; playing psychoeducation bingo).

Self-monitoring review: This intervention requires that participants have attended Session 1 and have started monitoring. Depending on your setting, the self-monitoring review can be implemented as described, or it can focus more on processing, validating, and normalizing the thoughts and feelings that may have come up as a result of eating higher-calorie food, eating avoided foods, and/or eliminating other eating disorder behaviors (e.g., self-induced vomiting, driven exercise, using laxatives). Sharing these thoughts and feelings with others going through a similar experience is often highly useful for patients. Patients can use one another for support in identifying strategies and approaches for coping. An entire group could be focused on this content.

Regular eating: Consider the usefulness of this intervention, depending on your service. Most inpatient and residential settings will already be implementing regular eating for their patients as a standard of care, typically closely facilitated by a team of dietitians. Patients benefit from understanding the reasons behind these regular eating meal plans through staff-provided psychoeducation. For patients that require weight regain in treatment, their therapeutic meal plan may include eating more frequently than typical regular eating patterns, or adding nutritional supplements to their meal plans, to accommodate for their nutritional needs. This can complicate regular eating education as the patient's eating plan while in treatment may be distinct from their meal plan once they are in lower levels of care and no longer require weight rehabilitation. Open communication and education about this is recommended, as well as utilizing the expertise of a dietitian team to help with educating patients about their individual needs.

For patients at partial hospital and intensive outpatient settings, parts of regular eating are likely incorporated into the times when the patient is in program. Supporting patients to engage in regular eating outside of the program, and when at home, is important and can be implemented as described.

Group Session 2

Handout 2.1 *Between-session Work Self-review – Session 2*

BETWEEN-SESSION WORK SELF-REVIEW – SESSION 2

Thoughts and Feelings about Starting Group
If you are completing this review, it means you have returned for Session 2. **Great work in attending and working towards your recovery!** Starting a new therapy can bring up a variety of feelings. Some folks may feel excited, others may be overwhelmed, some feel both, some feel not very much at all, or some feel something else entirely. All reactions are normal and expected. Take a moment to jot down some of your feelings and thoughts about the first week of treatment.

Complete the checklist below to indicate if you followed through with the between-session work.

Skill	Yes	Somewhat	No
Personalized formulation			
Reviewed my formulation	☐	☐	☐
Added in any missing information (boxes and arrows)	☐	☐	☐
Self-monitoring			
Started using my self-monitoring forms	☐	☐	☐

ANYTHING ELSE?

_____

_____

_____

_____

_____

Handout 2.2   *Self-monitoring Review*

SELF-MONITORING REVIEW

Did I....	Yes	Somewhat	No
Monitor every day?	☐	☐	☐
Monitor at every eating episode?	☐	☐	☐
Always monitor in real time?	☐	☐	☐
Make sure to be accurate/honest?	☐	☐	☐
Write down the time of eating?	☐	☐	☐
Write down foods and drinks I had?	☐	☐	☐
Use brackets for meals?	☐	☐	☐
Include the place of eating?	☐	☐	☐
Include asterisks when I thought that I had overeaten or felt a loss of control while eating?	☐	☐	☐
Mark when I vomited, used laxatives, or diuretics?	☐	☐	☐
Include exercise?	☐	☐	☐
Complete the context column with events, moods, or thoughts?	☐	☐	☐

Great work accomplishing what you have so far! For things that you marked as "somewhat" or "no," complete an Action Plan to help make some changes.

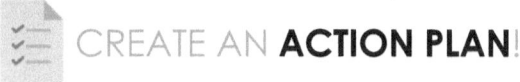

CREATE AN **ACTION PLAN**!

SAMPLE ACTION PLAN		DATE: **4/27**
PROBLEM:	I had a good start to self-monitoring but then have fallen off the last 3 days.	
CURRENT FREQUENCY (IF APPLICABLE):	Self-monitoring 4/7 days	
GOAL FOR UPCOMING WEEK:	Self-monitor 7/7 days	
SPECIFIC PLAN:	MY PLAN:	MY SUPPORT:
	To self-monitor every day this week.	Text my mother after the group to tell her my plan. Put my forms in my planner. Get a manicure as a reward after next group if I manage to do this.

ACTION PLAN		DATE:
PROBLEM:		
CURRENT FREQUENCY (IF APPLICABLE):		
GOAL FOR UPCOMING WEEK:		
SPECIFIC PLAN:	MY PLAN:	MY SUPPORT:

Handout 2.3   *Regular Eating*

REGULAR EATING

Regular eating is a skill that we will be working on throughout treatment. It is a pattern of eating in which you feed your body regularly throughout the day. It is one of the most effective tools in CBT-E designed to help eliminate eating disorder symptoms.

There are two steps to establishing regular eating:

1) Feeding yourself at regular intervals throughout the day
2) Ensuring that the amount is enough

At this point in treatment, the focus is on Step 1 (eating at regular intervals), but it is important to consider Step 2 (the amount) as treatment goes on.

Step 1: Eating at regular intervals

The pattern you choose is up to you. Many find that following the pattern in the box below works well. But not everyone! For example, some folks prefer to have a large meal just before bed and so their pattern might be meal, snack, meal, snack, snack meal. Here are the important parts to keep in mind:

Meal
Snack
Meal
Snack
Meal
Snack

- Eat 3 meals plus 2-3 snacks each day.
- Try your best to not skip any eating episodes.
- Try to eat every 3 hours and avoid going over 4 hours without eating.
- Give yourself a rest in between eating episodes and try to have times when you do not eat.
- What you choose to eat is up to you. Pick foods you are comfortable with and are unlikely to cause you to engage in an eating disorder behavior, like vomiting or taking laxatives

Step 2: Ensuring that the amount is enough

As you begin to establish a solid pattern of eating, consider that you may be undereating. Undereating is a major cause of eating disorder behaviors (request the *Underweight/Underfat* handout if you do not have it).

Regular eating gives you energy at intervals throughout the day. This can make sure that you have adequate energy and nutrition all day long.

Regular eating supports a healthy metabolic process.

Eating regularly can help to eliminate eating disorder symptoms (e.g., binge eating, self-induced vomiting, food restriction). If you are eating throughout the day, your body is less likely to be triggered to binge eat, which then may cause you to be less likely to vomit. Eating throughout the day encourages eating, which helps to decrease food restriction.

REGULAR EATING TIPS

Planning is key! Having a plan in place of <u>when</u> you will eat and roughly <u>what</u> you will eat makes it easier to stick to your plan (use the *Planning Ahead* handout).

Prioritize! For now, make regular eating a top priority. For at least the next several weeks, sticking to regular eating is one of the most important things you will be doing for your health and recovery. Try not to let other life responsibilities get in your way. You are worth it!

Ignore! Don't be guided by hunger and fullness cues for now. You have likely been overriding these cues for a while and they are no longer reliable. Regular eating will help restore the reliability of these cues. Eat according to the timings you've set for yourself.
    Tip: If you frequently feel hungry, including after eating, you may be undereating.

You choose! For now, choose the foods that you prefer and are comfortable with. These are foods that are not likely to cause you to binge or engage in behaviors like vomiting or laxative use.

Enough! You are enough and your food amounts should also be enough. Restricting your eating (in terms of amount, types of foods, and depriving yourself of foods you would enjoy eating) can lead to binge eating or keeping your body weight too low for optimal health. Focus now on the intervals of regular eating, and begin to consider if you may be undereating for your body to function optimally without eating disorder behaviors.

PLANNING AHEAD

Regular eating is a two-step process, and it takes time to get it fully established. Planning ahead is a useful tool that helps you to stick to your regular eating goals. Planning ahead can be helpful in the following ways:

- It can decrease anxiety and discomfort during or before eating. This is because deciding in advance <u>when</u> and <u>what</u> you will eat means not deciding in the moment when stress about eating may be more intense.
- It does not rely on using hunger and fullness cues to guide your eating, which are often unreliable at this point in treatment.
- It allows you to buy foods and prepare them in advance, if necessary
- It represents a commitment to yourself to implement regular eating to the best of your ability.

Remember, planning the times when you will eat is most important for now. Review the 'Tips' on the *Regular Eating* handout while making your plans.

MY EATING PLAN FOR TOMORROW		
Eating Episode	Time	Food and Drink Planned *Rough idea – do not add in specific amounts.*
		EXAMPLE
1	6:30am	Cereal and milk, fruit, coffee
2	10am	Cookie, tea
3	12:30pm	Peanut butter and jelly sandwich; carrot salad; roll; seltzer
4	3pm	Granola bar, water
5	6pm	Roasted chicken, vegetables, mashed potatoes; milk
6	9pm	Ice cream, herbal tea
1		
2		
3		
4		
5		
6		

Handout 2.5 *Dieting*

DIETING

Dieting is one of the main behaviors that keep eating disorders going. It is no surprise that so many people engage in dieting. We are surrounded by diet culture that promises that achieving your ideal body shape and weight through eating, or not eating, in certain ways is possible and morally superior.

DEFINITIONS

Dieting Behaviors	There are many kinds of dieting behaviors. For example, some dieting behaviors involve eating a certain number of calories (usually far below what is needed by the body), avoiding certain types of foods, or having rules about when to eat. Dieting behaviors sometimes go undercover as "healthy" eating or "clean" eating.
Diet Culture	Is a system of beliefs that through dieting (and often exercise), one can achieve their ideal body shape. Diet culture idealizes certain body shapes and weights. This can be anoverall thin shape/weight; particular body shapes, like a small waist and large thighs and buttocks; low body-fat percentage; or achieving a toned or "ripped" look. Diet culture not only pushes the idea that one can achieve the ideal desired shape/weight, it also encourages the thinking that those that do not are morally inferior to those that do – leading to weight stigma.

DIETING BEHAVIORS

Look at the list below. Do you recognize any of these? There are many, many more.
You may have been dieting for so long that it is impossible to spot some dieting behaviors. Consider "healthy eating" or "clean eating" behaviors that are promoted by diet culture and may be hiding dieting behaviors.

Counting calories and keeping to a low number	Exercising to allow myself to eat something
Avoiding certain types of foods I would enjoy or used to enjoy eating	Drinking lots of coffee
Ignoring hunger	Taking diet pills
Eating late in the day to avoid eating	Eating a plant-based diet as a way to have an excuse to avoid lots of foods
Not eating close to bedtime	Using a dieting app
Only eating whole grain carbs	Eating some types of fats (olive oil) and avoiding others (cheese)
Counting macronutrients	Fasting for a certain number of hours per day

There are **many** myths about dieting. Let's debunk a few:

Thinness is healthy; fatness is unhealthy	"Healthy" is a difficult concept to define on its own. But paired with thinness and fatness it's even more complicated. What is healthy is different for all bodies and what it looks like is different too. The idea that only thinness is healthy is incorrect and leads to weight stigma.
There are good foods and bad foods	Usually this is referring to certain macronutrients. For example, lean proteins are "good," carbohydrates are "bad," and depending on what diet is being promoted, fats can go either way. All bodies require these three nutrients in balance, they each play hugely important roles. For example, did you know that not only do carbohydrates help us to feel satisfied, low intake of carbs can lead to brain fog, sluggishness, and low mood? Labeling food as good/bad or healthy/unhealthy places a moral judgment on foods which is very risky. You are not good or bad based on the foods that you are craving, eating, or have available. Food is just food – it is nourishment that is neither good or bad.
Diets work, you just need to try hard enough	Much of our body shape and weight is determined by our genetics. We can make small changes, or changes that last for a short period of time, but pushing our bodies to achieve an "ideal" look is likely difficult and may be impossible in many cases.
Eating after a certain time/late at night will cause weight gain	Our bodies do not metabolize foods differently overnight. Bodies need energy (calories) 24 hours a day, including when we are sleeping.

Take a look at your formulation, how does dieting keep your eating disorder going? Let's explore the two main ways this works.

Physiological pressure	When you diet and prevent your body from getting the amount of energy (through calories) that it needs, the body responds by trying to get the needed energy in. It does this by releasing hormones to stimulate appetite which can increase feelings of hunger (but if you have been ignoring hunger sensations for a long time, you may not notice, but your body does!). When food is available, the body responds to this physiological deprivation to get the food in a quickly as possible, which can cause binge eating.
Psychological pressure	Dieting also puts great psychological pressure on you to eat. Have you ever noticed that the more you deny yourself something (food or other things), you think about them more? Dieting keeps your brain more preoccupied with food and eating. Dieting also involves denying yourself foods you might otherwise enjoy eating. This psychological deprivation can be extremely uncomfortable and hard to ignore and once you are around these foods, you may be more likely to binge on them.

Learning that all bodies require and deserve food is essential to overcoming an eating disorder. Making a commitment to go "diet-free" and instead feed your body regularly with nutritious, enjoyable, and satisfying foods is one of the most helpful ways to overcome an eating disorder. This includes eating carbs, fats, and proteins. It also includes choosing foods that you enjoy that may be labelled as "unhealthy" due to their "lack of nutrition." It is scary to make a change like this – but well worth it to overcome your eating disorder. Take a moment to think of all of the reasons why changing what you eat may be worth it. What motivates you?

Write down all of the reasons why you want to overcome your eating disorder. Include why you want to be free from dieting and instead feed your body regularly. Be as specific as possible.

1) Recognize how dieting behaviors keep the eating disorder going.

2) Consider some of the following:
- Take a stand against diet culture and move away from its control. Look for information about anti-diet approaches (e.g., blogs, websites, social media).
- Assess if you are undereating and increase total calories.
- Allow yourself to eat the foods you have been denying yourself – at first this may trigger binge eating. Be sure to use your alternative activities and urge tolerating to support your goals and review the *Binge Eating* handout.
- Seek to eat balanced meals and snacks – eat carbs, fats, and protein at each eating episode.
- Consider meeting with an eating disorder-informed dietitian to get specific nutrition guidance.

3) Make an Action Plan (below) and commit to addressing your dieting behaviors (Session 6 will cover this topic in more detail).

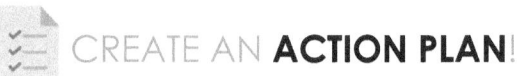 CREATE AN **ACTION PLAN**!

SAMPLE ACTION PLAN		DATE: **3/19**
PROBLEM:	Not allowing myself carbs	
CURRENT FREQUENCY (IF APPLICABLE):	Hardly ever	
GOAL FOR UPCOMING WEEK:	I will have some form of carbs at 2 of my eating episodes each day.	
SPECIFIC PLAN:	MY PLAN:	MY SUPPORT:
	My mid-morning snack – I will eat a handful of goldfish crackers. Before bed – I will have a piece of toast with my snack.	I am telling the group and will tell my support person. I will also think about why I am making this really scary change and review all of the reasons on this handout about how eating as I have been is keeping me sick. I will focus on the future and stay motivated by focusing on getting my degree and being a teacher when I am no longer struggling with my eating disorder.

Handout 2.6   *Binge Eating*

BINGE EATING

Binge eating is a common eating disorder symptom which involves eating a large amount of food and feeling a loss of control over eating. Binge eating typically involves: eating very quickly/in a short period of time; eating in secret/alone due to embarrassment about eating; eating a large amount of food when not feeling hungry; eating until feeling uncomfortably full; and feeling guilt/shame/sadness after eating. Sometimes the start of a binge can feel pleasurable or like a relief. Binge eating can be a consequence of dieting behaviors, or can be a soothing technique for intense emotions. Binge eating can impact mental and physical states.

SELF-CHECK

I have episodes of eating where I:			
☐	Feel out of control.	☐	Eat a large amount when not feeling hungry.
☐	Eat very quickly/in a short period of time.	☐	Eat until feeling uncomfortably full.
☐	Eat much more food than others eat in the same period of time.	☐	Feel guilt/shame/sadness after eating.
☐	Eat in secret/alone due to embarrassment about eating.		

EXAMPLES OF EFFECTS OF BINGE EATING

Decreased self-esteem	Depression
Thinking a lot about food, eating, shape, and weight	Gastrointestinal symptoms - acid reflux, heartburn, bloating, diarrhea, constipation, abdominal pain
Irritability	Anxiety
Fatigue	Sleep problems
Isolation	

When working toward stopping binge eating, review your personalized formulation to see if there is a connection between dieting (not eating enough for your body) and binge eating. If so, stopping binge eating may mean eating enough food, and allowing yourself to have the foods regularly that you may typically only allow yourself to have when you are bingeing. These foods likely taste good, give your body energy, and are foods that you may see at social occasions. Starting to incorporate these foods into your regular eating patterns may be helpful to reduce any deprivation experienced by restricting these foods and to learn how to have these foods in controlled ways. Use the support of the group to brainstorm strategies to help support yourself with this.

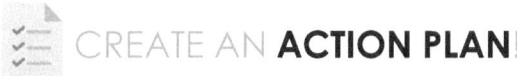 CREATE AN **ACTION PLAN**!

IDEAS TO CONSIDER INCORPORATING INTO MY ACTION PLAN

Make sure to prioritize regular eating throughout the day!
Plan ahead meals in order to support regular eating and to decrease triggers for binge eating.
Use all other strategies for regular eating, including alternative activities and urge tolerating.
If my binge eating is related to a shift in my mood, try addressing that shift in mood by using skills to work through the emotion (e.g., deep breathing, journaling, talking to a support person) or alternative activities until the emotion passes.
Make environmental changes to help decrease binge eating, such as making food less accessible during a triggering time for binge eating (e.g., leave the house, go upstairs to be further from the kitchen) and avoid engaging in activities that are typically accompanied by binge eating (e.g., watching television, laying down).
Consider having the foods that you may only allow yourself to have when binge eating in planful ways as a part of your regular eating plan. Make sure to have individual portions available regularly in typical portions.
Remember binge eating is a soothing technique for many. If it is for you, consider planning an alternative activity for soothing (e.g., listening to music while wrapped up in your favorite blanket). Alternative activities likely will not work as well as binge eating, especially in the beginning, but will bring you closer to your recovery goals.

SAMPLE ACTION PLAN		DATE: 2/16
PROBLEM:	Binge eating	
CURRENT FREQUENCY (IF APPLICABLE):	4 x a week	
GOAL FOR UPCOMING WEEK:	2 x this week	
	MY PLAN:	MY SUPPORT:
SPECIFIC PLAN:	Add alternative activities in the evening. Make sure to eat breakfast every day.	After eating dinner, I will try: 1) Taking a shower 2) Writing one card 3) Watching one television show upstairs I will go grocery shopping this afternoon to have available a couple of breakfasts to choose from. I will then set my alarm for 7:00 each morning so that I have plenty of time to eat breakfast. I will plan to have time to listen to my favorite AM news show while eating breakfast.

ACTION PLAN		DATE:
PROBLEM:		
CURRENT FREQUENCY (IF APPLICABLE):		
GOAL FOR UPCOMING WEEK:		
SPECIFIC PLAN:	MY PLAN:	MY SUPPORT:

Handout 2.7   *Underweight/Underfat*

UNDERWEIGHT/UNDERFAT

Many individuals with eating disorders are underweight or underfat for their bodies to function optimally. This informational handout will explore these terms and how reversing both of these states, when present, is essential to fully overcome an eating disorder.

DEFINITIONS

Underweight	In Group CBT-E, we use this term to describe a body that is a lower weight than it needs to be to function optimally without eating disorder behaviors. Some individuals may be at a weight that is a little bit below where their body ideally needs to be and others may be significantly below where their body needs to be.
Underfat	In Group CBT-E, we use this term to describe a body that does not have enough body fat to function optimally without eating disorder behaviors.

ASSOCIATED EATING AND WEIGHT CONTROL BEHAVIORS

The following behaviors may be associated with being underweight/underfat. Check any that you recognize for yourself and add others.

☐	Food restriction (low total number of calories)
☐	Avoiding many foods
☐	Prioritizing protein consumption
☐	Frequent weighing or measuring my body
☐	Pushing myself with exercise despite feeling tired or being injured
☐	
☐	
☐	
☐	

CONSEQUENCES

Being underweight/underfat keeps the eating disorder going. You can see this on your *My Formulation* handout. In addition to this, there are also many other consequences to maintaining an underweight/underfat body. Many of these are caused by being in a constant state of starvation or semi-starvation. Check any of the following you experience:

☐	Increased irritability
☐	Poor sleep
☐	Fatigue/tiredness
☐	Low mood
☐	Increased anxiety
☐	Feeling cold
☐	Lots of thoughts about my shape, weight, and/or eating
☐	Decreased concentration/attention
☐	Dreaming about food
☐	Extreme fear about changes to my body weight
☐	Increased obsessive thinking
☐	Low/no sex drive
☐	Loss of periods/irregular periods
☐	Cutting food into small pieces/taking small bites
☐	Eating around my plate in a particular pattern (e.g., clockwise)
☐	Narrowed interests that tend to be on topics of weight loss, cooking, muscle building, etc.
☐	Counting calories/checking food labels for fat or calorie content
☐	Missing out on socializing with family/friends

WHY CHANGE?

It is impossible to overcome an eating disorder while being underweight/underfat. If part of your eating disorder is being maintained by either or both of these, take time to consider this information and the impact on your life. While you are in Group CBT-E treatment, it is an ideal time to practice being flexible with your eating and being open to the possibility that your body and mind may need more overall calories and/or body fat to live the life that you want. Making changes to your body in this way may be one of the scariest things you have ever done and it may also be one of the most important things you can do.

The reasons why I want to overcome my eating disorder are (be as specific as possible):

STEPS TO CHANGE

1) Be open to the possibility that your body may be underweight/underfat. This contributes to keeping your eating disorder going and semi-starvation/starvation symptoms.

2) Consider one of the following:
    1. Going against the eating disorder and eating something from your avoided foods list several times each week (more direct support for this in Session 6).
    2. Give your body permission to increase in weight and eat additional calories.
    3. Reduce driven exercise each week.

3) Make an Action Plan below and commit to addressing being underweight/underfat.

SAMPLE ACTION PLAN		DATE: 3/20
PROBLEM:	Not eating a variety of macronutrients	
CURRENT FREQUENCY (IF APPLICABLE):	N/A	
GOAL FOR UPCOMING WEEK:	I will have a more balanced lunch 4/7 days this week (instead of salad only).	
SPECIFIC PLAN:	MY PLAN:	MY SUPPORT:
	Monday – Ham, cheese, and mayo sandwich, pretzels, apple Tuesday – Chicken and cheese burrito, tortilla chips Friday – Cheese, avocado, and mayo sandwich, chips, cookie Saturday – Dinner leftovers	I am telling the group my plan and will ask my coworker to have lunch with me during the weekdays so that I have a support person during the meals. I will plan to sit outside for at least 10 minutes after each weekday lunch and will plan to go to the library after my Saturday lunch.

ACTION PLAN		DATE:
PROBLEM:		
CURRENT FREQUENCY (IF APPLICABLE):		
GOAL FOR UPCOMING WEEK:		
SPECIFIC PLAN:	MY PLAN:	MY SUPPORT:

Handout 2.8 *Self-induced Vomiting and Medication Misuse*

SELF-INDUCED VOMITING & MEDICATION MISUSE

Oftentimes, compensatory behaviors start as a way to gain control when feeling out of control related to breaking a diet-related rule, eating in a different way, feelings of fullness, or experiencing a weight change. These behaviors become a way to compensate for perceived or actual overeating, or are used more routinely to attempt to lose weight. Compensatory behaviors become a part of the vicious cycle of eating disorder behaviors. There are a variety of compensatory behaviors. This handout will focus on self-induced vomiting (SIV) and the misuse of medications (MM) to control weight (e.g., abuse of weight loss medications, laxatives, diuretics, insulin). If you are struggling with other compensatory behaviors that have not yet been addressed in group therapy, make sure to alert your group therapist. There are several physical consequences of compensatory behaviors, and some that can be life-threatening. There are also many misconceptions about compensatory behaviors. Read below to learn more about the facts related to compensatory behaviors.

MYTHS/REALITIES

Myth	Reality
SIV and MM are helpful to get rid of food intake/calories	SIV and MM are relatively ineffective: • Vomiting: Does not get rid of the majority of food/calories consumed • Laxatives: Have very little impact on food absorption • Diuretics: Do not impact food absorption This is because absorption begins in the mouth, is retained by the stomach, and/or passed through to the small intestine.
SIV and MM are helpful for long-term weight loss.	Typically weight loss that is a result of SIV & MM is more related to dehydration and water loss and not long-term weight change.
SIV and MM help to control my eating behavior.	Believing that SIV and MM can "get rid of" binge eating maintains binge eating and makes it more likely to occur.
They don't impact me that much.	SIV and MM are often highly impairing. They lead to secrecy, dishonesty, guilt, shame, embarrassment, anxiety, depression, and loneliness. They can impact social and occupational activities. MM can be expensive.

EXAMPLES OF PHYSICAL EFFECTS OF SIV

Electrolyte disturbances, such as potassium and sodium, which can lead to fainting, confusion, fatigue, nausea, blood pressure changes, heart palpitations, irregular heartbeats, headaches, seizures, cardiac arrest, and death
Salivary glands can become enlarged causing cheeks to look swollen and puffy.
Dental erosion, brittleness, and thermal sensitivity from gastric acid. Repairing these conditions can be very expensive.
Impaired hunger and fullness cues
Peptic ulcers and pancreatitis (inflammation of the pancreas)
Esophageal burning
Swelling of hands and/or feet
Frequent sore throat
Red dots on the face, acne around the mouth
Mouth ulcers
Vomiting blood
Abdominal bloating

WHY DO I WANT TO CHANGE?

☐ I am worried about what it is doing to my body, in particular, it causes me to feel:
☐ I hate the feeling.
☐ I am worried about how it is affecting my relationships.
☐ I am worried about how it affects work/ school.
☐ I don't want to think about vomiting/medication misuse so much.
☐ It doesn't help me lose weight.
☐ It causes me to overeat/ binge.
☐ My vomiting/medication misuse makes me feel out of control.
☐
☐

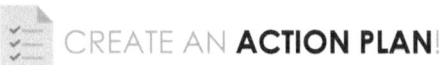 CREATE AN **ACTION PLAN**!

IDEAS TO CONSIDER INCORPORATING INTO MY ACTION PLAN

Call my primary care doctor about my SIV and/or MM behavior.
Ask my primary care doctor about setting up a withdrawal schedule for my laxative/diuretic use.
Make sure to be prioritizing regular eating throughout the day!
Plan ahead meals in order to support regular eating and to decrease triggers for binge eating.
Use all other strategies for regular eating, including alternative activities and urge tolerating.
Make sure to address my binge eating. Remember binge eating can often lead to SIV and MM.
Throw away pills/Give pills to a support person.
Delete online drugstore account.
Use my supports for accountability!
Identify what triggered my behaviors and address THAT trigger.
Avoid using the bathroom one hour after eating to decrease environmental cues attached to vomiting (i.e., toilet).

SAMPLE ACTION PLAN

DATE: **3/20**

PROBLEM:	Self-Induced Vomiting	
CURRENT FREQUENCY (IF APPLICABLE):	6x a week	
GOAL FOR UPCOMING WEEK:	4 x this week	
	MY PLAN:	MY SUPPORT:
SPECIFIC PLAN:	Decrease binge eating Add in alternative activities after eating dinner.	Commit to regular eating and implement my plan for completing breakfast each day to start off with my plan. Add in urge tolerating in the evenings when I have an urge to binge. I usually vomit after dinner. After dinner I will: Monday – Finish my paper Tuesday – Visit my sister Wednesday – Take a bath & get to bed early Thursday – Go for a drive Friday – Plan with friend Saturday – Work in evening Sunday – Start reading my new book

ACTION PLAN

DATE:

PROBLEM:		
CURRENT FREQUENCY (IF APPLICABLE):		
GOAL FOR UPCOMING WEEK:		
	MY PLAN:	MY SUPPORT:
SPECIFIC PLAN:		

Handout 2.9   *Driven Exercise*

DRIVEN EXERCISE

Exercise can be fun, reduce stress, boost mood, and improve cardiovascular health. Unfortunately, for individuals with eating disorders, exercise can sometimes become driven and can further contribute to the eating disorder. Driven exercise can have many side effects, including worsening preoccupation with weight and shape; increased eating disorder behaviors; anxiety and shame when not exercising; dangerous physical consequences; and negative impacts on other important areas of life. The goal is to evaluate your own exercise and find a movement routine that promotes wellness, is rejuvenating, and avoids increased stress.

SELF-CHECK

In the box below, list the types of exercise that you engage in (e.g., walking, running, going to the gym, participating on a team, hiking, stretching, biking).

Now, check the boxes below if you relate to the statements about exercise.

☐	I exercise to change my shape and weight.
☐	I feel driven to exercise and/or it creates anxiety/ shame when my exercise rules are not followed.
☐	I exercise to compensate for food eaten.
☐	My energy levels are depleted by the amount of exercise I engage in.
☐	I exercise at a frequency that is much more than others.
☐	I exercise even though I am sick or injured.
☐	I feel worried about my safety when exercising.
☐	Exercising takes away from doing other life activities.

ADVERSE EFFECTS OF DRIVEN EXERCISE

Driven exercise can have significant negative side effects, including:

- Being at a weight lower than your body needs/underfat which can lead to:
    - Cardiovascular damage
    - Vital organ damage
    - Bone damage
    - Reproductive system damage
- Risk of stress fractures
- Muscle damage
- Continues to maintain my eating disorder
- Takes away from other important areas of life

> If experiencing any of the below, please schedule an urgent visit with your medical provider:
> - Heart palpitations
> - Dizziness
> - Lightheadedness
> - Chest pain

IDEAS TO CONSIDER INCORPORATING INTO MY ACTION PLAN

Try a different form of joyful movement that allows me to focus on something fun and that doesn't have me thinking about shape and weight.
Call my primary care doctor to tell them about negative physical symptoms when I exercise.
Put away equipment that encourages driven exercise (e.g., running sneakers, home gym equipment).
Discontinue memberships that encourage driven exercise (e.g., online exercise class subscription, gym membership).
Tell a support person my goal related to exercise.

ACTION PLAN		DATE: 8/23
PROBLEM:	Driven exercise	
CURRENT FREQUENCY (IF APPLICABLE):	4 x a week	
GOAL FOR UPCOMING WEEK:	2 x this week + try a new joyful activity!	
SPECIFIC PLAN:	MY PLAN:	MY SUPPORT:
	Wednesday: Pilates class (no gym after!)	Do this right before I am meeting my friend at the dog park so I can't do additional exercise. Make sure to follow my regular eating!
	Friday: 45-minute run	I will be alone so I will make a specific plan to write in my journal once I get home and use urge tolerating if needed.
	Saturday: Try a new joyful movement.	I always go for a 6+ mile run on Saturdays. I will go for a walk with a friend and see about trying to stay present.

Chapter 8

Group Session 3
Regular Eating and Alternative Activities

Overview

Session 3 aims to further establish regular eating by introducing a valuable tool: the practice of engaging in alternative activities. Alternative activities are any activities that make it less likely that a patient will engage in an eating disorder behavior. When planned in advance, they are highly effective in helping patients stick to their regular eating plans. The first part of this session explores individual factors that are interfering with adopting a regular pattern of eating and supports patients in creating relevant Action Plans. The second part is on creating alternative activities and understanding how and when to use them.

Therapist Preparation

☐ Review this chapter in advance. Pay close attention to pages XY–XY which have useful information related to the regular eating review.
☐ Review accompanying handouts and have copies available for patients.

Handouts

- Standard Weekly Handouts
  - *1.3 Self-monitoring Form*
  - *1.6 Between-session Work Log*
  - *3.1 Between-session Work Self-review – Session 3*

- Session-specific Handouts
  - *3.2 Regular Eating Review*
  - *3.3 Alternative Activities*

Group Session Agenda

1. Setting the agenda and orienting to the session (2 minutes)
2. Between-session work self-review (5 minutes)
3. Reviewing regular eating (35 minutes)
4. Introducing alternative activities (15 minutes)
5. Group wrap-up (3 minutes)

DOI: 10.4324/9781003450849-10

1. Setting the Agenda and Orienting to the Session

Begin with a positive, encouraging welcome. Share that this is Session 3, Stage 1 with 11 sessions remaining. Clearly list the session agenda.

2. Between-session Work Self-review

Handout: *Between-session Work Self-review – Session 3*

Patients should begin by completing the *Between-session Work Self-review – Session 3* handout. This self-review focuses on self-monitoring forms, using similar questions to those in the *Self-monitoring Review* handout from Session 2. It also briefly checks in on starting regular eating and reviewing the informational handouts (e.g., *Dieting, Binge Eating, Underweight/ Underfat, Self-induced Vomiting and Medication Misuse,* and *Driven Exercise*). Reviewing regular eating is one of the primary agenda items for this session and a detailed in-session review is conducted following the between-session work self-review.

In this, and all subsequent sessions, once patients have had the opportunity to complete the handout, praise patients for areas that are going well and support patients in creating Action Plans for areas that need additional focus (using the extra Action Plan copies supplied in Appendix E). Sometimes during the self-review patients will need to update their Action Plans to make for a more challenging plan or to alter the current plan to address barriers. Other times patients will create new Action Plans to address a new skill that they are ready to tackle or to more appropriately address a previous goal. Make sure that this review time is an opportunity for patients to organize themselves (using Action Plans) around which goals have been achieved, which are longstanding, and which need to be updated.

For this particular review, check in on whether patients are following through with self-monitoring. If a patient is struggling to implement self-monitoring regularly, return to strategies discussed in Session 2, and remind patients of the critical importance of self-monitoring to successfully reach their treatment goals. Be sure to ask about any thoughts group members had about reading the informational handouts or progress with relevant Action Plans. Encourage group members to write relevant Action Plans on their *Between-session Work Log* handout.

3. Reviewing Regular Eating

Handout: *Regular Eating Review*

Establishing a regular pattern of eating can be difficult for patients and takes practice to implement with ease. It is essential to jointly evaluate with patients how they are progressing with adopting this new eating pattern. Using the *Regular Eating Review* handout, ask the group to identify places where they struggled to implement the regular eating guidelines, consider factors that may have led to these struggles, and identify Action Plans for change. The focus of the discussion will be on how closely the patients' eating patterns fit with regular eating guidelines. Start by engaging a volunteer in a discussion about regular eating and then incorporate the rest of the group, both for support and to share their own experience.

After completing the Regular Eating Review handout, I will ask you to share what you learned from completing the checklist. Were there areas where you struggled with regular eating patterns? What do you think is causing the difficulties and how might you make changes to address this?

I would like to invite a volunteer to share a day from your week – perhaps a day that you felt was particularly challenging to stick to regular eating patterns. I know that sharing your eating patterns aloud with others may be new to you and may bring up feelings of embarrassment. I encourage you to try to challenge yourself in this way. I also encourage the group to make sure that we keep this a safe space for others to share in this way. Please take us through your day and let us know where you noticed a time when you struggled to implement regular eating, and together we can think about what may have happened. We can brainstorm how you might address these challenges for the coming week.

Therapist Insight

It can be emotionally challenging for patients to share aloud information from their self-monitoring forms about their eating behaviors and symptoms. Patients can hold much judgment related to their food choices and experience feelings of guilt and shame reading back the information to themselves, and certainly sharing it with the group. Make sure to create a safe and non-judgmental space. Normalize this difficulty for patients and consider surveying the group to determine how many group members experience worries about sharing their eating patterns. Often, when multiple patients have this same experience, they find comfort in knowing that they will be facing their fears together as a group.

To help guide your review of the *Regular Eating Review* handout, the following questions and accompanying psychoeducation (adapted from Individual CBT-E, Fairburn 2008 will likely be useful.

- *Did I have 3 meals plus 2–3 snacks daily?* If the answer to this question is 'no,' further exploration is needed to identify factors that may be getting in the way (see items below). It also allows for a reminder about the purpose of regular eating.

  Let's go back to your Regular Eating handout and review the reasons why regular eating is so important. Remember, eating regularly throughout the day can help to significantly reduce (or eliminate) certain eating disorder symptoms. If you are nourishing your body throughout the day, this will reduce the pressure to binge eat and reduce symptoms of maintaining a weight lower than one's body needs/being underfat, caused by dieting and not getting enough energy. If there are decreases in binge eating, then likely there will be decreased compensatory behaviors to "get rid of" the energy consumed during binge eating. Remember, this is a process and won't change overnight. Let's celebrate the days/times when you were able to get closer to regular eating and learn from those too.

- *Did I roughly plan the times and content of meals ahead?* Planning ahead is very useful for patients that struggle to adhere to regular eating guidelines. Encourage patients to continue to complete the plan on the *Planning Ahead* handout daily to keep up the practice.

> *You may remember from your Planning Ahead handout that planning ahead can help to decrease anxiety and discomfort during or before an eating episode because decisions about what food to eat have been made ahead of time. Deciding ahead of time means that you do not have to make a challenging decision at a time when you are hungry, or possibly feeling anxious, about the upcoming meal/snack. It also means that you will have the food you need available as planning ahead also allows for shopping ahead or packing meals/snacks when necessary. In general, it is helpful to have a sense of when and what you will be eating during your next meal or snack. Planning ahead takes time and quite a lot of effort, so keep practicing!*

- *Did I take a break from eating in between my meals and snacks?* Eating in between meals and snacks can be problematic. Many patients find this highly distressing as it can cause increased focus on food throughout the day. In these situations, it is helpful to understand the function of this eating to determine how to address it. For example, if a patient engaged in having an extra snack in a socially enjoyable way and maintained regular eating throughout the rest of the day, this would not be worthy of clinical attention (other than to celebrate that flexibility!). On the other hand, if a patient is picking on food throughout the day without a structure to their meals, supporting patients to reduce this will better help them to overcome the eating disorder. Engaging in distracting, alternative activities is a valuable practice and will be discussed later in the session. If eating in between meals and snacks is due to the patient not eating enough total calories earlier in the day, encourage the patient to consider that they increase the amount they are eating at meals and snacks. Highlight on their formulation the impact of maintaining a weight too low for their body and dieting and how this leads to further eating disorder behaviors. Provide them with the *Dieting* and *Underweight/Underfat* handouts; and encourage patients to make relevant Action Plans about increasing the overall amount they are eating.

- *Did I eat enough food to have enough energy between eating episodes?* While eating at regular intervals is the first step to establishing regular eating, it is imperative that patients are also learning that they need to have adequate amounts of food at each eating episode (Step 2 on the *Regular Eating* handout). As mentioned, this allows for stable amounts of energy throughout the day and avoids triggering binge eating episodes. The same guidance from the point above applies here too.

- *Did I follow hunger/fullness cues over my regular eating plan?* Remind patients that hunger and fullness cannot be relied on at this stage of treatment. Because of their eating disorder, hunger and fullness cues have not been responded to appropriately over a sustained period of time, which has impacted the accuracy of these cues.

- *Were there more than 4 hours between eating episodes?* Remind patients about how long gaps between eating puts them at risk of binge eating and sustained undereating.

- *Did I prioritize eating over other activities?* Struggling to prioritize eating can commonly occur for patients new to CBT-E. It can feel like a dramatic change to prioritize eating in this way. At times, the realities of other life demands can distract from regular eating recommendations, and it can seem unnecessary to rearrange priorities to follow the pattern in this way. At other times, focusing on other life activities can provide a way to avoid eating. It can be helpful to remind patients of the following:

  For now, it is essential to prioritize regular eating. You will not always need to follow the plan so closely and will be able to be more spontaneous with your eating and other life activities in the future. At the moment, it is one of the most important pieces of treatment. Sometimes it can help to think of food as your medicine. In the same way that you would prioritize taking a critical medication and not missing any doses, you must do the same with your eating. For example, when you are out and busy, this includes packing an easy to eat snack to help you to stick with regular eating in these situations.

- *Did social eating impact regular eating?* Work with patients to identify any negative thoughts/feelings that occur related to eating with others, or avoidance of eating with others. Oftentimes eating socially can impact the choices that are available to patients and the lack of control over making choices can increase anxiety. Strategies such as planning ahead and applying the use of breaks can be helpful in these situations.

- *Did I engage in behaviors like binge eating, vomiting, misusing medications, or driven exercising?* In these situations, the first recommendation is to help support patients to find times where they struggled to implement regular eating and provide support. If regular eating was implemented and followed, then additional specific focus in these areas may be needed. Ask patients to take out the handout that accompanies the behavior that they experienced (i.e., *Binge Eating, Self-induced Vomiting and Medication Misuse, Driven Exercise* handouts). Ask patients to share aloud the Action Plans that they identified related to these behaviors and the outcome of the plans this week. Support patients that are struggling in one of these areas to identify an updated Action Plan that is realistic and that will likely set them up for success. For example:

  I know that some people endorsed that they experienced binge eating behaviors this week. Let's take out the Binge Eating handout and talk today about the Action Plan that you put in place to help reduce this behavior. Would someone be willing to share what they tried and what was helpful and what was not so helpful?

Evaluation of what was happening before engaging in an eating disorder behavior, and any consequences of these behaviors, is worthwhile. At times, identifying triggers for the behavior is necessary to then choose a course of action.

- *Did my feelings, events, or situations impact my eating?* Commonly, eating disorder urges and behaviors are impacted by thoughts, feelings, and situations, as shown on the formulation. When this occurs, it can be a great opportunity to engage the group to help to support one another in assessing if eating disorder behaviors are useful in these situations, taking a short and long term perspective.

I noticed that you mentioned that you struggle with feelings of sadness when you are alone in the evenings and that when you are feeling sad, you are more likely to binge. Does anyone else relate to that? Let's take a moment to think more about this. It is likely that your eating disorder does help in these moments. Does it help with the emotion long term? Take a look at your personalized formulation. Does responding to emotions in this way maintain eating disorder symptoms? Would it be worthwhile for you to try to respond to these emotions or events in a new way? We will talk about some alternative activities that could be applied when experiencing emotion dysregulation in the session today. [If patients report that feelings, events, or emotions caused eating disorder behaviors, but do not have this reflected on their formulation, be sure to encourage them to consider adding it.]

- *Did I sit for the meal?* It is best to have a place to sit when eating to help encourage a beginning and end to eating and increase mindfulness during the meal.

- *Did I eat from packages?* It is helpful to plate the food ahead of eating as eating from packages can be associated with feeling a loss of control. For some patients struggling with binge eating, it can be useful to talk about how to have individual portions of foods available and make environmental modifications to support regular eating (e.g., cutting a pan of brownies into portions and placing brownies in the freezer to take out one at a time or purchasing individual servings of ice cream until the patient is comfortable working their way up to having more standard sizes available at home).

- *Did I eat while distracted?* Patients are recommended to focus on eating while eating and minimize distractions that can impact following through with regular eating plans. The exception to this recommendation is for patients who are experiencing a high level of discomfort, which can lead to avoidance, at mealtimes. For these patients, sometimes distraction can be a temporary strategy that can help with eating success. Once a patient is more accustomed to regular eating, the goal is that less distraction will be necessary.

> **Therapist Insight**
>
> Remember to stick to the agenda's time allocation related to regular eating in this session. There will likely be a lot to talk about regarding regular eating and not every behavior will be addressed in this timeframe. The next session also reserves time to focus on regular eating. The aim for this session is that each patient will create at least one Action Plan to support regular eating patterns.

- *Did I have difficulties with my speed of eating (eating very slowly or quickly)?* Pacing is often difficult for patients. Start making recommendations for normalizing eating pace, which may need to occur through small incremental changes session by session, with an end goal of taking at least 15 minutes, but not an extensive amount of time, to complete a meal. Strategies such as setting a timer, or pacing eating behaviors with a support person, can be helpful.

At the conclusion of the regular eating review, ask each patient to complete at least one Action Plan to address a struggle with their regular eating.

4. Introducing Alternative Activities

Handout: *Alternative Activities*

As suggested in many of the considerations reviewed above, engaging in alternative activities is a critical skill to help support regular eating recommendations. Patients will need to have other activities to engage in to distract from a variety of eating disorder-related urges (e.g., the urge to binge eat or take laxatives). Having a list of alternative activities can be helpful in three ways: 1) to plan in advance during increased times of distress (e.g., a stressful family event) or times with an increased likelihood of engaging in eating disorder behaviors (e.g., eating a snack when one usually does not have snacks); and 2) to have a pre-created list of activities to utilize in moments when urges to engage in behaviors occur unexpectedly and 3) to have prepared a list of activities that can be used in moments of stress or emotional dysregulation to manage these feelings in new, more functional ways (i.e. in ways that do not contribute to the eating disorder).

Engage the group in a brainstorming process to identify alternative activities. As group members start to list personal ideas for alternative activities, ask them to record these ideas on their *Alternative Activities* handout. Using a whiteboard [see Table 8.1], record the group's ideas so that all members can view each other's responses. Ask the group to provide feedback to one another and to challenge themselves to consider activities that they may not currently be engaged in but are willing to try.

Let's take out your Alternative Activities handout. Alternative activities are distracting activities that can help you to follow your regular eating habits, including eating at the planned eating times and avoiding eating between eating episodes, driven exercise, binge eating, medication misuse, and self-induced vomiting. Let's think creatively as a group about

Table 8.1 Sample Whiteboard – Alternative Activities

Activities with others:

Call my cousin
Text my sister and make plans to get together
Go for a walk with my partner

Changing the environment:

Go to my room and listen to music
Go to the library
Sit on my front stoop

Other activities:

Play an online game
Journal
Take a shower or bath
Play with my dog
Play my guitar
Crochet
Dance
Watch TV

alternative activities to add to your list. Please share aloud ideas that you have. In order to have a full list with options that can be used in a variety of situations, think of interpersonal activities with others, activities that help to remove you from a triggering situation/environment, and anything else that might be helpful. If you hear something that another group member has shared – something that you are already practicing or are curious about practicing – and would like to add it to your list, please do so.

Once a solid start to an alternative activities list is created, let patients know that this list will be a work in progress and will continue to be something to add to following the session and throughout treatment. Ask group members to share their Action Plan describing which alternative activities they plan to engage in over the coming week.

It is also important that patients have easy access to their list. Ask patients to identify where they will store their alternative activities list so that they have it available when they need it. Ask patients to consider if sharing these with a support person may be useful.

I encourage you to keep your alternative activities list at the forefront of your mind during times when you have urges to act on symptoms. Where could you post this list? What do you need to do to remember these during moments of need? Would it be helpful to share this list with a support person?

We have seen patients post these lists in their bedrooms, carry them in their wallets, or take a picture of the list and include it as a background on their mobile devices.

Using your Alternative Activities handout, let's also create one Action Plan related to increasing the use of alternative activities this week. Plan for how and when to best incorporate these. Consider also planning these during typically challenging days, times, or events, when possible. Make sure to add your alternative activities to your self-monitoring forms for this week.

5. Group Wrap-up

Session Review

Today we continued to focus on regular eating and the importance of adopting this pattern of eating. We identified some of the challenges you encountered implementing regular eating and considered strategies to help increase your regular eating patterns. In particular, we listed alternative activities that may be helpful to practice in a variety of situations to help you to stick with regular eating.

Between-session Work

Remember to encourage patients to write the between-session work on their *Between-session Work Log* handout. The between-session work for Session 3 is:

- Continue work from Sessions 1 and 2:
  - *Self-monitoring* – to be completed daily, in the moment.
  - *Regular Eating* and *Planning Ahead* – continue to practice following a regular pattern of eating.
- New work from Session 3:
  - *Alternative Activities* – review and implement at least one Action Plan. Record on self-monitoring forms when alternative activities are used. If useful, consider posting and sharing with a support person a list of alternative activities.

Higher Level of Care Adaptations: Modular Implementation

When this session is used modularly, the following adaptations are suggested.

Regular eating: Working toward regular eating patterns is a primary goal in all HLOC treatment. At inpatient and residential programs, the eating plan is typically determined by the treatment team, as opposed to being decided by the patient. The aim is to quickly support eating disorder behavior elimination and renourish the body to repair any associated medical consequences. In these situations, patients do not typically have choices related to the timing, portions, and types of foods that are provided for them and are expected to consume the food as served. Though patients do not have a choice related to the content of the meals, they do have a choice related to whether or not to eat the meals and snacks provided and whether or not to engage in other eating disorder behaviors (e.g., self-induced vomiting, driven exercise). When meal refusal or other eating disorder behaviors occur, patients are usually expected to replace the missed energy with nutritional supplements or another form of caloric intake. For patients at these levels of care, some of the regular eating review is not relevant; however, other aspects might be useful to consider in these environments. For patients who are not able to complete the meals and snacks as prescribed, assessing certain aspects of their eating may be useful to help identify strategies for better complying with the meal plan. For patients who are struggling with significant eating disorder urges at meals, some of the regular eating review can be useful to better understand their urges. Aspects of the regular eating review to consider in both these situations include:

- *Did I have 3 meals plus 2–3 snacks daily (without relying on meal replacement nutritional supplements)?*
- *Did I follow my regular eating plan (i.e., meal plan) rather than hunger/fullness cues (which are not reliable currently)?*
- *Did I engage in behaviors like binge eating, vomiting, misusing medications, or driven exercising?*
- *Did my feelings, events, or situations impact my eating?*
- *Did I eat while distracted (and was this helpful or not helpful for meal/snack completion)?*

Patients at partial hospital and intensive outpatient settings likely have a combination of meals and snacks prepared while in treatment and then opportunities to choose their own meals during time away from treatment. Some intensive outpatient programs, as well as virtual partial hospital programs, will ask patients to prepare all of their own meals. Planning for time away from the program, or planning for prepared meals while in the program, using the regular eating principles, is important and can be implemented as described.

Alternative activities: Guidance on the use of alternative activities to apply in the place of engaging in eating disorder behaviors is useful at all levels of care and could serve as content for a complete group at HLOCs. Some programs will reserve leisure time following meals and snacks to practice planned alternative activities (e.g., journaling, listening to music, completing word games, reading, playing a group game) and as such, patients may use an alternative activities group to practice these skills.

While implementing some of the activities, a group member may describe an activity that is not possible at inpatient and residential settings (e.g., many patients will say that calling a friend is a helpful alternative activity but the logistics of calling a friend while in HLOC treatment may not always be an easily accessible activity). Encourage patients to consider listing activities they can do while in treatment and once they get home and be flexible with how they implement alternative activities (e.g., while in treatment, talking to a fellow patient in the program after a meal, as opposed to a personal friend). Alternative activities can be implemented as described in partial hospital or intensive outpatient programs.

Group Session 3

Handout 3.1   *Between-session Work Self-review – Session 3*

BETWEEN-SESSION WORK SELF-REVIEW – SESSION 3

Did I….	Yes	Somewhat	No
Self- Monitoring			
Monitor every day?	☐	☐	☐
Monitor at every eating episode?	☐	☐	☐
Always monitor in real time?	☐	☐	☐
Make sure to be accurate/honest?	☐	☐	☐
Write down the time of eating?	☐	☐	☐
Write down foods and drinks I had?	☐	☐	☐
Use brackets for meals?	☐	☐	☐
Include the place of eating?	☐	☐	☐
Include asterisks when I thought that I had overeaten or felt a loss of control while eating?	☐	☐	☐
Mark when I vomited, used laxatives, or diuretics?	☐	☐	☐
Include exercise?	☐	☐	☐
Complete the context column with events, moods, or thoughts?	☐	☐	☐
Regular Eating			
Get started with regular eating? *More in-depth review will happen in session.	☐	☐	☐
Optional Information Handouts			
Read and consider the information on these handouts?	☐	☐	☐

Which skills are going well? Great work, keep practicing them! Which skills am I struggling to use and need to prioritize? Plan to take action this week – write an **Action Plan** to address these.

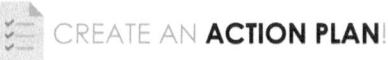 CREATE AN **ACTION PLAN**!

Handout 3.2   *Regular Eating Review*

REGULAR EATING REVIEW

Did....	Yes	Somewhat	No
I have 3 meals plus a couple of snacks daily?	☐	☐	☐
I roughly plan ahead the content and times of meals and snacks?	☐	☐	☐
I eat enough food to have enough energy between eating episodes?	☐	☐	☐
I prioritize eating over other activities?	☐	☐	☐
I sit down for meals?	☐	☐	☐

Keep track of the items above that you marked as **somewhat** or **no.** These are areas that require more focused work.

I eat in between my 3 meals plus a couple of snacks?	☐	☐	☐
I follow hunger/fullness cues over my regular eating plan?	☐	☐	☐
I go more than 4 hours between eating episodes?	☐	☐	☐
Social eating interrupt regular eating?	☐	☐	☐
I engage in behaviors like binge eating, vomiting, misusing medications, or driven exercise?	☐	☐	☐
Feelings, events, or situations impact my eating?	☐	☐	☐
I eat from packages?	☐	☐	☐
I eat while distracted?	☐	☐	☐
I have difficulties with my speed of eating (eating very slowly or quickly)?	☐	☐	☐

Keep track of the items above that you marked as **yes** or **somewhat**. These are areas that may require more practice.

Great work accomplishing what you have so far! For things that you have struggled with, complete an **Action Plan** to help make some changes.

SAMPLE ACTION PLAN		DATE: **4/27**
PROBLEM:	Skipping meals	
CURRENT FREQUENCY (IF APPLICABLE):	I am eating 2 meals a day most days.	
GOAL FOR UPCOMING WEEK:	I will have 3 meals a day plus 2-3 snacks, 5/7 days this week.	
	MY PLAN:	MY SUPPORT:
SPECIFIC PLAN:	I will have 3 meals plus 2-3 snacks a day on Monday, Wednesday, Thursday, Friday, & Sunday.	After group, plan ahead my week. Plan to read my new book after each meal. Tell my friend my goal so that I can call them when feeling nervous about eating.

ACTION PLAN		DATE:
PROBLEM:		
CURRENT FREQUENCY (IF APPLICABLE):		
GOAL FOR UPCOMING WEEK:		
	MY PLAN:	MY SUPPORT:
SPECIFIC PLAN:		

Handout 3.3   *Alternative Activities*

ALTERNATIVE ACTIVITIES

Alternative activities are distracting activities that may help you to avoid acting on an eating disorder urge (e.g., binge eating, out of control eating, vomiting, driven exercise, food restriction). Alternative activities can be particularly useful if you are struggling with eating between planned eating episodes or are experiencing emotional dysregulation that is impacting eating disorder symptoms. Alternative activities can be used in moments of stress/uncomfortable emotions to manage feelings in new, more functional ways that don't contribute to your eating disorder. For example, as opposed to responding to anxiety after completing a challenging meal by vomiting, calling a friend to cope with that anxiety may help to avoid vomiting, and help you to stay on track with recovery!

IDEAS FOR ALTERNATIVE ACTIVITIES

Activities with others	Getting out of the situation/ Changing the environment	Other alternative activities
☐ Talking with a friend	☐ Going for a drive	☐ Reading a book
☐ Making plans to see a friend	☐ Going outside	☐ Listening to music

I will plan to post my list here:
(e.g., as a background on my phone, on my closet door)

_____

Write on your self-monitoring forms when you practice alternative activities!

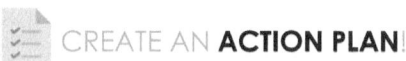

ALTERNATIVE ACTIVITY TIPS

1. Delaying

Delaying is one strategy to help you engage in alternative activities. It is the practice of planning to delay acting on an urge until after a particular time expectation and activity has occurred. This will help you to feel more in control of your behaviors. For example, Ray is experiencing the urge to binge eat. They try setting an expectation for themselves to step outside for 5 minutes, or to listen to one song, or watch one segment of their favorite television show BEFORE binge eating. Following that activity, Ray can decide if they would still like to binge eat, if they are able to engage in another delaying alternative activity, or if they have decided not to binge eat. The delaying can continue for as long as Ray requires. Even if Ray does binge after delaying, they have just had the opportunity to have a bit more control over their behaviors and have slowed down their behaviors to make that decision. This has now offered Ray the opportunity to have more control over their urges.

2. Reaching out to others

It is often very useful to reach out to others when struggling. Whether you engage with supports about your particular emotions, thoughts, or urges in the moment, or if you use supports to help as a distracting activity, reaching out to others tends to be useful. You may have more limited social support and it may be helpful to spend some time brainstorming who might be available in your life in this way.

CREATE AN **ACTION PLAN**!

SAMPLE ACTION PLAN		DATE: **10/10**
PROBLEM:	Needing to add more alternative activities	
CURRENT FREQUENCY (IF APPLICABLE):	N/A	
GOAL FOR UPCOMING WEEK:	I will plan to try 3 new alternative activities on the weekends when I typically am more likely to binge eating.	
SPECIFIC PLAN:	MY PLAN:	MY SUPPORT:
	Play the piano.	I will get out one of my old piano books and plan to play for at least 10 minutes (I will set a timer) after each meal this weekend.
	Go for a drive.	After dinner, I will go for a drive and consider driving to an activity (going to the movies).
	Call my friend who lives far away.	I will plan to call myfriend on Saturday and Sunday morning while making breakfast. I will let him know this plan and that I plan to make breakfast while talking.

Chapter 9

Group Session 4

Regular Eating, Urge Tolerating, and Feelings of Fullness

Overview

Session 4 is the final session of Stage 1. The focus of this session is on continuing to strengthen regular eating. In the last session, the use of alternative activities was introduced as a way to distract from, and not engage in, eating disorder behaviors. Two further CBT-E interventions are presented in this session to support patients in adopting a regular pattern of eating:

1. The use of *urge tolerating* to sit with and accept urges to engage in eating disorder behaviors, without acting on the urges.
2. Better understanding *feelings of fullness* and their impact on the eating disorder using CBT-E's RAD Approach, described in detail below.

Therapist Preparation

- ☐ Review this chapter in advance.
- ☐ Review regular eating therapeutic strategies discussed in Session 3 (pp. 67–69).
- ☐ Review accompanying handouts.
- ☐ Have copies of handouts available for patients, including an EDE-Q and CIA.

Handouts

- Standard Weekly Handouts
  - *1.3 Self-monitoring*
  - *1.6 Between-session Work Log*
  - *4.1 Between-session Work Self-review – Session 4*

- Session-specific Handouts
  - *3.2 Regular Eating Review*
  - *4.2 Urge Tolerating*
  - *4.3 Feelings of Fullness*
  - *EDE-Q and CIA (available at www.cbte.co)*

DOI: 10.4324/9781003450849-11

Group Session Agenda

1. Setting the agenda and orienting to the session (2 minutes)
2. Between-session work self-review (5 minutes)
3. Reviewing regular eating (20 minutes)
4. Introducing urge tolerating (10–15 minutes)
5. Introducing feelings of fullness (10–15 minutes)
6. Preparation for Session 5 (5 minutes)
7. Group wrap-up (3 minutes)

1. Setting the Agenda and Orienting to the Session

Begin with a positive, encouraging welcome. Share that this is Session 4 of Stage 1 with 10 sessions remaining. Clearly list the session agenda.

2. Between-session Work Self-review

Handout: *Between-session Work Self-review – Session 4*

Ask patients to complete their *Between-session Work Self-review – Session 4* handout. This review briefly covers self-monitoring, regular eating, and alternative activities. Let patients know that the self-monitoring section does not contain the same questions as the full review used in previous sessions. Anyone who found the full review useful is encouraged to return to the *Self-monitoring Review* handout and create an Action Plan related to this. The regular eating review is short since an in-depth review occurs again in this session. As always, the idea is to praise patients for the things that are going well, identify barriers and how to address such obstacles, and build on the existing interventions by identifying increasingly challenging ways to tackle eating disorder symptoms. For this session in particular, make sure to check in with patients about their progress with alternative activities. This includes any goals the patients have to continue, or augment, their practice of these activities in the coming week, as well as any new alternative activities that patients have identified. At the end of the review, encourage patients to create updated Action Plans to reflect goals for the week, and include these on their *Between-session Work Log*.

3. Reviewing Regular Eating

Handout: *Regular Eating Review*

As in Session 3, continue supporting the group in identifying ways to strengthen regular eating patterns and implementing Action Plans. Make sure to recognize things that are going well with regular eating and praise patients for their hard work in making changes. To help patients progress with regular eating, encourage volunteers to share occasions when they struggled to follow a regular pattern of eating during the week. This may be sharing particularly challenging days, and/or symptoms or urges that occurred. Make a list on a whiteboard [see Table 9.1] of areas that have gone well, areas where patients can see an opportunity for change, and ideas for interventions to support change. Use the list of considerations in Session 3 (page 68) to help support patients.

Just like in the last session, we will start by completing the Regular Eating Review handout. Once this is complete, I want to hear about how regular eating has gone this week. And also about the Action Plan goals that you identified last week to help support your regular eating. I'd like us to focus on three areas: 1) Things for us to celebrate. What are some things that have gone well this week?; 2) Challenges that you are encountering to regular eating; and 3) Identify some new Action Plans for helping to address these challenges. Would anyone like to volunteer to share first?

Table 9.1 Sample Whiteboard – Regular Eating Successes, Challenges, and Ideas for Change

Successes:

- Increased to 2 meals plus 2 snacks a day.
- Ate at my dining room table 5 times this week.
- Decreased my self-induced vomiting to 2 x this week.
- Added in 2 snacks every day.
- Only binged 2 x this week.

Challenges:

- I was unable to decrease my binge eating.
- I had 3 days when I engaged in driven exercise.
- I am vomiting 2 x a week at night.
- I am finding that I need to eat a couple of snacks between lunch and dinner.
- I can't seem to stop using laxatives even though I have started to work toward eating more regularly throughout the day.

Action Plan Ideas for Change (each point addresses a related challenge from above):

- Planning ahead eating times, food, and alternative activities.
- Tell my partner I want to decrease exercising to only one day this week and will plan alternative activities with them (night-time board games) to help stick with this plan.
- Recognize that decreasing vomiting to 2 times this week is a great change! Think back to how binge eating leads to vomiting and return to trying to eliminate that – eat breakfast every day this week and set an alarm to do so.
  - If not related to mood/events, try adding increased energy to lunch to better sustain energy during this time. Try adding another food item every day to lunch this week.
- Throw away laxatives. Engage a support person (my roommate) in knowing that I have a goal to eliminate laxative use. Put a plan in place to engage in 3 alternative activities (that take me physically away from laxatives) before considering using.

Some patients may be frequently weighing themselves and may share that they have noticed that their weight has gone up as they have adopted a regular eating pattern or reduced other eating disorder behaviors (e.g., self-induced vomiting, driven exercise). Other patients may report that they are noticing their clothes are feeling tighter. At times these changes might be quite minimal, but feel significant due to the over-evaluation of shape and weight, which will be addressed in Stage 3. Remember that the goal of CBT-E is to reduce and eliminate eating disorder symptoms, not to lose weight. This focus is the same for all patients of any body size. Some patients will gain or lose weight during treatment, while others will have no change to weight. In outpatient treatment, as the therapist, you will want to project a neutral and open stance about weight changes during treatment. In HLOC settings, underweight patients will have particular weight range goals and working toward this will be an important part of their treatment plan.

4. Introducing Urge Tolerating

Handout: *Urge Tolerating*

Urge tolerating will be introduced as another specific skill, along with engaging in alternative activities, that can be used to help strengthen regular eating. While alternative activity engagement is a strategy used to distract to avoid acting on urges, urge tolerating is a tool used to confront, accept the urge, and give it time to pass. Urge tolerating relies on the knowledge that urges will grow in intensity, peak, and ultimately diminish. Using the *Urge Tolerating* handout, guide the group through education about urge tolerating and think through how this tool might be useful in recovery. Try sketching out the urge tolerating process using a whiteboard.

Alternative activities are very useful strategies for helping to distract yourself to avoid acting on urges. Another skill, called urge tolerating, can also be helpful. Urge tolerating is the act of accepting the urge and allowing it to exist as is, rather than acting on it or responding to it. By accepting the urge and tolerating it, you will see that over time the strength of the urge decreases.

Let me draw this out for you. [draw out just the curved line of the Urge Tolerating graph in Figure 9.1]. *This curve represents the life of an urge, see how its intensity strengthens, peaks, and weakens?*

Now let's use an example. Say you start noticing that an urge is triggered [draw Box 1 from Figure 9.1]. *Your urge begins and it starts to rise in intensity* [Box 2 from Figure 9.1], *causing you to feel more and more uncomfortable. At some point, usually quite quickly, the urge feels intolerable, and you act on the urge (e.g., engage in an eating disorder behavior) to stop the intolerable feelings* [draw out the curve of the eating disorder in Figure 9.2 on top of this curve], *causing the intensity of the emotions to fall. In the short term, this works – you feel better in the moment, In the long term, however, you learn that the way to deal with the urge is to use eating disorder behaviors – and that is understandable since eating disorder behaviors do reduce the distress.*

Let me propose a different strategy. Instead, it might be possible that if you can tolerate the urge long enough to get to its peak [Box 3 in Figures 9.1 and 9.2], *you may learn that the urge will eventually fall* [Box 4 in Figures 9.1 and 9.2] *without needing to resort to eating disorder behaviors. It will naturally fall, just like it naturally rose, but it decreases more slowly than when you engage in an eating disorder behavior. Over time, if you tolerate the urge and allow it to peak, you will not have to rely on eating disorder symptoms to respond to the urge, instead you will learn how to accept such urges. With repeated practice, eventually you will find that the peak will be less intense over time. The urge will rise, but over time will not rise with as much intensity, as you start to respond differently (see Figure 9.3 where Line*

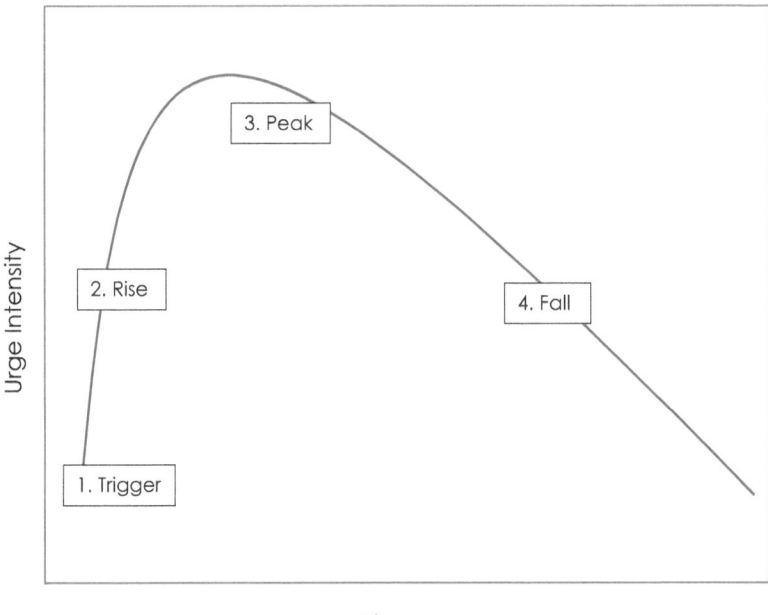

Figure 9.1 Urge tolerating psychoeducation graph.

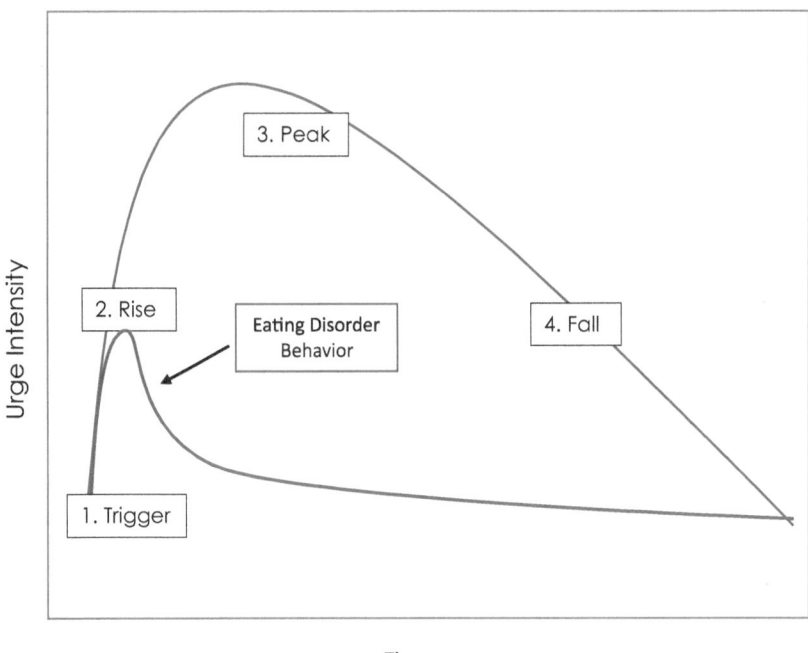

Figure 9.2 Urge tolerating graph with eating disorder behavior.

1 represents earlier efforts to tolerate urges and Line 4 represents later efforts). Does anyone have a recent example of an urge that they were or were not able to tolerate and what happened?

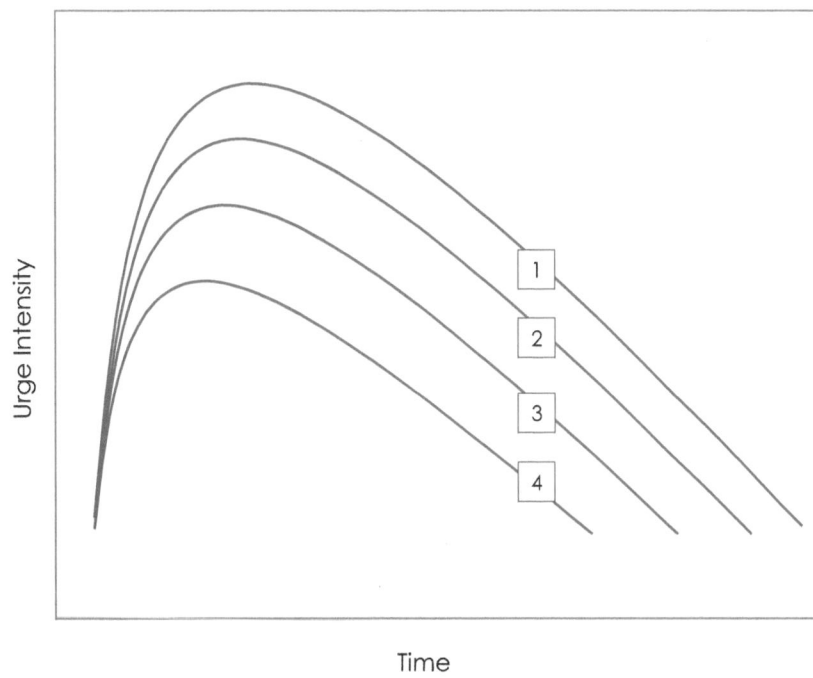

Figure 9.3 Long-term urge tolerating graph with decreased peak intensity.

After the group has a chance to reflect on the idea of urge tolerating, consider asking a volunteer to provide a recent example of an urge and draw this on the whiteboard. Ask patients to review their Urge Tolerating handout and create an Action Plan for how to use this skill moving forward. Encourage patients to consider using urge tolerating when they are having particularly strong urges. Ask patients to record moments when they use urge tolerating on their self-monitoring forms as a part of their between-session work this week and moving forward.

5. Introducing Feelings of Fullness

Handout: *Feelings of Fullness*

The final skill introduced in this session focuses on evaluating feelings of fullness. Despite feelings of fullness being quite a normal and typical human experience of having eaten a satisfying amount of food, these feelings are often significantly uncomfortable sensations for individuals with eating disorders. For these individuals, these feelings are frequently misinterpreted as indications of something else, often something negative about their shape, weight, or eating (e.g., having eaten too much food, a change in weight, and/or a sign that one is eating in an out-of-control way). These misinterpretations elevate discomfort and/or anxiety, often causing patients to engage in eating disorder behaviors (e.g., food restriction, self-induced vomiting) to reduce or avoid experiencing the sensation. For those who engage in binge eating, the sensation of fullness may accurately reflect the large amount of food consumed. This fullness can feel overwhelming and uncomfortable, often experienced as distressing and physically painful. Aside from fullness caused by binge eating, we typically see the following scenarios when a patient describes feelings of fullness:

- Patient has eaten a meal and is physically satiated (i.e., satisfactorily full), though judges this experience critically, impacting thoughts and feelings about shape, weight, and eating (e.g., "I have eaten too much food.", "I have gained weight.").

- Patient has eaten a small amount of food and feels full due to slowed digestion related to undereating. This fullness is judged negatively.

- Patient has eaten a small amount of food and feels full due to other factors (e.g., breaking a diet-related rule, telling themselves they have eaten too much food, thinking clothes are fitting tighter on their body after eating). This experience is judged negatively.

- A combination of the above. For example, a patient may complete a typical-sized meal and describes a feeling of being "completely overstuffed." In this scenario, it may be that the patient is experiencing typical satiation (which the patient is judging), as well as negative thoughts about having eaten an avoided food, both of which are leading to an uncomfortable feeling of fullness.

Feelings of Fullness Psychoeducation

To introduce feelings of fullness, start by asking patients to compile a list of thoughts and feelings that occur when feeling full. After that, you will ask the patients to consider: 1) their impressions about how a typical physical sensation (i.e., fullness) is interpreted negatively; 2) if feelings of fullness are reliable; and 3) how negatively labeling feelings of fullness maintains eating disorder symptoms. To start, you may say:

Feelings of fullness are typical sensations that all humans experience – usually several times a day when finishing meals. Similarly to urges described above, they rise in intensity after eating and then pass. Often for patients with eating disorders, feelings of fullness can feel scary and you may want to avoid them. Does anyone relate to this? Today, we are going to think about fullness, what it means to you, what else it could indicate, and what other factors, other than physical fullness sensations, may cause it. Please use your Feelings of Fullness handout during this discussion. Let's start by creating a list on the whiteboard of what feeling full means to you. [(see Table 9.2 sample whiteboard)]

Table 9.2 Sample Whiteboard – What Feeling Full Means to Me

1. I have eaten too much
2. I need to get rid of this food (vomit/exercise)
3. I've definitely gained weight
4. Just an overall gross feeling
5. It makes me feel slowed down, rounder
6. That I am unattractive

Following the creation of this list, highlight to the group how the eating disorder has labeled a normal bodily sensation as something negative.

It is really interesting to see how in many situations, the eating disorder is negatively interpreting what is a normal bodily sensation, one that can even be pleasurable or satisfying for many people. Have you ever heard someone remark after a meal, "That was delicious and 'hit the spot.'"? That expression is typically associated with feeling full or satiated. But when we look at the list we just created, feeling full here is associated with many different negative thoughts and feelings. What does everyone think about this?

After discussing patients' thoughts, emphasize that for some group members, feeling full may be a particularly unreliable indicator of having eaten enough/too much. This may be related to under-nourishing one's body, but also may be related to uncomfortable thoughts and feelings.

I'd also like to stress that when we do not feed our bodies enough food, our body slows down how we digest and pass food through. When this happens, one can feel full even after eating only small amounts of food. Is anyone aware of this happening for them?

Also, does anyone have the experience that your thoughts and feelings about your shape, weight, and eating ever cause or enhance feelings of fullness? For example, have there ever been times when you have eaten differently than intended and this alone has led to fullness? For example, eating a very small snack before dinner and then suddenly feeling too full to eat dinner, despite not having eaten much? Is it possible that some of this fullness may be related to judgments about eating differently (and perhaps breaking a diet-related rule), and the anxiety that goes along with that?

Finally, consider with the group how these negative thoughts and feelings keep the eating disorder going:

On our list (Table 9.2), there is an item that feelings of fullness cause urges to vomit or exercise. Do others relate to this? Do feelings of fullness make you want to engage in an eating disorder behavior? Does anyone have a desire to restrict their food as a result of feelings of fullness? It makes sense that someone would want to engage in a behavior to get rid of this unpleasant feeling. In this way, feelings of fullness can keep the eating disorder going.

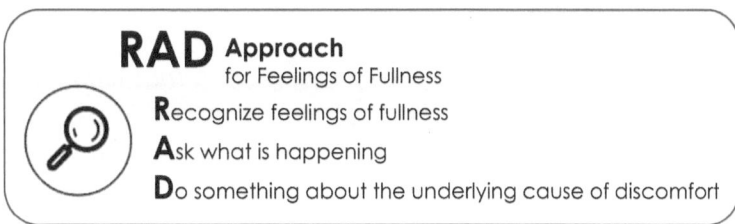

RAD Approach
for Feelings of Fullness
Recognize feelings of fullness
Ask what is happening
Do something about the underlying cause of discomfort

Figure 9.4 RAD Approach for feelings of fullness.

After providing this psychoeducation, introduce patients to the RAD Approach (share Figure 9.4 on the whiteboard). The RAD Approach is a three-step tool to support patients in better understanding their feelings of fullness and considering what is happening at these times. Being able to recognize feelings of fullness, and what may be causing them, will allow patients to address the underlying cause or tolerate the feeling of food being in their stomach.

To reduce the current negative impact of feelings of fullness, we will use the RAD Approach. RAD is a three-step tool to help you address feelings of fullness and reduce their impact on keeping the eating disorder going. And most importantly, to help return the experience of feelings of fullness to a reliable, and possibly even pleasurable, sensation in the future. Let's use your Feelings of Fullness handout to apply the RAD Approach.

 ## Recognize feelings of fullness

The first step is to recognize when feelings of fullness are occurring. For patients who endorse distressing feelings of fullness, encourage them to record these feelings on their self-monitoring records.

 ## Ask what is happening

Once these feelings are identified, the next step is to evaluate what may be going on when a patient experiences feelings of fullness. At times, the only answer to this is that the patient has eaten a full meal and is physically satiated. In these situations, encourage patients to consider if they are negatively evaluating a common physical sensation. This sensation can be caused, or intensified, by a variety of other thoughts, events, or emotions.

Engage the group in a brief brainstorming session to identify what tends to trigger feelings of fullness. Some examples of triggers are listed in Table 9.3.

 ## Do something about the underlying cause of discomfort

Once patients have created a list of triggers, you can help the group to identify new ways of responding to these triggers that do not involve eating disorder symptoms, using some of the suggestions listed in Table 9.3. As seen in the table, the recommendation is for patients to ask themselves if the feelings of fullness are purely caused by having enough food in one's body. If so, strategies to tolerate this feeling and challenge negative appraisals or assumptions about this may be warranted. If the feelings of fullness can be attributed to something else, ask patients to address that trigger.

In many cases, feelings of fullness are caused by eating food that leads to satiety. In these situations, the goal is to work on tolerating this experience and addressing any negative thoughts or feelings that you may have about the fact that your body experiences fullness. In many other situations, as we just noticed, there is also a long list of triggers, outside of eating to satiety, that can also lead to feelings of fullness. Addressing these triggers directly can be much more helpful and can be useful in avoiding eating disorder symptoms. Let's look back at our list and

Table 9.3 Examples of Triggers of Feelings of Fullness

Trigger	How to Address
Eating food (any food – even "safe" foods)	Remind patients that this is a normal sensation and one that does not indicate any other body changes and is not a sign of anything concerning. Support patients in creating a key phrase they can repeat to themselves when they experience feeling full after eating: e.g., "*This is my body letting me know there is food in my belly, it does not indicate anything else and the intensity of this feeling will pass.*"
Breaking a diet-related rule, eating an avoided food, or thinking that one has eaten too much	This can be identified through self-monitoring review. Use the support of the group to examine if the feelings of fullness are well aligned with the eating event, or if it is the thoughts or feelings the patient is having about the food that are impacting their fullness. For example, is the patient telling themselves they have eaten too much, which is leading to feelings of guilt, which ultimately causes them to feel fuller than they really are? This will be addressed more in Stage 3.
Feeling one's clothes fitting differently on one's body	For some patients in treatment, their clothes may start to fit differently due to changes in shape as they are regularly eating. This is not related to levels of fullness; however, does indicate that there may be body changes that warrant wearing loose-fitting clothes for a couple of weeks to be more comfortable in the recovery process. There may also be natural changes (e.g., tighter-fitting pants feeling tighter after a meal) that occur following eating, which is typical and can be helpful to normalize for patients.
Emotions (e.g., anxiety, sadness, guilt)	This will be addressed further in Stage 3. At this point in treatment, we recommend engaging the patient in a discussion about alternative activities or urge tolerating if fullness is in response to a particular emotion.
Comparing food intake to others	This may also require some psychoeducation and engagement with the group to assess how one's food intake compares to someone else's and if that assessment is reliable. Remember, we never know what someone's energy intake or output has looked like in a day and comparing one meal to another's meal is not a reliable measurement of overall intake. You may want to ask patients to provide examples of instances when fullness related to comparison to others has seemed irrational.
Feeling as if one's abdomen is sticking out	Help to avoid equating bloating, or perceived abdominal changes, with weight changes. Recommend strategies such as choosing comfortable clothing or experimenting with assessing whether or not abdominal changes following eating are noticeable (by asking patients to assess this phenomenon in others). Additionally, provide education that bloating is a normal sensation, particularly after eating certain foods.
Negative thoughts about one's body, body checking/ avoidance, or body dissatisfaction spikes	This will be more fully addressed in Stage 3. At this point in treatment, the recommendation is to focus on alternative activities to distract from these negative body image thoughts.

Table 9.3 (Continued)

Trigger	How to Address
Eating until uncomfortably full as a part of binge eating	Encourage patients to consider what may be triggering binge episodes, including their eating patterns and events/emotions. Remind patients that tolerating the physical discomfort of binge eating without engaging in a subsequent eating disorder behavior (e.g. dieting, self-induced vomiting) is an important step in eventually stopping binge eating completely. That is because this helps to break the vicious cycle between binge eating and other eating disorder behaviors to compensate for binge eating. Ask patients to review the Binge Eating handout and identify specific strategies to address binge eating.

add ways of addressing these triggers to the list. From now on, when you notice discomfort related to feelings of fullness, I want you to try to identify the possible cause (self-monitoring forms can be helpful for this) and then address that cause directly. Please start adding to your self-monitoring forms when you are noticing discomfort related to feelings of fullness, what the cause might be, and how you plan to address that cause.

For between-session work, ask patients to apply their findings from the *Feelings of Fullness* handout when they are noticing such sensations. Ask patients to start adding feelings of fullness (and their triggers) to their self-monitoring forms as a means to start evaluating the possible triggers for feelings of fullness and to identify plans for how to respond.

6. Preparation for Session 5: Reviewing Progress

In the last few minutes of this group ask patients to complete the EDE-Q and CIA. Asking patients to complete these before the end of the session will allow you time before the next session to review their scores and compare them to pre-session scores on these measures. Provide a brief reminder of what these measures are for and how to complete them.

Before we end, I'd like to ask everyone to complete two assessment measures. You may remember completing them just before starting Group CBT-E. These two measures consider how things have been going for you over the past month – more or less since treatment started. These measures help to give an idea of the progress you are making in treatment and will be used as part of our review session next week.

7. Group Wrap-up

Session Review

Today is our last session of Stage 1. We continued to talk about regular eating and ways to strengthen it. We talked about two important tools to use to help keep you on track with regular eating and avoid eating disorder symptoms: tolerating urges and planning to respond to feelings of fullness differently. These two skills, plus alternative activities, will be important to continue to practice throughout treatment and beyond in order to better stick with regular eating and your recovery. Next week we will move to Stage 2 and will be reviewing progress.

Between-session Work

Remember to encourage patients to write the between-session work on their *Between-session Work Log* handout. The between-session work for Session 4 is:

- Continue work from previous sessions:
  - *Self-monitoring* – to be completed daily, in the moment.
  - *Regular Eating* and *Planning Ahead* – continue to practice following a regular pattern of eating.
  - *Alternative Activities* – continue to record on self-monitoring forms when alternative activities are used.
  - Follow through with Action Plans identified during the session related to regular eating and symptoms (e.g., binge eating, driven exercise, self-induced vomiting).

- New work from Session 4:
  - *Urge Tolerating* – review and implement Action Plans and add urges to the self-monitoring forms.
  - *Feelings of Fullness* – review and implement Action Plans, add any times when feelings of fullness occur to the self-monitoring forms, and use the RAD Approach.

Higher Level of Care Adaptations: Modular Implementation

When this session is used modularly, the following adaptations are suggested.

Regular eating: Consider the usefulness of continuing to reinforce this intervention in your particular setting. Regular eating reviews at inpatient and residential settings may be limited as patients are likely not in charge of their intake (see the Higher Level of Care Adaptions section of Session 3 for more detailed information). However, reviewing the reasons for adopting a regular pattern of eating is important and bears repeating at these levels of care. This can be used as a way to support patients by providing a rationale for following eating patterns set by the program. For patients at partial hospital and intensive outpatient settings, continuing to support these patients to implement regular eating when in charge of planning their own food is important and can be implemented as described.

Urge tolerating: Education on urges to engage in eating disorder behaviors and implementing urge tolerating is useful at all levels of care and can serve as content for a complete group at HLOCs. Patients at inpatient and residential settings are likely being supported in urge tolerating through the program structure and environment (e.g., not having access to the bathroom after eating, or having program rules about exercise). Education on urge tolerating can be particularly useful in these situations to provide patients with a rationale for these aspects of their treatment. Urge tolerating can be implemented as described in partial hospital or intensive outpatient programs.

Additionally, at HLOCs, patients often struggle with urges to engage in other behaviors related to emotional dysregulation (e.g., refusing aspects of treatment, self-harm behaviors). Practicing urge tolerating for these urges may also be useful for patients. As with many CBT-E skills, it can be very useful for all HLOC staff to receive training in urge tolerating in order to help support patients to implement this skill in the moment, while in the program.

Feelings of fullness: Addressing feelings of fullness is useful at all levels of care and can serve as content for a complete group at HLOC. Feelings of fullness can be very intense and frequent for patients at HLOCs, especially patients who are undergoing the refeeding process. Much of this fullness is related to the physical discomfort of refeeding, and strategies (e.g., using a heat pack, wearing loose-fitting clothes) can be applied to help with this discomfort. It is important to validate patients' experiences related to this physical cause of fullness and remind patients that this is a natural consequence of refeeding that is out of a patient's control. In these situations, engage patients in a conversation about what else might be going on, above and beyond this significant physical fullness, that may be contributing to their fullness sensations. Patients may struggle initially to be able to recognize these factors, but it can be helpful to remind them that some feelings of fullness are due to factors outside of physical fullness and these factors may be within their control. Better understanding and addressing these fullness triggers is very useful for tolerating HLOC treatment and more consistently following regular eating expectations. Also, at HLOCs, consider adding to the feelings of fullness trigger list "not being in control of the foods I eat," in settings where the patient does not choose food items or amounts.

Administration of EDE-Q and CIA: Obtaining updated scores on these measures is encouraged, even if patients will not be returning to the next session. In these cases, where possible, meet with patients individually to share their scores, use the information to inform their care, and provide the information to providers at the next level of care. In HLOCs, we also recommend using the Eating Problem Checklist (EPCL), which measures symptom change in a shorter timeframe (i.e., week-by-week changes).

Group Session 4

Handout 4.1   *Between-session Work Self-review – Session 4*

BETWEEN-SESSION WORK SELF-REVIEW – SESSION 4

Did I....	Yes	Somewhat	No
Self- Monitoring			
Use my records daily?	☐	☐	☐
Complete my records "in the moment"?	☐	☐	☐
Regular Eating			
Eat 5–6 times a day?	☐	☐	☐
Not eat in between planned eating times?	☐	☐	☐
Plan ahead?	☐	☐	☐
Alternative Activities			
Keep an up-to-date list of alternate activities to use?	☐	☐	☐
Use my activities to displace eating disorder behaviors?	☐	☐	☐
Plan in my alternate activities on challenging days or during difficult events?	☐	☐	☐

Which skills are going well? Great work, keep practicing them! Which skills am I struggling to use and need to prioritize? Plan to take action this week – write an **Action Plan** to address these.

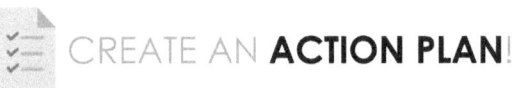

CREATE AN **ACTION PLAN**!

URGE TOLERATING

Urge tolerating is the practice of being aware of your urges to engage in a particular behavior and rather than following through with these urges, feeling the urges without acting on them until they reduce in intensity. After an urge is triggered (e.g., to binge eat, to restrict eating), the urge rises in intensity and eventually peaks in intensity. Then, with time, the intensity begins to decrease.

Learning to recognize these urges and tolerate them, without attempting to suppress them, will provide you with valuable information that the urge will peak and then decrease in intensity. With practice of not reacting to urges, they will likely not be as strong when they occur in the future.

Check out this image illustrating urge tolerating:

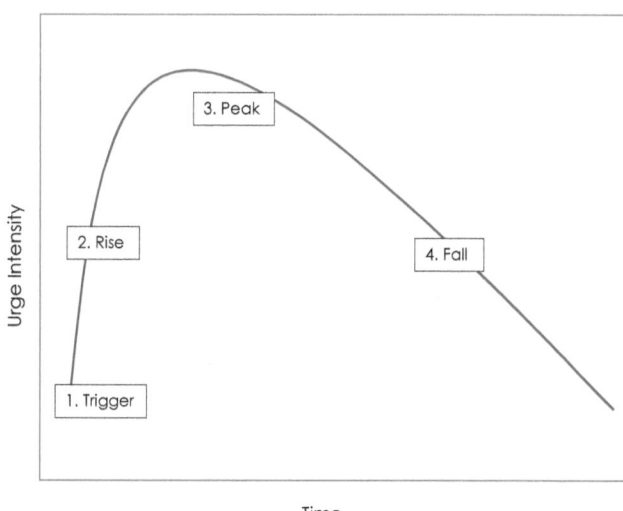

1. <u>Trigger</u>: Something (e.g., an argument with a friend, a negative appraisal at work) triggers an urge (e.g., to engage in driven exercise).
2. <u>Rise</u>: The urge rises in intensity which may happen gradually or suddenly.
3. <u>Peak</u>: The intensity reaches its highest peak and it may feel completely intolerable.
4. <u>Fall</u>: If you allow yourself to feel that peak without engaging in the eating disorder behavior, the urge will start to decrease in intensity and eventually go away.

Tolerating urges by sitting with unpleasant emotions that occur and not responding to the urge can be very difficult to do. This is because the behavior that you are wanting to do (e.g., engage in driven exercise) is likely highly effective at quickly reducing the urge, though this tends to only be helpful in the short term, not in the long term. Be gentle with yourself as you begin the practice of urge tolerating. It does get easier with time.

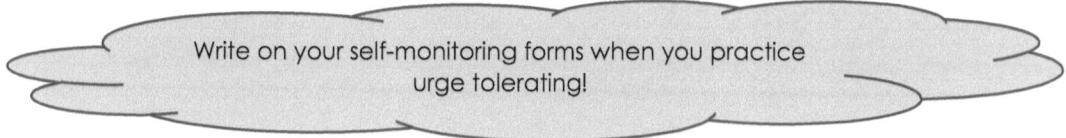

Write on your self-monitoring forms when you practice urge tolerating!

SAMPLE ACTION PLAN		DATE: 12/20
PROBLEM:	Needing to incorporate more urge tolerating.	
CURRENT FREQUENCY (IF APPLICABLE):	N/A	
GOAL FOR UPCOMING WEEK:	Daily urge tolerating	
SPECIFIC PLAN:	MY PLAN: I will plan to practice urge tolerating after each dinner in order to help with urges to self-induce vomit.	MY SUPPORT: I will make a sign and post it in my kitchen and dining room with the urge tolerating graph. I will set an alarm to remind myself. I will tell my mother about this skill so that she can help support me in these moments with tolerating my urge.

ACTION PLAN		DATE:
PROBLEM:		
CURRENT FREQUENCY (IF APPLICABLE):		
GOAL FOR UPCOMING WEEK:		
SPECIFIC PLAN:	MY PLAN:	MY SUPPORT:

FEELINGS OF FULLNESS

Despite feelings of fullness being a normal and typical experience in our lives, they are often significantly uncomfortable sensations for individuals with eating disorders. Fullness can be interpreted as evidence of eating too much, a change in weight, an intensification of body dissatisfaction, and/or feelings of being out of control, all of which lead to increased feelings of discomfort and/or anxiety. To reduce the discomfort or anxiety, many individuals engage in eating disorder behaviors (e.g., food restriction, vomiting). As a result, this misinterpretation of fullness can keep the eating disorder going. A helpful way to address feelings of fullness that cause eating disorder behaviors/urges is to determine what is causing the feeling or discomfort, and address the underlying cause. The three steps of the RAD Approach can be a helpful guide.

ASSESSING FEELINGS OF FULLNESS

What feeling full means to me (e.g., "feelings of fullness mean that I have eaten too much"):

_____

_____

_____

_____

_____

_____

My current thoughts about my feelings of fullness...

☐	Cause me to judge fullness (a sensation that is a normal body sensation) as scary and unpleasant.
☐	Lead me to worry that I have eaten too much even if I have only eaten a small amount.
☐	Can be based on thoughts and feelings that may have nothing to do with the amount of food in my stomach.
☐	Can trigger wanting to engage in eating disorder behaviors (e.g., driven exercising, vomiting, delay eating).
☐	
☐	
☐	

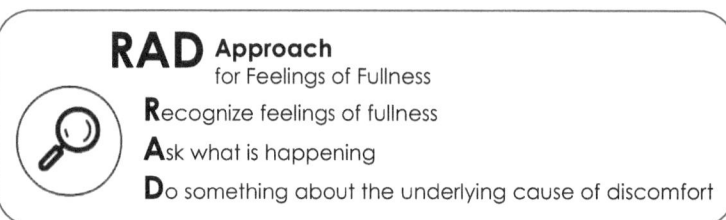

RAD Approach
for Feelings of Fullness
Recognize feelings of fullness
Ask what is happening
Do something about the underlying cause of discomfort

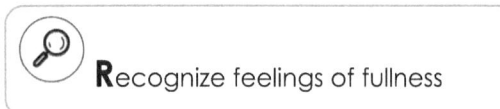

Recognize feelings of fullness

Write on your **self-monitoring forms** when you notice particularly strong feelings of fullness.

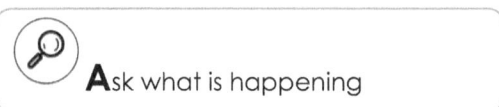

Ask what is happening

What might be going on when you are experiencing feelings of fullness? List examples generated together with the group that you relate to below.

Do something about the underlying cause of discomfort

Write on your self-monitoring forms when you practice the RAD Approach!

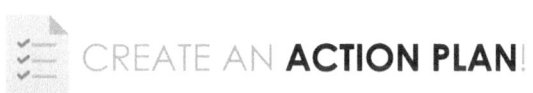 CREATE AN **ACTION PLAN!**

IDEAS TO CONSIDER INCORPORATING INTO MY ACTION PLAN

Overall Tips
Remember that feelings of fullness are normal bodily sensations. The feeling passes and in time, you will be able to view this feeling more naturally with less distress.
Sometimes the best option may be to sit with the discomfort using urge tolerating. Alternative activities can be helpful too.

SAMPLE ACTION PLAN		DATE: **7/7**
PROBLEM:	Feeling overly full and sure that this means I overate.	
CURRENT FREQUENCY (IF APPLICABLE):	Right after eating my lunch	
GOAL FOR UPCOMING WEEK:	Use RAD to support me in not using ED behaviors in response to feeling so gross.	
SPECIFIC PLAN:	MY PLAN:	MY SUPPORT:
	Practice urge tolerating when I have this feeling.	Remind myself it will pass.
		Reread the Urge Tolerating handout when I need to.
	Plan in alternative activities to use.	This week I will call Bo right after I eat to help take my mind off the feeling.
		Remind myself why I am doing this – I want to stop throwing up!!
		Review this Action Plan.

Reviewing Progress

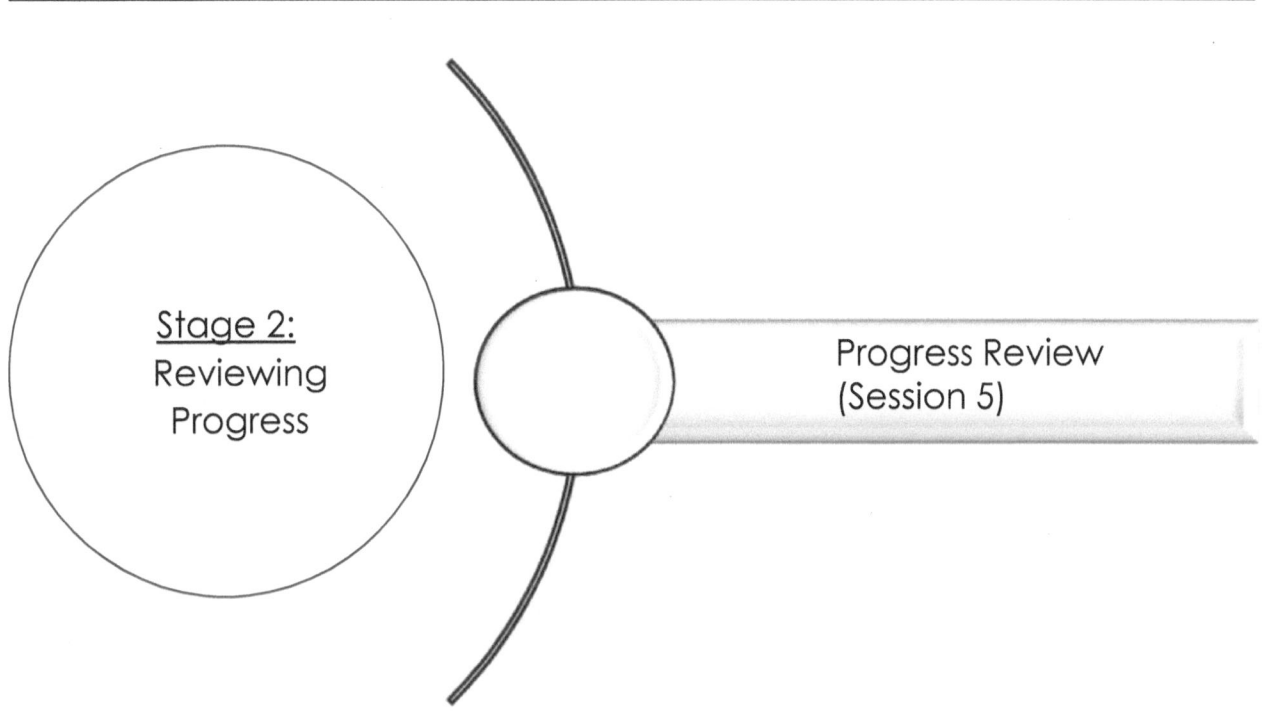

Stage 2:
Reviewing
Progress

Progress Review
(Session 5)

Chapter 10

Group Session 5

Progress Review

Overview

Stage 2 of treatment consists of one vital session focused on jointly reviewing progress in Group CBT-E thus far. The review aims to highlight areas that are going well and should be continued, and areas that require more practice. Specific attention is given to exploring the barriers that a patient may be encountering. For some patients, this review session is a time to decide if Group CBT-E is the appropriate treatment or if an alternative recommendation should be considered. Guidance for changing or stopping Group CBT-E is provided. The final part of this session is to prepare the group for Stage 3.

Reviewing one's progress in treatment is essential. Early progress is a robust indicator of response to therapy and so identifying any barriers allows for the best outcome. This response is related to how well the therapy is implemented: both the patient's ability to implement the therapy in their own lives and the therapist's ability to adhere to the therapy program with competence. This review session offers an opportunity for patients to evaluate their response to treatment and guidance for therapists to assess their adherence.

Therapist Preparation

☐ Review this chapter in advance.
☐ Review accompanying handouts and have copies available for patients.
☐ Have a copy of each patient's EDE-Q and CIA from timepoint 1 (pre-group administration) and timepoint 2 (Session 4 administration) available for patients.
☐ Score and compare patients EDE-Q and CIA from timepoint 1 to timepoint 2.
  ○ At the end of the last session, you will have administered the EDE-Q and CIA. In between sessions, score these questionnaires so that you can share the information with patients during group. Guidance on scoring can be found in *Cognitive Behavior Therapy and Eating Disorders* (Fairburn, 2008) and the CBT-E website (www.cbte.co). Scoring and reviewing the measurements provides information on how each individual is progressing in the group and alerts you to issues that may not be voiced in group. Some patients are more comfortable reporting symptoms on a questionnaire rather than verbally in a group.

DOI: 10.4324/9781003450849-13

Handouts

- Standard Weekly Handouts
  - *1.3 Self-monitoring Form*
  - *1.6 Between-session Work Log*
  - *5.1 Between-session Work Self-review – Session 5*

- Session-specific Handouts
  - *EDE-Q and CIA from timepoints 1 and 2*
  - *5.2 Progress Review – Treatment Components*
  - *5.3 General Barriers to Change*
  - *5.4 Ways to Overcome Barriers to Change*
  - *5.5 Therapist Self-review*

Group Session Agenda

1. Setting the agenda and orienting to the session (2 minutes)
2. Between-session work self-review (5 minutes)
3. Conducting a joint review of progress (35 minutes)

    a. Reviewing patient implementation of treatment components
    b. Reviewing eating disorder symptoms
    c. Reviewing global impairment

4. Identifying and addressing barriers to change (10 minutes)
5. Preparing for Stage 3 (5 minutes)
6. Group wrap-up (3 minutes)

1. Setting the Agenda and Orienting to the Session

Begin with a positive, encouraging welcome; share that this is Session 5, Stage 2, with nine sessions remaining. Clearly list the session agenda.

2. Between-session Work Self-review

Handout: *Between-session Work Self-review – Session 5*

Ask patients to complete their *Between-session Work Self-review – Session 5* handout. This review focuses on the main elements of Stage 1: self-monitoring, regular eating, alternative activities, urge tolerating, and addressing feelings of fullness. As always, the idea is to praise patients for the things that are going well; identify barriers and how to address such obstacles; and build on the existing interventions by identifying increasingly challenging ways to tackle eating disorder symptoms. At the end of the review, encourage patients to create updated Action Plans to reflect goals for the week, and include these on their *Between-session Work Log*.

3. Conducting a Joint Review of Progress

Progress in group is assessed in two ways:

1. Patient's implementation of treatment components (e.g., attending sessions, regular eating).
2. Patient's current eating disorder symptoms.

a. Reviewing Patient Implementation of Treatment Components

Handout: *Progress Review – Treatment Components*

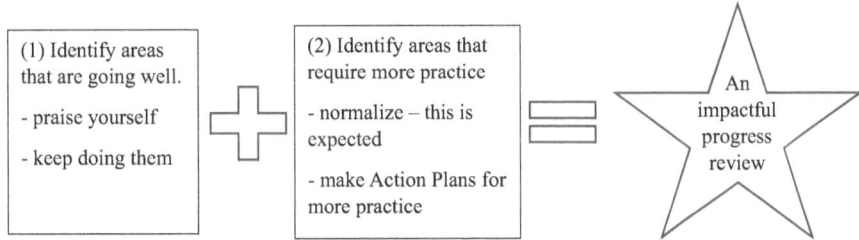

Figure 10.1 Components of an impactful progress review.

Using the *Progress Review – Treatment Components* handout, the first part of the review helps patients to consider progress with the practical elements of the treatment (e.g., coming to group, completing between-session work, regular eating). The aim is to identify which skills or practical elements of treatment are going well, and which items require further focused practice (see Figure 10.1). In some ways this review overlaps with the between-session work self-review, but contains extra items and, unlike the self-review, the ratings on this review are shared together in the group.

> *Today we will review how you are progressing in therapy. Reviews are helpful as they can identify areas that are going well – these are actions or skills to continue. Reviews also help us to spot areas where you may be able to improve what you are doing to get more benefit from treatment. Let's first begin with rating some of the practical aspects of group so far using the Progress Review – Treatment Components handout. I will read these aloud and we can share our ratings. Be as honest with yourself as possible. We can do this simply by giving a thumbs-up for 'going well;' thumbs down for 'not going well;' and a thumb in the middle pointing sideways to indicate 'somewhat of a problem.'*

In addition to the items provided on the handout, be sure to ask patients if there are other items they would like to include. Frequently, group members like to add areas where they see a peer doing well. Support patients to recognize their accomplishments in applying skills and praise changes that have been made. After identifying areas that are going well, and those that need more practice, the next step is to create an Action Plan. The Action Plan incorporates a commitment to:

1. The continued use of skills practiced thus far.
2. Further practice in areas that are going less well, or where there is limited progress.

Therapist Insight

Peer support is particularly useful during the progress review. Encourage group members to praise one another for areas of success and brainstorm action steps for areas that require additional work.

The group can be particularly helpful in brainstorming Action Plans together. We have often seen times when a patient is not sure how to improve an area and group members join in supportively to share what helps for them or other ideas they have for their peers.

Let's create a list on the whiteboard of areas where continued practice is needed. You can come up to the board to add your own, or I can write it for you. If you have an Action Plan to put in place, add it, and if you need some support in creating one, we will work on them as a group. [see Table 10.1]

Therapist Insight

Encourage patients to share the outcome of their progress reviews and Action Plans with a support person.

Table 10.1 Sample Whiteboard – Treatment Components Needing Further Practice and Action Plans

Areas I need more practice	Action Plans
I have been late to most groups.	Make treatment a priority, set a phone alarm, leave work a little early.
I have not been completing between-session work.	I am going to ask my support person to sit with me each evening to work on these.
I am missing snacks most days.	I'm making a commitment to start having at least one snack per day and will increase it to 2 next week. I will share this with my partner so they can check in with me. I'll text them now from group so I don't back out of this!

b. Reviewing Eating Disorder Symptoms

Handouts: *EDE-Q from timepoints 1 and 2*

After reviewing the practical aspects of treatment, review specific eating disorder symptoms using the original and updated EDE-Q. The focus is again on highlighting areas of progress and offering praise, while also identifying areas where further progress can be made. Patients will have completed this measure prior to Session 1 and in the previous session, so there is an opportunity to compare scores from these two timepoints. Share with patients their overall scores and allow them time to review the individual responses. Encourage patients to share general impressions from comparing their pre-group ratings to their current ratings. Remind the group that everyone progresses at different rates.

Let's now think about some of the specific symptoms and behaviors of your eating disorder. I will give you a couple of minutes to review both copies of your EDE-Q. You may recall completing this just prior to starting treatment and then again at the end of the last session. What are your overall impressions? Do you see any changes in your scores?

Typically, patients will find that some areas are improving, while others have worsened or have had no change. It is important to normalize this result as an expected outcome and explain why it occurs.

Often, we find that at this point in treatment some areas are starting to improve while other areas start to get worse or stay the same. Typically, the areas that start to improve (such as binge eating, self-induced vomiting) are directly related to the treatment skills you have already put in place and are working hard on, while the areas that are worse, or show no improvement, are areas that we have not yet covered in treatment (such as body image). This suggests that areas you are working hard on in treatment are already benefiting you and that you will likely experience similar positive benefits in the other areas once we get to those parts of treatment, which are coming soon in the next stage of CBT-E.

At this stage in treatment, it is quite common for patients to have remaining eating disorder symptoms. If you notice that certain symptoms are not being reported in the group, but are likely still a struggle for some patients, specifically mention this in group. It is important to recognize when a patient is not progressing and also when a patient is having difficulty sharing their lack of progress.

Self-induced vomiting was not mentioned by the group today but is often still a problem at this point. If this, or any other symptom, is occurring for you regularly and it was difficult to raise this in group, I'd like to stress that eating disorder behaviors are common at this point in treatment and it can take a while for them to reduce or stop. At the same time, I'd like to support you in meeting your treatment goals. I encourage everyone to think of this group as a safe space to share your struggles, and if that feels too overwhelming, please do check in with me at the end.

Sometimes group members have difficulty in accurately assessing their progress. They may be overly harsh in their judgments, or they may view things as going better than they are. It is important to help patients come to accurate views on progress so they can fully benefit from treatment. Table 10.2 provides guidance on supporting patients to form accurate impressions of their progress.

Table 10.2 How to Respond in Situations When Patients Inaccurately Report Progress

<u>What to do when progress review ratings inaccurately indicate little progress</u>

In cases where a patient views everything as having worsened, but this does not match clinical reality, it is important to check in on their ability to self-rate and provide some objectivity in supporting them with their rating. There are two ways to do this, either through direct interaction with the group leader or via an interaction or "call-out" from another group member.

Therapist-led

When led by you, support the patient to reassess their ratings using objective information. This may look like this:

Therapist: *It is interesting to hear that you rated nearly everything worse. Let's start by looking at your report that binge eating is worse. At the start of treatment, you said you were binge eating 5 times per week. Looking at your records, you binged 3 times this week. What do you make of this change?*

Patient: *Well, I know that 3 times is less than 5 times, but I am still binge eating 3 times per week and lots of other group members are no longer binge eating at all.*

Therapist: *I can hear your disappointment that you are binge eating 3 times per week and at the same time, you have reduced your binge eating by 2 binges per week. That is impressive! What do you think has helped with those reductions and what might be things to keep doing? Next, we are going to review the things that might be getting in the way of progress. As we do, let's come back to your remaining 3 binges per week and see if there are further places to help you make changes to your eating.*

Peer-led

Sometimes a peer may be able to convey the same information in a different and helpful way:

Therapist, same scenario as above: *I am hearing that Patient B is thinking that they have made no progress at all. Does anyone have any reactions to that?*

Patient A: *I am really surprised that you think you are making no progress! When we started in group you were binge eating 5 times a week and now you are down to just 3. I am really proud of you!*

Patient B: *Yeah, but you stopped binge eating completely and so did Patient C. I'm doing the worst in the group.*

Patient A: *I hear that, but I know for me, that whenever I compare to others, it is not helpful for me. We are all doing the best we can and it seems like you are doing really great work – you have almost decreased your binge eating by half!*

<u>What to do when progress review ratings inaccurately indicate a good amount of progress</u>

Sometimes a patient may rate their progress as better than it actually is. When you notice this occurring, help the patient create a more accurate view of their progress. Depending on the group and the patient, it may be best to wait until after the group or arrange a separate brief one-on-one meeting.

I noticed that you rated your attendance and participation with a green light. I agree that when you come to session you are really engaged and supportive to others. There have been a couple of times, though, that you have come late to session and once when you did not attend at all. In order for you to get the most out of treatment, let's think about what got in your way on those occasions and see if we can come up with ways to help you get to group each week and on time. How does that sound?

c. Reviewing the Impact on General Functioning

Handouts: *CIA from timepoints 1 and 2*

Next, review the CIA in a similar way as described above for the EDE-Q. Provide background information that the CIA is a measure that assesses the impact of the eating disorder on life in general. Share with patients their scores from timepoints 1 and 2, and consider their overall impressions of change. Remember that in this early phase of treatment, a patient may not yet experience changes to their quality of life. If this is the case, normalize this experience.

4. Identifying and Addressing Barriers to Change

Handouts: *General Barriers to Change, Ways to Overcome Barriers to Change*

Where there is limited change, it is essential to help patients identify what is getting in the way of fully engaging in treatment. Some barriers, like those just reviewed in the previous section, are related to specific aspects of treatment (e.g., not completing between-session work), while other barriers are more general. Reviewing these general barriers can be done as a group using the *General Barriers to Change* handout [see Table 10.3].

Table 10.3 Sample Whiteboard – Collaboratively Created Barriers to Change List

- I am scared to lose my eating disorder.
- I am worried that I will dislike myself even more if I allow myself to eat enough food.
- I don't have enough time to work on between-session work.
- I can't seem to get to sessions on time.
- I need to focus on my relationship with my partner now rather than my eating disorder.

Let's now think through other barriers that may be getting in your way of fully engaging in treatment. Please take out your General Barriers to Change handout. Would someone like to read the listed barriers? We'll go around and everyone can indicate if they are struggling with the particular barrier. While we are reviewing barriers, please also add other personal barriers to the bottom of your General Barriers to Change handout.

Next, ask a volunteer to share more about one or two of their general barriers. As a group, you can then help the patient to challenge a barrier by reviewing related items on the *Ways to Overcome Barriers* handout. In parallel, patients can create an Action Plan to overcome their specific barriers, using the *General Barriers to Change* handout.

Changing or Stopping Treatment

The review serves as a time for the therapist and patient to consider if continuing in Group CBT-E is appropriate.

- *What to do if eating disorder symptoms are worsening*: Frequently at this point in treatment, symptoms related to distress about body shape and weight have not improved and may be worse. This is because the first part of treatment targets eating behaviors and not yet the over-evaluation of shape and weight. If a patient has made progress with starting regular eating and reducing other eating disorder behaviors (e.g., binge eating, self-induced vomiting, laxative use, driven exercise), but is reporting increased distress regarding their body image, this may actually be a good sign! It shows that they are highly engaged and that the areas that are improving are those that have been targeted in treatment. It further suggests that they are likely to continue to respond well to treatment and will benefit from interventions focused on body image. If symptoms related to eating are occurring at the same frequency as the start of treatment or worsening with no clear cause (e.g., they are attending and completing between-session work) or with a clear cause (e.g., they are not engaged and missing sessions), it is time to consider if this is the best treatment for this individual. Where possible, an individual session can be helpful to determine if there are ways to get the person back on track or if stopping their involvement in the group at this point is the best option for them.

In addition to limited progress with eating disorder symptoms, there are additional barriers to change that indicate treatment needs to be modified or stopped (Fairburn, 2008). Often these concerns (reviewed in Chapter 3) are an intensification, worsening, or emerging of other mental health symptoms, including safety concerns and/or substance misuse. While the review serves as an opportunity to specifically consider these barriers, any indication of concern should be addressed when issues arise and not delayed until the review.

> Eating disorder symptoms are not expected to be eliminated at this stage of treatment or significantly reduced for all patients. If there is some reduction in symptoms, it suggests the treatment is beneficial and should continue.

- *Other mental health concerns*: If other mental health symptoms develop or intensify during the treatment (e.g., clinical depression, grief/loss), which cause a disruption to the patient's ability to respond to Group CBT-E, it is recommended for the patient to discontinue the group intervention and address the concern (e.g., starting antidepressant medication, undergoing grief/loss therapy). The patient would be recommended to return to Group CBT-E once there is improvement with symptoms. This likely would mean joining a different group in the future. If this does not work logistically, consider Individual CBT-E which could potentially pick up where the patient left off with their group work.

- *Safety concerns*: If at any point in Group CBT-E a patient discloses a new onset, or increased frequency or intensity of suicidal ideation or self-injurious behaviors, a one-on-one check-in is required. Intensification of suicidal thinking or self-injurious behaviors should be considered potential acute safety concerns and may indicate that continuing with Group CBT-E for this individual is no longer appropriate.

- *Substance misuse*: The degree of severity and the function of the substance misuse is important to assess. For patients with a comorbid substance use diagnosis, we recommend that this be treated first. If a group member is arriving to group intoxicated, they should be asked to not attend group on this occasion and an individual check-in should be arranged. If their substance use is minimal but is associated with the eating disorder behaviors (e.g., more binge eating when drinking or high), these behaviors should be incorporated into the formulation and reviewed in detail during Session 13 (Events, Emotions, and Eating).

If it is determined that a patient needs to stop treatment, use your judgment to determine the best course of action and what level of care is appropriate, based on safety and treatment needs. Options include, but are not limited to: Individual CBT-E; another evidence-based treatment for eating disorders; an evidence-based treatment for a comorbid condition; a HLOC treatment; a break in treatment; and/or the addition of other services (e.g., dietitian counseling, psychiatric medication management). If scheduling demands are the issue, guided self-help for eating disorders or an evidence-based app program can be useful alternatives.

5. Preparing for Stage 3

The next session marks the start of Stage 3 of treatment. Stage 3 focuses on identifying and addressing the majority of the maintaining mechanisms of the eating disorder. For most patients, these remaining maintaining factors are some combination of 1) dieting behaviors and diet-related rules, 2) body image, and 3) emotions and events. We recommend addressing these mechanisms in this order. If this ordering does not fit the group of patients you are working with (e.g., the group could benefit more from body image being a focus first), the order is flexible and can be adjusted.

Next week, we will start Stage 3 of treatment. This stage includes the next seven sessions and focuses on the factors that are maintaining eating disorder symptoms that we have not yet addressed directly. These sessions will focus on dieting and diet-related rules, then body image, and finally how events and moods impact eating.

6. Group Wrap-up

Session Review

In today's session, we assessed your progress in treatment so far. Progress reviews are helpful in letting us know where we are doing well – it is important to praise our efforts – and where we need to continue to focus to get the most benefit from treatment. We looked at progress in terms of the practical aspects of treatment, like coming to sessions on time, and also the status of various eating disorder symptoms. With the latter, we compared ratings you provided before starting Group CBT-E to ratings from last week to provide you with valuable information about the change to your symptoms since the start of treatment. We also looked at barriers that may be getting in your way of fully engaging in treatment. For the reviews and assessment of barriers, you set clear Action Plans to work on for next time. We wrapped the group up by briefly outlining what the next treatment stage will cover.

Between-session Work

Remember to encourage patients to write the between-session work on their *Between-session Work Log* handout. The between-session work for Session 5 is:

- Continue work from previous sessions:
  - *Self-monitoring* – to be completed daily, in the moment.
  - *Regular Eating* – continue to prioritize regular eating using *Planning Ahead, Alternative Activities, Urge Tolerating*, and *Feelings of Fullness* to support this work.
  - Follow through with any Action Plans identified during the session.

- New work from Session 5:
  - *General Barriers to Change; Ways to Overcome Barriers to Change* – review this material. Create and act on relevant Action Plans.
  - Share progress with support person.

Higher Level of Care Adaptations: Modular Implementation

When this session is used modularly, the following adaptations are suggested.

> *Reviewing progress*: Reviewing individual progress is useful at all levels of care. Reviews at HLOCs tend to focus more on general aspects of one's treatment (i.e., treatment plan goals), rather than specific treatment interventions. Match the review to elements that the patient has encountered in their treatment (e.g., attending all available groups, completing 100% of the meal plan). The principles of the review remain the same: 1) to identify what is going well and should be continued; and 2) to identify areas that require further practice and make specific plans to address these. Use the review handouts for inspiration to identify barriers and ways to address these; ask patients to rate their progress aloud in the group; create shared ideas on a whiteboard; and allow adequate processing time.

Therapist Progress Review

Handout: *Therapist Self-review*

One barrier not included in the handouts is to do with the therapist's ability to lead the group and effectively implement treatment interventions. It is important to assess your own ability in providing this therapy. We want to ensure that you provide patients with all of the ingredients, tools, and skills described in the treatment. How you convey the information will be somewhat different based on the patients in the group, but it is important that each group and patient receives the full dose of treatment (i.e., the complete content). One of the best ways you can ensure this is by checking that you have covered the content as described in this treatment guide. Ideally, clinical supervision is a helpful place to get support with this. However, obtaining expert supervision can be difficult and acts as a barrier due to cost and lack of available supervisors. Peer supervision can be a useful alternative. Tools that help improve adherence to treatment models (providing the therapy as intended to achieve maximal results) can be useful. We have created a *Therapist Self-review* handout. This can be used in conjunction with the *Group CBT-E Components Checklist* found in Appendix E. The *Therapist Self-review* handout is in three parts: 1) content assessment; 2) barrier assessment; and 3) setting action steps. Give yourself adequate time to complete this review in a space free of distractions.

Therapist Content Assessment

The content assessment lists all of the skills and interventions that have been covered in the group so far. The list provides a quick way to assess if you have covered the main treatment elements at this point, both elements common to each session (e.g., sharing the agenda) and specific CBT-E skills (e.g., regular eating).

Therapist Barrier Assessment

Just as you consider what barriers patients encounter in treatment, you want to consider the barriers that you encounter in implementing the therapy. Take a moment for self-reflection on what may be getting in the way of implementing all components of the treatment and then create positive action steps to increase your treatment adherence going forward. Below are some common reasons therapists provide for changing the delivery of the therapy.

- *Not enough time in the sessions to cover the content.* This is a commonly reported challenge to effective implementation. There is a lot to cover each group session! Sometimes running out of time cannot be helped – perhaps there has been a safety-related crisis for a group member and it is not possible or appropriate to redirect the group back to the agenda. Most times though, a therapist's ability to keep the group on course and organized will become easier with time and practice. Facilitating groups can be more challenging than individual sessions as the therapist is attending to the needs of several patients at once. We have found that practicing responding to patients in a validating way that guides them back to group content is useful. Be conscious of other factors (e.g., not being prepared, believing that other material unrelated to the agenda takes priority, not understanding the material, difficulty interrupting group members to help get back on track) that may be pushing the time expectations for group, and consider if there are opportunities to improve in any of these areas.

- *Anxiety regarding the usefulness of content.* Sometimes therapists have reported feeling anxious about using some of the skills. For example, therapists have voiced worries about asking patients to change their eating habits and follow a regular pattern of eating, or speaking openly about self-induced vomiting. It is normal to feel anxious when having conversations about typically private topics or topics that patients feel shameful about. At the same time, we know that talking openly about eating disorder symptoms is the best way to try to confront the disorder and help a patient work toward recovery. Equally, providing firm, yet friendly, guidance on the importance of changing one's eating habits can allow patients to feel empowered to overrule the eating disorder thinking and engage with regular eating.

- *Leaving material out or using material from other therapies.* CBT-E is made up of many different skills and components. It is not known which components are the most effective and which could be modified. When delivered together these elements collectively contribute to a higher percentage of patients improving from their eating disorder. Therefore, it is essential to include all components to ensure that patients receive all critical elements. The delivery of each component is flexible and can be adjusted based on the specific needs of your patient group. For example, teaching the group a 5-minute mindfulness exercise in Session 3 may be an in-vivo activity to practice an alternative activity, if time allows. However, including a full session on mindfulness would take away from session time devoted to the rest of the Group CBT-E content and could potentially dilute its effects. Overall, when considering a modification, it is best to assess the intention behind the change and have a high threshold for doing so.

- *Disagreeing with content.* There are times in delivering a guided treatment when you may find that you do not agree with a particular intervention. This can be especially challenging for therapists if they believe that the skill could be harmful for patients. Where possible, it is best to be familiar with the therapy before starting the group. Not all therapies will align with previous clinical experience and personal preferences. If Group CBT-E feels to you to be impossible to implement as suggested, it is probably best not to offer it.

Taking Action

Once you have assessed your progress and identified any barriers to change, it is time to identify action steps. Your plan may be as simple as: "*I am on course and have covered all treatment skills so far, I will continue to do so.*" Or you may have found an obstacle: "*I am behind where I need to be for this point in treatment, my sessions have been running over and I am not covering the content fully. I will set aside time to review content in advance and practice running a session to see if I can rein session focus in.*" Or "*I will practice redirecting patients and tolerating any discomfort I feel in not letting the patient fully express their view during group.*" Problem-solving (introduced in Session 12) can be a helpful tool in creating action steps for yourself.

Reviewing our own progress as therapists is not something that many of us have regularly done. It can feel uncomfortable or frustrating when thought of as a useless, time-consuming task. If you have taken the time to complete the *Group CBT-E Components Checklist* and have completed this therapist progress review, well done!

Group Session 5

Handout 5.1 *Between-session Work Self-review – Session 5*

BETWEEN-SESSION WORK SELF-REVIEW – SESSION 5

Did I....	Yes	Somewhat	No
Self- Monitoring			
Use my records daily?	☐	☐	☐
Complete my records "in the moment"?	☐	☐	☐
Regular Eating			
Eat 5–6 times a day?	☐	☐	☐
Not eat in between planned eating times?	☐	☐	☐
Plan ahead?	☐	☐	☐
Alternative Activities			
Keep an up-to-date list of alternate activities to use?	☐	☐	☐
Use my activities to displace eating disorder behaviors?	☐	☐	☐
Plan in my alternate activities on challenging days or during difficult events?	☐	☐	☐
Urge Tolerating			
Notice when I have an increased urge to use an eating disorder behavior?	☐	☐	☐
Make the decision to not act on the urge?	☐	☐	☐
Sit with the urge?	☐	☐	☐
Feelings of Fullness			
Identify fullness triggers and response to the trigger?	☐	☐	☐

Which skills are going well? Great work, keep practicing them! Which skills am I struggling to use and need to prioritize? Plan to take action this week – write an **Action Plan** to address these.

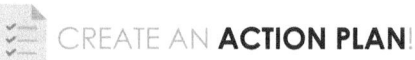 CREATE AN **ACTION PLAN**!

Handout 5.2   *Progress Review – Treatment Components*

PROGRESS REVIEW – TREATMENT COMPONENTS

Actions and Skills	👍	So-so	👎
Attending all groups	☐	☐	☐
Arriving on time	☐	☐	☐
Minimizing distractions while in group	☐	☐	☐
Staying focused while in group	☐	☐	☐
Participating in group	☐	☐	☐
Being open and honest in group	☐	☐	☐
Completing between-session work	☐	☐	☐
Self-monitoring	☐	☐	☐
Eating regular meals and snacks	☐	☐	☐
Using alternative activities	☐	☐	☐
Tolerating urges to engage in eating disorder behaviors (vomiting, restricting eating)	☐	☐	☐
Addressing feelings of fullness	☐	☐	☐
Making treatment (and myself!) a priority	☐	☐	☐
	☐	☐	☐
	☐	☐	☐
	☐	☐	☐

- Take a look at your Thumbs Up – these are the things to keep doing! Give yourself praise for all your Thumbs Up!
- So-so are areas that need more practice and support.
- Thumbs Down need extra attention.

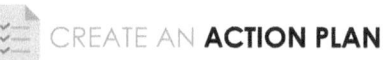 CREATE AN **ACTION PLAN**!

SAMPLE ACTION PLAN		DATE: 5/5
PROBLEM:	I am not participating very often in group. I really only say something if the group leader calls on me.	
CURRENT FREQUENCY (IF APPLICABLE):	N/A	
GOAL FOR UPCOMING WEEK:	Participate more without the group leader prompting me.	
SPECIFIC PLAN:	MY PLAN: I will challenge myself to say at least 1 thing in group each session.	MY SUPPORT: I will attempt to tolerate my anxiety before, during, and after to see what happens. The first time I say something, I will introduce it by saying that I am feeling nervous to share. For the first time, I will plan to saying something about my between-session work and will plan that ahead of time since I know what to expect there.

ACTION PLAN		DATE:
PROBLEM:		
CURRENT FREQUENCY (IF APPLICABLE):		
GOAL FOR UPCOMING WEEK:		
SPECIFIC PLAN:	MY PLAN:	MY SUPPORT:

Handout 5.3 *General Barriers to Change*

GENERAL BARRIERS TO CHANGE

Place a checkmark next to any of the barriers you are encountering:

☐ I am scared to change.

Common fears: What will the future look like without my eating disorder?, My eating disorder makes me feel special – what if there is nothing else special about me without it?, What if making these changes makes me hate my body even more?

☐ I don't have time to make treatment a priority.

Common competing responsibilities: Work deadlines, caring for children/elderly parents.

☐ I struggle with planning and being organized.

Common difficulties: completing between session work, making treatment a priority, missed groups or arriving late to group.

☐ I am dealing with a major life stress.

Examples: Breakup/divorce, ill child, job loss.

☐ I cannot afford my copay or session fee.

☐ I am encountering other financial-related stress, including food insecurity.

Examples: Paying for childcare while I am in therapy, cost of transportation to attend session.

☐ I do not like CBT-E.

☐ I feel too depressed.

☐ I am not worth it.

☐ I am using substances to self-medicate.

Other barriers for me:

_____

_____

_____

_____

Ways to overcome my barriers:

_____

_____

_____

_____

Handout 5.4 *Ways to Overcome Barriers to Change*

WAYS TO OVERCOME BARRIERS TO CHANGE

1) I am scared to change.

In general, a fear of change is common. When someone is struggling with an eating disorder, there is often an intense fear that their shape and weight will change. This is to be expected. You may not like your current body shape and weight and fear that you may not be able to tolerate any change. One way to support yourself with this fear is to share it with group members. Other members of the group likely also have this fear and it can help to talk with others who can truly relate to your intense worry. Another way is to allow the worry to come into your mind, accept that it is a common worry, and allow the thought to be. Finally, creating a list (or piece of artwork) of all of the reasons why you want to engage in change, even though it is scary, can be helpful. Make an Action Plan about this and share it with a support person and/or the group.

2) I don't have time to make treatment a priority.

Making treatment a priority is actually making **YOU** a priority! Treatment lasts for a few months and at the end, your eating disorder will likely be interfering with your life less and taking up less time. As much as possible, give yourself the time needed to fully engage with treatment sessions and between session work. You are worth it. And treatment will not work if you miss sessions or do not complete the between-session work. There are occasions in life when competing responsibilities cannot come second (e.g., a family crisis). If this is the case for you, speak with your group therapist and give yourself permission to stop the group. Making a collaborative decision to stop therapy will allow your group therapist to wrap things up for you. Even if you cannot finish treatment, you can finish where you got to with strength (i.e., taking time to review progress with the therapist and make a solid plan for the future). Later on, when life settles down, you can restart. And hopefully that is what you will do!

3) I struggle with planning and being organized.

Setting phone alarms or using an app-based reminder tool can be really helpful in this case. Asking for help from supports can also greatly help.

4) I am dealing with a major life stress.

Some life stress makes engaging in treatment impossible and it may be more helpful to stop treatment for now. See comments under point 2. In other situations, taking time to identify ways of helping you to handle the stress, while also continuing in group, can work (e.g., taking a leave of absence to care for an ill child; making a calendar to schedule time for applying for jobs while also scheduling in your treatment goals and sessions; asking for help).

5) **I cannot afford my copay or session fee and/or I am encountering other financial-related stress, including food insecurity.**

Be sure to raise these issues with your group therapist. There may be ways to reduce some of your financial burden associated with treatment costs and/or ideas to support you in accessing nutritious foods.

6) **I do not like CBT-E.**

Short-term, focused psychotherapies are not for everyone. If possible, try sticking the course and remain fully engaged if you are able to. You may find that even if you do not like this style of treatment that you are still able to make progress with your eating disorder. If, however, you feel strongly that treatment is not a good match for you, speak with your group leader about possible referrals and alternatives.

If you are experiencing any of the following, it is crucial that you share this with your group leader:

7) **I feel too depressed.**

Depression and eating disorders frequently co-occur. Sometimes low mood improves as the eating improves, but not always. If you are struggling with low mood, thoughts of ending your life, or urges to harm yourself in any way, it is crucial that you share this with your group leader immediately.

8) **I am not worth it.**

Feelings of worthlessness can be associated with depression, low self-esteem, and other factors. Often with improvement to eating disorder symptoms these feelings improve, but not always and they should not be ignored. Talk to your group leader if you are experiencing feelings of worthlessness.

9) **I am using substances to self-medicate.**

If you are using substances to deal with anxiety, low mood, or emotional dysregulation, you are likely not getting the most benefit out of treatment. At times, as the eating disorder improves, a reliance on substances increases. This makes sense as the eating disorder had likely been playing an important role in helping (or at least appearing to help) deal with anxiety, low mood, and emotional dysregulation. If you are struggling in this way, make sure to talk to the group leader.

Handout 5.5   *Therapist Self-review*

THERAPIST SELF-REVIEW
REVIEWING PROGRESS

Content.

For each session, I have:	Yes	Most of the time	No	MY PLAN		
				Make a plan for change	Consult with a professional support (e.g., colleague, supervisor)	Praise myself for working hard on this!
Shared the agenda	☐	☐	☐	☐	☐	☐
Oriented the group to the current session number & number of remaining sessions	☐	☐	☐	☐	☐	☐
Reviewed the between-session work self-review	☐	☐	☐	☐	☐	☐
Provided a group summary	☐	☐	☐	☐	☐	☐
Asked patients to complete their between-session work log	☐	☐	☐	☐	☐	☐
Completed the group CBT-E CC	☐	☐	☐	☐	☐	☐
I have covered:						
Personalized formulations	☐	☐	☐	☐	☐	☐
Self-monitoring forms	☐	☐	☐	☐	☐	☐
Regular eating	☐	☐	☐	☐	☐	☐
Alternative activities	☐	☐	☐	☐	☐	☐
Urge tolerating	☐	☐	☐	☐	☐	☐
Feelings of fullness	☐	☐	☐	☐	☐	☐

Barriers.

Barriers I have encountered when trying to implement the group are:

☐	Not having enough time to complete all material
☐	Not keeping to the agenda
☐	Not preparing in advance of each session
☐	
☐	
☐	

Actions.

Based on my review, I plan to take the following step(s) to help support me in implementing the treatment:

☐	I'll set aside time each week in my calendar to review materials in advance. (20 mins)
☐	I'll use a gentle-sounding phone alarm to alert me when it is time to wrap up one section on the agenda.
☐	
☐	
☐	
☐	

Anything Else?

_____

_____

_____

_____

_____

_____

Stage Three

Maintaining Mechanisms

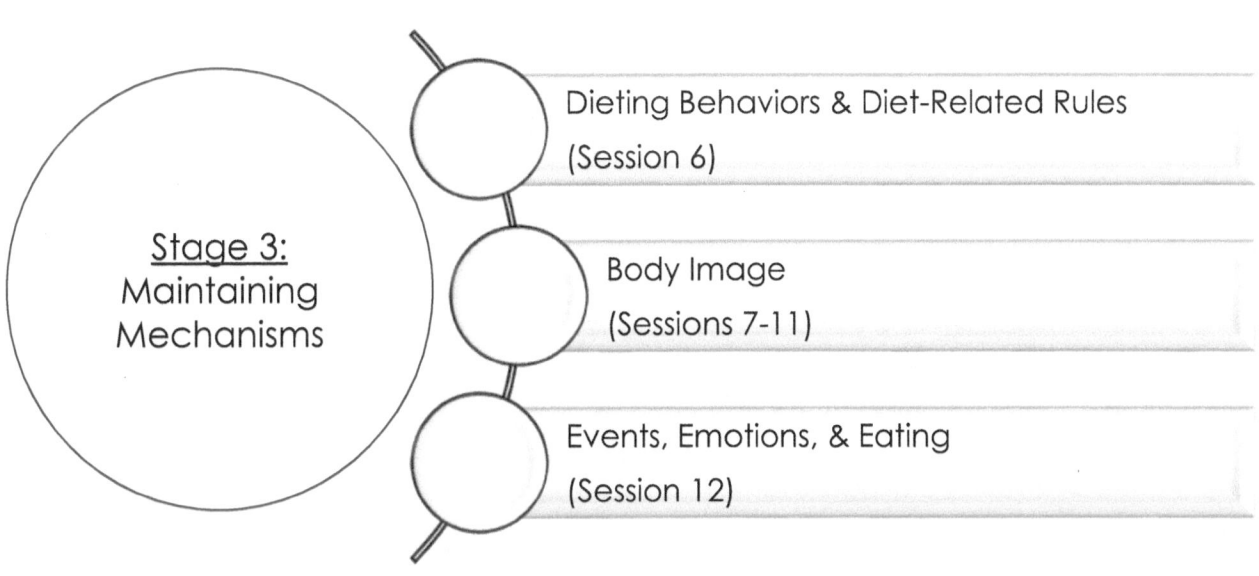

Stage 3:
Maintaining
Mechanisms

Dieting Behaviors & Diet-Related Rules
(Session 6)

Body Image
(Sessions 7-11)

Events, Emotions, & Eating
(Session 12)

Chapter 11

Group Session 6

Dieting Behaviors and Diet-related Rules

Session 6 is the first session of Stage 3 of Group CBT-E. Stage 3 focuses on the main remaining mechanisms keeping the eating disorder going. Session 6 focuses on dieting behaviors and diet-related rules, Sessions 7–11 focus on body image, and Session 12 focuses on events and emotions.

Overview

Encouragement to diet is ubiquitous in our society. The dieting industry is a multibillion-dollar enterprise. Direct and indirect messages are everywhere that weight loss and achieving one's ideal body are possible, promising increased attractiveness, happiness, love, and success. It is not surprising, therefore, that individuals with eating disorders, who place great emphasis on their shape and weight, are particularly vulnerable to diet messaging.

In this group, we will consider the impact that dieting has on maintaining disordered eating. Thinking back to the personalized formulations completed in Session 1, engaging in dieting behaviors or having diet-related rules is one of the primary maintaining mechanisms that we target in CBT-E. CBT-E focuses on reducing dieting behaviors and diet-related rules and encourages flexible eating, making it an anti-diet approach. By targeting the cycle of restrictive eating and challenging the diet mentality, CBT-E promotes a more sustainable relationship with food.

The main goals of this session are to support patients in considering the pros and cons of dieting and provide education about how reducing diet-related rules is necessary to overcome their eating disorder. The group starts by engaging the patients in a discussion to acknowledge the presence and impact of diet culture (which includes exercise). Then, the focus is on providing specific education about how dieting and diet-related rules maintain eating disorders. Finally, specific skills to break diet-related rules and eat more flexibly are identified.

> Throughout many of the Stage 3 chapters, "Social Media Alert" boxes are included to provide additional education on the impact of social media on particular interventions and strategies for addressing these impacts.

DOI: 10.4324/9781003450849-15

Therapist Preparation

☐ Review this chapter in advance.

☐ Review accompanying handouts and have copies available for patients.

☐ Have a copy of each patient's *My Formulation* handout as this will be used in session.

☐ Consider the diet culture messaging that you personally have internalized.

Handouts

- Standard Weekly Handouts
  - *1.1 My Formulation*
  - *1.3 Self-monitoring Form*
  - *1.6 Between-session Work Log*
  - *6.1 Between-session Work Self-review – Session 6*

- Session-specific Handouts
  - *6.2 Resetting My Thinking About Dieting*
  - *6.3 My Avoided Foods List*
  - *6.4 My Food Rules*
  - *6.5 Exposure*
  - *6.6 My Breaking Food Rules Plan*

In preparing for this group, it can be helpful to identify any diet culture messages that you have internalized and believe to be true. These can serve as interesting examples for the group and also help you to notice any biases that you may have. For example, it is not uncommon to hear therapists refer to "good" foods and "bad" foods, or "healthy" and "unhealthy" foods. Labeling foods in this way – with moral judgments – is unhelpful as it can lead to thinking that eating "good/healthy" foods makes someone good, and eating "bad/unhealthy" foods makes someone bad. Foods are not good or bad, nor does eating any particular food change our value. Additionally, these so-called "good foods" are often low-calorie, low-carbohydrate, high-protein, or diet-type foods, which may not actually be what patients require nutritionally to eat flexibly and overcome their disorder.

Group Session Agenda

1. Setting the agenda and orienting to the session (2 minutes)
2. Between-session work self-review (5 minutes)
3. Acknowledging diet culture and weight bias (10 minutes)
4. Exploring dieting behaviors (5–10 minutes)
5. Addressing dieting behaviors (5–10 minutes)
6. Identifying diet-related rules (10–15 minutes)
7. Addressing diet-related rules (15 minutes)
8. Group wrap-up (3 minutes)

1. Setting the Agenda and Orienting to the Session

Begin with a positive, encouraging welcome; share that this is Session 6, Stage 3, with 8 sessions remaining. Clearly list the session agenda.

2. Between-session Work Self-review

Handout: *Between-session Work Self-review – Session 6*

Ask patients to complete their *Between-session Work Self-review – Session 6* handout. You may notice that between-session work self-reviews begin to have less detail as more skills are added. This review checks in on the Stage 1 elements (self-monitoring, regular eating, alternative activities, urge tolerating, and addressing feelings of fullness). There is also additional space for patients to add in anything else they noted in the progress review (Session 5) as an area they wanted to work on. Ask the group to review their Action Plans from Session 5 and to add in specific items they were working on and then to rate their progress. Praise patients for the things that are going well; identify barriers and how to address such obstacles; and build on the existing interventions by identifying increasingly challenging ways to tackle eating disorder symptoms. At the end of the review, encourage patients to create updated Action Plans to reflect goals for the week, and include these on their *Between-session Work Log*.

3. Acknowledging Diet Culture and Weight Bias

Begin this session by exploring with patients their awareness of diet culture. Some patients may be quite aware, while others may be absorbing diet culture information without even realizing it. Diet culture places great positive emphasis on idealized versions of body shape and weight (i.e., the "thin ideal," a muscular or toned ideal, a small waist and large buttocks ideal) and equates these idealized bodies with attractiveness or being "good." Diet culture is related to and perpetuates fatphobia and weight bias (described in Chapter 5). Entire multi-session groups could be devoted to exploring and processing diet culture and weight bias. While this is not possible in the context of the focus of Group CBT-E, we encourage you to seek out education on these topics and consider their impact on yourself and your patients.

Starting the Conversation About Diet Culture

With the group, create a list of messages that patients have heard about dieting. If you have come prepared to the group with a recent dieting message that you have seen or heard, share this with the group. Ask patients to consider the impact of these messages on their self-worth, eating disorder behaviors, and body image.

Let's start the group today by thinking about our diet culture, specifically the messaging we receive about dieting and achieving our "ideal" body shape and weight. Is anyone aware of a recent dieting advertisement or social media post they have seen linking dieting and the promotion of attractiveness? What about messages from family members or loved ones about your body? Do you hear ideas from them that suggest that thinness, muscularity, small waist and large buttocks, or another certain body shape, is better than others? [Jointly create this list on a whiteboard. See Table 11.1]. *What do you think the impact of seeing messages like this has on your overall self-worth? How do these messages impact your eating disorder?*

The intention of this discussion is to help provide a strong rationale for why letting go (or at least beginning to be open to letting go) of a diet mentality is necessary for recovery. This discussion also allows you to provide validation to the group about their experience of living in our current diet-focused culture.

I can see here on the whiteboard a long list of diet messages that most of you believe and some of you have tried to follow. In our culture we are bombarded with diet messaging that falsely promises all sorts of benefits of dieting, weight loss, and our ability to change our bodies. I also know that each of you is in this group for a reason – your current eating behaviors are not working for you. In addition, we've created a long list of negative consequences of believing these messages. I wonder if holding onto these dieting messages is keeping you stuck in your disorder and making you feel worse about yourself. In a moment, we are going to examine further some of these negative consequences.

Table 11.1 Sample Whiteboard – Diet and Body Ideal Messages

Diet-Positive and Body Ideal Messages	How These Messages Make Me Feel
"You need to trim your waste and thicken your butt."	Sad, disgusted with my current shape – my butt is so flat and I barely have a waist.
"Pre-vacation workout and meal plans to get the body you want" (image of someone with really toned arms and abs).	I'll never look like that. Instead, I'll look gross on the beach and I won't go.
"You look so good now" (following weight loss that was achieved through not allowing myself enough food).	Obviously, I used to look bad at a higher weight. And so, starving myself and exercising for hours every day is worth it – even if it means being sick.
"Follow me for easy fat burning tips to get that chiseled look" (video of someone cooking in their bathing suit).	They look so good. I look terrible compared to them. I will try to follow their meal plan and lifting routine but I know I'll never look like them.
"Lose weight and feel great."	If only I could lose weight so that I would feel better about myself, but I'm not strong enough to stick to my diet.
"Eating sugar is like taking drugs."	I must avoid sugar at all times, but I have no willpower ever.

Providing this foundational information provides a context for understanding the pressures to change one's body and sets the group up to discuss dieting behaviors and diet-related rules.

4. Exploring Dieting Behaviors

After a general discussion about diet culture and the impact of body shape and weight ideal messaging, the next topic is on dieting behaviors (i.e., Box A on the *My Formulation* handout from Session 1). Diet culture promises that dieting will get someone to their desired shape or weight. This is false. Dieting and other weight control behaviors will not necessarily lead someone to achieve their "ideal" body shape/weight. The reality is, there is only so much control a person has over their shape and weight. While limiting intake can lead to changes, these changes are often short-lived and perpetuate cycles of "yo-yo dieting" or dieting and binge eating, which lead to negative feelings about oneself. For many patients with eating disorders, their attempts to restrict or restrain their eating are extreme and are associated with rigid rules about eating.

Social Media Alert

Social media is often a tool used to promote dieting. Social media promotes rapidly changing diet fads and can spread dieting messages at alarming rates. Assess with patients any social media behaviors that they may be engaged in that promote dieting, such as watching video content about what others are eating; following pro-weight loss or eating disorder sites; posting diet-related cooking advice; "liking" posts about other people's weight loss; posting images of self only when they were at their lowest weight; and following friends/pages that are wrought with diet comparisons (e.g., dieting, food, cooking, or clean eating sites). Ask patients to consider the impact of these diet behaviors and support patients in any strategies to decrease these behaviors.

Additionally, a highly engaging exercise can be viewing in the group an advertisement or social media content that promotes a dieting trend.

The aim is to help patients begin to view their dieting as unhelpful and begin to question the usefulness of dieting. Again, given the diet-positive environment we live in, this can be extremely challenging. This perspective goes against years of internalized messages about "good" food and "bad" food. Many patients believe dieting is beneficial and necessary. They falsely believe that if only they were better at it, or had more willpower, they would be able to stick to these diets and achieve their desired weight and shape.

Ask patients to share any dieting behaviors they engage in or believe they should engage in and create a shared list on the whiteboard. Remind patients to not share specific calorie amounts aloud in the group but to include them on their *My Formulation* handout.

5. Addressing Dieting Behaviors

Handouts: *My Formulation; Resetting My Thinking About Dieting*

Table 11.2 Sample Whiteboard – Benefits and Harms of Dieting

<u>Benefits of dieting</u>

It helps me to maintain the weight/shape I want.

I am good at it.

It helps me to feel in control.

It helps me to compensate for binges.

It helps me to eat less in advance of large meals (during holidays, birthdays, parties, meals at restaurants).

<u>How dieting harms me</u>

It causes some of my binges.

It keeps me distracted with thoughts about eating, and my weight and shape.

It causes anxiety (about eating out with others, about breaking rules, about fear of gaining weight).

I don't get to eat the foods I really like.

What it promises is a lie!

To address dieting, start by exploring with patients their beliefs about the benefits of eating in this way.

I'd like to spend some time thinking about the ways that dieting may not be as beneficial as we have been led to believe that it is. But before we do this, let's first consider the ways you believe dieting is helpful. We will use the Resetting My Thinking About Dieting handout and will create a shared list of examples on the whiteboard. [see Table 11.2].

Take time to allow patients to think through their beliefs, validating where possible, and then exploring the belief further. For example, if someone in the group were to share that a benefit of dieting is to help lose weight, your response may include providing education about the ineffectiveness of dieting long term, asking to share more about their personal experience, and encouraging them to consider that their dieting may be less helpful than it initially appeared.

While it is true that limiting our intake can change our weight, at least in the short term, what has been your personal experience with dieting? You shared that you have been on every diet there is. It sounds like they have worked for you in the short term, but have any worked in the long term? When these diets no longer work or "fail," how does that end up making you feel? What about for others?

Therapist Insight

In supporting patients to reconsider their view on dieting (and hopefully moving away from thinking that dieting is a helpful tool), we have found the group format to be particularly useful. Group members are often extremely validating and supportive to one another in understanding the challenges in changing these long-held beliefs.

In cases where a patient describes that dieting does allow them to be the weight they prefer, it is important to explore the costs of their dieting. Gentle probing using some of the questions below can be helpful:

- *Does your dieting ever lead to episodes of out-of-control eating?*
- *Do you have limited 'brain space' because many of your thoughts are focused on eating, weight, and/or shape?*
- *When you feel that a diet has worked, has it ultimately stopped working at some point? Do you blame yourself for this – for example, 'If only I had just stuck to it closer, it would have worked because it was working initially.'?*
- *Does dieting prevent you, or make you feel uncomfortable engaging in, certain social events that involve eating?*

Next, provide education on the harms of dieting and specifically its relationship to keeping the eating disorder going. Looking back at the *My Formulation* handout, remind patients that dieting behaviors and diet-related rules lead to other eating disorder behaviors. One behavior common to many in the group will be binge eating. Binge eating is a consequence of dieting behaviors in two main ways:

1. Undereating (i.e., not eating enough calories) causes *physiological* hunger. When we restrict our eating, the brain, wanting to maintain homeostasis or an equilibrium, produces hormones that increase the natural drive to eat. After a period of undereating, it is not uncommon to respond by eating quickly and having larger amounts of food than typical. We can see this following being ill with a stomach flu. Caloric intake is greatly reduced while one is unwell, often causing weight loss (some of this weight loss is dehydration), and when the virus passes, most people return quickly to their pre-illness weight due to eating and drinking larger quantities after a period of not eating much.

2. Dieting behaviors also encourage binge eating via *psychological* or *emotional* deprivation. Often the more someone denies themselves a food they would like to eat, the more likely they are to overeat it when they eventually gain access to it. Sometimes food avoidance and food rules are so strong and rigid that even having a bite of an avoided food can trigger a binge.

It is essential to highlight both of these mechanisms to the patients. Highlighting these on their individual *My Formulation* handouts and drawing the mechanisms on the whiteboard helps patients to visualize the pressure from the eating disorder to engage in further eating disorder behaviors. Table 11.3 provides information about several ways dieting is problematic.

For patients who do not engage in binge eating, highlight how dieting and diet-related rules keep *their* eating disorder going. For some there will be a line from dieting (Box A) straight back to the over-evaluation of shape and weight box (Box F). For others, the dieting box causes them to maintain a weight too low for their body (Box C). And for others, it may greatly impact – and be impacted by – events, emotions, and eating (Box E). Be sure to individualize this information for all members of the group and update personalized formulations as needed.

Table 11.3 Dieting is Problematic

Similar to Individual CBT-E (Fairburn, 2008), Group CBT-E emphasizes that dieting is problematic in several ways.

1. *Dieting keeps the eating disorder going.* The formulation highlights this mechanism. When we can remove the middle box of dieting rules and behaviors (Box A, *My Formulation*), other eating disorder behaviors can be reduced. For example, when someone stops limiting their intake and avoiding specific foods they otherwise would enjoy, their binge eating often greatly reduces (binges related to emotion regulation and binges related to ongoing compensatory mechanisms remain. These are removed with other skills described in Chapter 12.) It is essential to help patients to see the connection between dieting and ongoing binge eating and other eating disorder behaviors.

2. *Dieting takes up "brain space" and keeps one preoccupied with thoughts about food and eating, which is distracting and often distressing.* Limiting the overall amount of calories eaten and denying oneself certain foods makes the brain far more likely to think about these foods. Many patients who are undereating or avoiding certain foods report very busy brains. They think about the next time they will eat or what they will have to eat. If they are denying themselves a specific food they often think about this food with great intensity.

3. *Having so many rules is exhausting and anxiety provoking.* A brain that is always thinking about what foods can be eaten and which ones cannot, is a tired brain. In fact, such brain busyness is a frequently mentioned reason why a patient has come in for treatment. Patients also share how rules negatively impact meal-centered holidays and special occasions, bringing excessive worry and anxiety instead of enjoyment.

4. *Having so many rules gets in the way of social events and spontaneity.* It is often impossible for patients to enjoy a meal out with friends, especially when they do not know what will be served. Being spontaneous and "living in the moment" is nearly impossible when diet-related rules are so strong. Many patients will either make detailed plans to "allow" themselves to eat out (e.g., dieting in advance of the meal, planning in exercise after the meal) or avoid the meal entirely and withdraw from friends and family.

5. *Dieting causes negative feelings.* It is impossible for someone to follow all their dieting rules all the time when there are so many and they are often extreme. As a result, these rules are inevitably broken. When these rules are broken, many patients experience strong negative feelings about themselves. They may feel tremendous guilt, or intense feelings of self-disgust.

Helping patients to view dieting as unhelpful and likely harmful can be even more challenging for those who are "successfully" maintaining a weight lower than their body needs without engaging in out-of-control eating. For these patients, it is hugely important to provide education about maintaining a weight too low for their body or being underfat (provide the *Underweight/Underfat* handout).

If you have not already done so, provide relevant optional information handouts (found in Session 2) on any related behaviors that emerge during the conversation: *Dieting; Binge Eating; Underweight/Underfat; Self-induced Vomiting and Medication Misuse;* and *Driven Exercise.*

Now, using the Resetting My Thinking About Dieting handout, let's think about the ways that dieting may be harmful to you. Together we will create a list on the handout and also on the whiteboard. Looking at your formulation, we can see how dieting puts pressure both physiologically (not eating enough which causes the body to need to make up energy) and psychologically (not choosing foods that I would like to eat and feeling deprived and/or out of control when I do eat them) to binge eat. I'll start our list with: "Dieting puts pressure on me to binge eat."

Continue the list with the group. Take time to process what group members think seeing the perceived benefits and harms next to one another.

6. Identifying Diet-related Rules

The next agenda item is to help group members identify specific types of dieting they engage in. Do this by helping patients to create a list of food and eating rules, which includes a list of avoided foods. As mentioned, some of these rules may have already been identified on their personal formulations (Box A – *My Formulation* handout).

Now we are going to start identifying specific rules that you have about food and eating. Let's look at your formulation. In the middle box, you likely listed some of the rules you follow or believe that you should follow. For example, you may try to stick to a calorie limit that is too low, or deny yourself certain foods. Rules like these are very common when someone has an eating disorder. To fully overcome your eating disorder, it is helpful to be aware of your food/eating rules and foods that you avoid or deny yourself.

Avoided Foods

Handout: *My Avoided Foods List*

To begin the exploration of food rules in group, start by first helping patients to identify foods or food groups that they avoid eating or plan to avoid eating. Avoiding or planning to avoid entire food groups or specific types of foods is common for individuals with eating disorders. Support patients in identifying their rules and what is motivating them to stick to, or attempt to stick to, these rules. It is important to explore what the patients believe will happen if they break their rules. Many patients believe that eating avoided or feared foods (or breaking a dietary rule) will lead to changes in their weight. These fears are often extreme. For example, a patient can believe that having one ice cream cone will immediately result in weight gain.

Therapist Insight

When creating dietary and avoided foods lists be sure to ask patients about sensory-related food rules and avoided foods. For example, some patients may avoid foods that they find slimy or sharp. This may indicate an avoidant/restrictive food intake disorder presentation; be related to heightened sensory awareness experienced by many neurodivergent individuals; or be a general preference. There is often a different approach to introducing sensory-related avoided foods.

Let's create a list on the whiteboard of foods that each of you avoids or tries to avoid. These are sometimes described as feared, forbidden, or challenge foods. There may be some similarities among some of you and there likely will be differences that are personal to each of you. You will have time to complete this as between-session work so you do not need to rush now, as your list likely will not be completed by the end of group today. In addition to the foods themselves, I'd also like you to share what you fear will happen if you break the rule and one thought about how having the rule limits your life [Group members can be excellent in helping peers to identify how the fear limits life – so do encourage them to help out] [see Table 11.4].

This is a really helpful start. We can already see how many foods everyone is trying hard each day to not allow themselves to eat. There are a lot on the list. What a lot of work and pressure to put on yourself. We can also see the reasons you put such effort into following these rules, as many of you described fear about breaking them. And you've also done a great job thinking

Therapist Insight

Be sensitive to culturally informed food rules. Ask patients if there are foods that they cannot, or do not eat, due to cultural or religious beliefs. Check in about holidays that may also inform food choices.

Therapist Insight

Some patients will share that there are particular foods that they consider "binge foods" (i.e., foods that they only allow themselves to eat when binge eating, often depriving themselves of these foods at other times). If relevant, help patients to identify these foods and encourage them to consider planning these foods in as a part of addressing avoided foods.

Table 11.4 Sample Whiteboard – Avoided Foods, Fears About Breaking the Rule, and How the Rule is Limiting

Avoided Foods List	My Fear About Breaking the Rule	How the Rule Limits Me
Cake	My weight will go up.	I missed out on my daughter's first birthday cake.
Fries	The transfats will clog my arteries.	I really like fries and miss the taste.
Cookies	My weight will go up.	I can't resist them and so it just makes me feel awful and guilty when I do eat them.
BBQ	It will cause me to binge.	I haven't attended a family reunion (my family always BBQs) in 6 years.
Sauces	I'll end up eating more calories total as a result – and my weight will go up and they have a lot of chemicals in them.	They taste good. I miss out.

about what life might be like without these rules. At times, it was challenging to identify how missing out on these foods is negatively impacting your lives. Well done on supporting each other with this! It makes sense that it is difficult to know how missing out on these foods harms you as you have been doing it for so long. Having so many rules is really limiting your enjoyment in life, placing a great deal of pressure on you, and keeping the eating disorder going.

After identifying some initial ideas as a group, ask patients to take a couple of minutes to start their own personal avoided food lists and to categorize the avoided foods into three categories on the *My Avoided Foods List* handout. The categories ("Foods that I am absolutely terrified to eat," "Foods that I am scared to eat," and "Foods that I might consider trying but would find it really hard to do") are helpful for the patients to identify where they would like to start in making change, which will be addressed later in the session.

You will see on your My Avoided Foods List handout that there are three categories. I will give you a couple of minutes here to start listing your avoided foods right on the handout. We won't have enough time to complete these today, so for between-session work, spend time completing the boxes. You will want as comprehensive a list as possible. Remember to include foods that you primarily avoid but eat when binge eating. There may be foods that you have been avoiding for so long that you no longer remember that you once liked them. A helpful way to create the most detailed list as possible is to go to your grocery store and walk up and down the aisles and jot down the foods you are avoiding. Or you can do some online grocery shopping. Or you can ask a trusted support person to help in remembering foods you used to enjoy before your eating disorder.

Other Diet-related Rules

Handout: *My Food Rules*

As Fairburn (2008) describes in *Cognitive Behavior Therapy and Eating Disorders*, in addition to having rules about avoiding specific foods, many individuals also have rules regarding eating in general. Typically, these rules revolve around:

• What to eat and what not to eat
• When to eat
• How much to eat
• Not eating in front of others
• Not eating more than anyone else present
• Certain textures and shapes

Helping patients to identify other dietary rules is an essential component to moving towards flexible eating. Often these rules are so ingrained that patients may struggle to even identify them as rules. Using the *My Food Rules* handout, start to have a group discussion about food rules.

Great job coming up with the avoided foods list. Now let's think together about all of the other rules that you each try to follow regarding your eating. Before we do, is anyone aware of a rule that we as a group have already started to challenge? I am thinking about how regular eating has likely broken some rules for you. For example, following a regular pattern of eating, which you have been working on since group Session 2, challenges any rule about needing to eat just a limited number of times a day. Nice job to those who broke a food rule by eating 5–6 times per day instead. Using your My Food Rules handout, let's list your food rules on the handout and share them aloud as a group. Let me know which food rule category it fits under for you. Some examples to get us started are: 'delaying eating for as long as possible' and 'sticking to a too low calorie limit' [see Table 11.5].

> **Therapist Insight**
>
> The goal is to be able to eat flexibly. Eating flexibly allows patients to be back in control of their eating rather than food and food rules being in control.

Table 11.5 Food Rules

Rules concerning what to eat and what not to eat
Fill up on coffee and ice water. Don't eat fried food.

Rules concerning when to eat
No food before 12 noon.

Rules concerning how much to eat
Only have one carbohydrate per day.

Rules concerning not eating in front of others
Avoid going out to eat with others.

Rules concerning not eating more than anyone else present
Make sure I eat less than my sister.

Rules concerning certain shapes or textures
Avoid all sharp or slimy foods (chips, oatmeal).

Take time to understand and discuss each rule. If time is limited, choose a few to focus on and encourage group members to spend more time between sessions thinking about the implications of each rule. Be sure to highlight, again, how having multiple rules regarding eating can keep the eating disorder going. If a patient has strict rules about the overall amount of food or calories they eat and this amount is suggestive of undereating, encourage them to review both the *Underweight/Underfat* handout which describes the importance of eating enough food for one's body.

7. Addressing Diet-Related Rules

Handouts: *Exposure; My Avoided Foods List; My Food Rules; My Breaking Food Rules Plan*

At this point, patients have identified their rules (both avoided food rules and other dietary rules) and have started to consider how attempting to follow these rules is leading to more disordered eating and feeling badly about themselves. It is now time for patients to devise a plan to address them. The main way we tackle rules is through exposure to breaking the rules. Exposure is a potent tool to help decrease anxiety that is felt around a feared stimulus. Exposure-based therapies are well grounded in the treatment for anxiety disorders where avoidance of the fearful event or circumstance is common. By encouraging patients to expose themselves to a feared food, or break a dietary rule, and tolerate any associated anxiety (without engaging in a behavior to reduce the anxiety), they learn that their feared outcome does not occur or that if it does, they can tolerate associated distress. When introducing the concept of exposure, review the *Exposure* handout with patients.

Between now and the next session, and likely between all the sessions until the end, encourage patients to practice breaking food rules.

You've all done a great job starting to identify your food rules and avoided foods. And you will continue to add to your lists between sessions. You've also been open to considering how following these rules plays a role in keeping your eating disorder going. It is now time to make a plan to break these rules and start learning to eat flexibly. It will likely be scary at first and you may believe that you will lose further control of your eating. This may happen occasionally. With practice, however, you will likely find that no longer having these rules is truly freeing. And over time, you will become less preoccupied with thoughts about your shape, weight, and eating. Take a look at your My Avoided Foods List and My Food Rules and think about which foods you could plan into your eating for the next week and which food rule(s) you would like to practice breaking. Ideally you will plan to have an avoided food and break a food rule three times over the week. Choosing a specific food and a specific time will help you to stick to breaking the food rule. When you decide, please fill out the My Breaking Food Rules Plan handout.

Therapist Insight

For patients who struggle with binge eating, sometimes the idea of breaking diet-related rules related to foods that they typically eat during binges can be particularly anxiety provoking. For example, we have heard patients say "I do not allow brownies in my house. When I do, I eat the whole pan." This type of statement highlights the vicious binge-diet cycle. To interrupt this cycle, patients need to learn to eat brownies regularly, in ways that do not lead to binge eating. In these situations, we find it to be sometimes useful to have gradual exposure to these foods. Using the brownie example, suggest that the patient incorporates brownies into their home in steps. Perhaps the first step is buying a single brownie to bring home to eat as a part of a dessert. The next step may be baking a pan of brownies and putting individual brownie slices into a freezer, thawing out the necessary number each day according to their regular eating plan. Eventually, patients will work toward having an entire pan of brownies on their kitchen counter at home to eat in typical portions as a part of their regular eating plan. Other initial strategies, such as portioning food from larger bags into individual serving bags (e.g., potato chips) and preparing food to share with others, can be implemented. In many cases, these exposure interventions will generalize to other avoided foods.

Some important points related to rule breaking/exposure:

- For some, breaking the avoided food rules is easier than breaking other dietary rules and for others, the opposite is true. Allow patients to choose for themselves in which order to break the rules and how fast to go.

- Avoid encouraging patients to go too slow as that can serve to worsen anxiety and decrease learning from the exposure. We typically encourage rule breaking about 3x/week in between sessions.

- Take the patient's lead in knowing how much to eat to break the rule. Let's use the example of chocolate as an avoided food. For one person, a bite of chocolate may be all they can tolerate and enough to break their rule. For another, it would need to be a whole chocolate bar. Encourage patients to be brave and push themselves, and also remind them that they know better than anyone else what amount would be the 'correct' amount to break their rule. They can build up from there.

- Patients should work toward identifying challenging exposure goals that do produce anxiety, but not goals that are so challenging that they will be impossible to follow through with. This will look different for each patient. For example, some patients may be able to start by challenging themselves to have foods in their most difficult avoided food category and others will only be able to have foods in their "might consider" category.

> **Therapist Insight**
>
> When possible, schedule the group at a time of day most consistent with eating. It can be a wonderful opportunity to include a snack to be eaten during a subsequent group as part of the breaking food rules intervention. See the In-Session Food Exposure guidance in Appendix E.

For many patients, the distress they feel following eating an avoided food or breaking a food rule can trigger them to engage in an eating disorder behavior (e.g., restrict their intake, binge eat, self-induce vomiting, exercise). Those feelings are likely to be present even when these foods are intentionally planned in. Provide patients with psychoeducation about this and also encourage them to use their skills to distract from, or tolerate, their eating disorder urges.

After you have eaten your planned avoided food or broken a rule, you are at increased risk of binge eating or compensating in some way. To protect against this, you will also want to plan in an alternative activity and/or remind yourself to engage in urge tolerating afterward. Here is an example: Dez planned to eat an ice cream sundae after dinner. He knew that eating a sundae usually would lead to more eating and then a full-blown binge. So, he planned to take a walk with his partner after the sundae and also remind himself that the urge to binge will increase and intensify and then, with time, start to go down. He also planned in a backup distraction of calling his friend if he still felt like binge eating after the walk. Think about which distraction activities work best for you and plan them in on your My Breaking Food Rules Plan. Consider if urge tolerating (discussed in Session 4) could be useful for you here and write into your plan how you will tolerate your eating disorder following breaking a food rule.

Remind patients that they are likely overriding years of internalized damaging diet messaging when they are breaking rules. It is understandable that it is anxiety provoking and scary. It will take time to break these rules and re-introduce foods they may not have eaten or may not have eaten outside of a binge in a long time. That said, despite all the discomfort in the short term, the long-term benefits will be worth it!

8. Group Wrap-up

Session Review

In today's session, we talked about how dieting behaviors and diet-related rules (inflexible eating) keep the eating disorder going. We started by thinking about diet culture that encourages the view that dieting will help someone to achieve the body they desire. We thought through how the eating disorder latches onto this thinking and takes it to extreme levels often causing many group members to undereat or attempt to undereat, follow a variety of diet rules, and avoid, or attempt to avoid, certain foods entirely. We thought about how these rules keep the eating disorder going and cause other eating disorder behaviors, like further negative body image thoughts, binge eating, and/or negative mood. We talked about how to address these rules and made Actions Plans to start breaking these rules this week.

Between-session Work

Remember to encourage patients to write the between-session work on their *Between-session Work Log* handout. The between-session work for Session 6 is:

- Continue work from previous sessions:
  - *Self-monitoring* – to be completed daily, in the moment.
  - *Regular Eating* – continue to prioritize regular eating using *Planning Ahead, Alternative Activities, Urge Tolerating*, and *Feelings of Fullness* to support this work.
  - Follow through with any Action Plans identified during the session.

- New work from Session 6:
  - Review *Resetting My Thinking About Dieting*.
  - Continue work on *My Avoided Foods List*.
  - Continue work on *My Food Rules*.
  - Review *Exposure*.
  - Follow *My Breaking Food Rules Plan*.

Higher Level of Care Adaptations: Modular Implementation

When this session is used modularly, the following adaptations are suggested.

It is important to note that for some patients at HLOCs, particularly those at inpatient and some residential settings, implementing Stage 3 interventions may not be practical. Due to the intensity of HLOC treatment and the significant amount of change that is made in a very short period, treatment can be overwhelming. At the highest levels of care, patients may benefit from focusing their efforts exclusively on making behavior changes related to regularly eating, improving the physical health consequences of their eating disorder (e.g., gaining weight, increasing fat intake), and eliminating other eating disorder symptoms (e.g., self-induced vomiting, binge eating, driven exercise, laxative or diuretic use). Patients who are maintaining a weight lower than their body needs/underfat may not be cognitively able to meaningfully engage with the material. As always, use your clinical judgment regarding who is appropriate for, and likely to benefit from, the group.

Exploring diet culture and dieting behaviors: This can be essential and implemented as described in all HLOCs. Depending on the nature of a patient's current level of dieting, and length of time in treatment, a patient's acknowledgment of the consequences of dieting as problematic may be difficult for some patients. If patients are new to an HLOC treatment they may be actively engaged in dieting, have had no consistent exposure to regular eating patterns, may have little motivation to change eating disorder symptoms, and may not yet recognize the disadvantages of dieting. As always, approach these situations with an open mind, knowing that the patient's perspective is important to their own experience. Allow other group members to share their perspectives. As the patient's treatment progresses, they may have new or altered perspectives.

Addressing diet-related rules: The first part of this intervention, identifying diet-related rules, can be implemented at all levels of care. Consider similar HLOC considerations to those mentioned in the diet culture/dieting behaviors section above. The second part of the intervention, breaking diet-related rules, will require planning and consideration of the availability of specific avoided foods at inpatient and residential levels of care. If this is not possible at these levels of care, then this piece of the intervention cannot be implemented. Instead, future planning (i.e., creating a list of current avoided foods to start introducing once the patient has access to such foods) could occur with the idea of implementation once the patient steps down to a lower level of care. For partial hospital and intensive outpatient programs, the intervention can be implemented as described.

Group Sesstion 6

Handout 6.1   *Between-session Work Self-review – Session 6*

BETWEEN-SESSION WORK SELF-REVIEW – SESSION 6

Skill/Goal	THIS IS GOING...			MY PLAN		
	Well	OK	Not Well	Make an Action Plan to address	Share with my support person for accountability	Praise myself for working hard on this!
Self-monitoring	☐	☐	☐	☐	☐	☐
Regular eating	☐	☐	☐	☐	☐	☐
Alternative activities	☐	☐	☐	☐	☐	☐
Urge tolerating	☐	☐	☐	☐	☐	☐
Addressing feelings of fullness	☐	☐	☐	☐	☐	☐
Items from the review last session that required additional focus. Write in and then rate (e.g., coming on time, completing between-session work).						
	☐	☐	☐	☐	☐	☐
	☐	☐	☐	☐	☐	☐
	☐	☐	☐	☐	☐	☐
	☐	☐	☐	☐	☐	☐
	☐	☐	☐	☐	☐	☐

Which skills are going well? Great work, keep practicing them! Which skills am I struggling to use and need to prioritize? Plan to take action this week – write an **Action Plan** to address these.

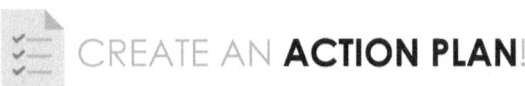 CREATE AN **ACTION PLAN**!

Handout 6.2 *Resetting My Thinking About Dieting*

RESETTING MY THINKING ABOUT DIETING

MY BELIEFS ON THE BENEFITS OF DIETING

☐	It helps me to maintain the weight/shape I want.
☐	I am good at it.
☐	It helps me to feel in control.
☐	It helps me to compensate for binges.
☐	It helps me to eat less in advance of large meals (e.g., during holidays, birthdays, parties, meals at restaurants).
☐	
☐	
☐	

HOW DIETING HARMS ME

☐	It puts pressure on me to binge eat.
☐	It keeps me preoccupied with thoughts about eating, and my weight and shape.
☐	It causes anxiety (about eating with others, breaking rules, gaining weight).
☐	
☐	
☐	

For more information about dieting, make sure to review the **Dieting handout**. If you don't have that handout, make sure to ask your group therapist for a copy.

Handout 6.3 *My Avoided Foods List*

MY AVOIDED FOODS LIST

Foods that I am **absolutely terrified** to eat:

Foods that I am scared to eat:

Foods that I might consider trying but would find it really hard to eat:

Handout 6.4   *My Food Rules*

MY FOOD RULES

Rules about what and what not to eat ("I will not eat fried foods."):

_____

_____

_____

_____

Rules about when to eat ("I will not eat until 12 noon."):

_____

_____

_____

_____

Rules about how much to eat ("I will only eat X amount of calories each day."):

_____

_____

_____

_____

Rules about how I eat ("I can only take tiny bites of food."):

_____

_____

_____

_____

Any other type of eating-related or food rules I try to follow:

_____

_____

_____

_____

How does trying to follow these food rules interfere with my life?

☐	It keeps me preoccupied with thoughts about eating, and my weight and shape.
☐	It causes anxiety (about eating out with others, breaking rules, gaining weight).
☐	I feel sad and guilty whenever I break a rule.
☐	
☐	

EXPOSURE

Exposure therapy is a highly effective treatment for anxiety and has been shown to be very effective in addressing fears for patients with eating disorders. Exposure means "facing your fears" and is the opposite of avoidance. When you avoid something that is scary, the fear gets stronger and the avoidance doesn't allow you to learn about your ability to cope. If you face your fears and learn that you can tolerate your fears, then you become more able to manage similar situations in the future. Exposureis applied throughout Group CBT-E as a part of particular interventions, such as facing fears about regular eating, breaking diet-related rules, and reducing body avoidance.

HOW EXPOSURE WORKS

Consider an example:

Steps	Example	Learning
Step 1: Learning to be afraid of something	Mary always used to love ice cream until she started to focus on her weight and shape. At a time when she was feeling particularly bad about her body, she read a social media post about the number of calories in ice cream. She feels very anxious when faced with an opportunity to have ice cream, or even when thinking about ice cream, and believes her shape and weight will change as a result of eating ice cream and will cause her to binge. Her avoidance has kept this fear strong as she has stopped having ice cream completely and therefore has not tried to cope with what it would be like to have ice cream again.	Ice cream= fear = avoidance
Step 2: The problem of fear	Thinking about having ice cream makes Mary feel afraid. She avoids situations where she could be around ice cream at all or could be asked if she wants ice cream. Eventually she starts to avoid eating all desserts. Mary has missed many social opportunities because of this and craves ice cream and birthday cake.	Desserts = fear = avoidance
Step 3: Exposure	As part of her treatment, Mary decides to gradually start eating desserts in a variety of different situations. She does not notice a change with her shape and weight – which she measures by if her clothes are still fitting, which they are. She learns that she can tolerate the distress following eating ice cream and challenge the belief that her weight has changed by reminding herself that weight cannot change so rapidly. She uses urge tolerating until the fear passes. She also learns that she can eat ice cream and desserts without it triggering a binge. By finding out that her fears do not become reality, and that she can tolerate the distress associated with challenging her fears, she starts to feel safer eating ice cream and eventually this generalizes to other avoided foods, including desserts. The more she challenges herself, the more her **anxiety is reduced**. She even notices some other benefits, like eating foods that taste good (i.e., desserts) and being able to eat desserts socially with friends.	Desserts = fear = exposure Long-term learning: Desserts = less fear

Handout 6.6   *My Breaking Food Rules Plan*

MY BREAKING FOOD RULES PLAN

This week I will reintroduce the following avoided food(s) (plan 1–2 foods):

_____

_____

And/or break the following food rule(s) (plan 1–2 rules):

_____

_____

I will eat the above food(s) **3** times before the next group:

    Date and time 1: _____

    Date and time 2: _____

    Date and time 3: _____

I will break the above food rule(s) **3** times before the next group:

    Date and time 1: _____

    Date and time 2: _____

    Date and time 3: _____

After eating the food/breaking the rule, I will use either/both:

    ☐ Distraction activities (specify): _____

    _____

    ☐ Urge tolerating (specify): _____

    _____

Remember:

- Stick to your plan (help yourself by setting a phone alarm or other notification).
- If the day is too difficult or stressful, replan to have your avoided food on another day.
- Be sure to plan in distraction activities and/or urge tolerating and use them!
- The goal is to move toward flexible eating. Flexible eating allows you to choose the foods that you prefer, based on taste and enjoyment, and not based on calories or the impact they will have on your shape and weight.

Chapter 12

Group Session 7

The Over-evaluation of Shape and Weight and Its Consequences

Overview

For many patients, the ability to control their body shape and weight is a primary way they assess and judge their self-worth. As described in Chapter 2, this phenomenon is referred to as the over-evaluation of shape, weight, and their control. This *over-evaluation of shape and weight* is the core psychopathology that maintains the eating disorder (i.e., keeps the eating disorder going). Implementing strategies to reduce this over-evaluation is a critical piece of Group CBT-E. It takes time to address the over-evaluation and therefore, the next five sessions of Group CBT-E are devoted to supporting patients in making these changes:

Session 7: The Over-evaluation of Shape and Weight and its Consequences
Session 8: Body Shape and Weight Checking I – Education, Evaluation, and Behavior Change
Session 9: Body Shape and Weight Checking II – Reflection Checking, Body Comparisons, and Social Media Body Checking
Session 10: Body Shape and Weight Avoidance
Session 11: Stage 3 Check-in and Body Dissatisfaction Spikes

> **Over-evaluation of shape and weight**: Judging self-worth on body shape and weight includes judgments based on appearance, muscularity, body composition, and the ability to control these characteristics, often to the minimization or exclusion of other values.

The current session, Session 7, has three main aims:

1. To identify the over-evaluation of shape and weight.
2. To consider the consequences of the over-evaluation of shape and weight.
3. To develop a strategy to begin to reduce the over-evaluation of shape and weight.

DOI: 10.4324/9781003450849-16

Therapist Preparation

☐ Review this chapter in advance.

☐ Review accompanying handouts and have copies available for patients.

☐ At the end of this session, specific between-session work needed for Session 8 (monitoring body shape and weight checking) is described. Be sure to have familiarity with this content to adequately explain the between-session work.

Handouts

- Standard weekly Handouts
  - *1.3 Self-monitoring*
  - *1.6 Between-session Work Log*
  - *7.1 Between-session Work Self-review – Session 7*

- Session-Specific Handouts
  - *7.2 Self-evaluation*
  - *7.3 Over-evaluation of Shape and Weight – Extended Formulation*
  - *7.4 Other Areas of Life*
  - *7.5 Body Shape and Weight Checking Self-monitoring*
  - *7.6 Body Shape and Weight Checking Self-monitoring Example*

Group Session Agenda

1. Setting the agenda and orienting to the session (2 minutes)
2. Between-session work self-review (5 minutes)
3. Identifying the over-evaluation of shape and weight and its consequences (15 minutes)
4. Assessing the impacts of the over-evaluation of shape and weight (15 minutes)
5. Identifying a strategy for addressing the over-evaluation of shape and weight (15 minutes)
6. Preparation for the next session, Session 8 (5 minutes)
7. Group wrap-up (3 minutes)

1. Setting the Agenda and Orienting to the Session

Begin with a positive, encouraging welcome. Share that this is Session 7, Stage 3, with 7 sessions remaining. Clearly list the session agenda.

2. Between-session Work Self-review

Handout: *Between-session Work Self-review – Session 7*

Ask patients to complete their *Between-session Work Self-review – Session 7* handout. This review continues to check in on the Stage 1 elements and for the first time, Stage 3 interventions appear (i.e., dieting behaviors and diet-related rules). Ask the group to review their ongoing progress with items like self-monitoring and regular eating and pay special attention to how they are progressing with breaking food rules. Breaking food rules can be scary and difficult. Praise any attempts at breaking rules or eating avoided foods. If breaking rules caused eating disorder behaviors (e.g., restricting, binge eating), support the patient to make Action Plans to address this (e.g., planning in a distraction activity after breaking a rule). Also, ask patients to identify new foods to try and rules to break that they will plan for this week. As you have been, praise patients for the things that are going well, identify barriers and how to address such obstacles, and build on the existing interventions by identifying increasingly more challenging ways to address eating disorder symptoms. At the end of the review, encourage patients to create updated Action Plans to reflect goals for the week, and include these on their *Between-session Work Log*.

3. Identifying the Over-evaluation of Shape and Weight and Its Consequences

Handout: *Self-evaluation*

The start of this session focuses on identifying all the ways in which patients evaluate themselves (i.e., how they judge their self-worth). Identifying the ways in which patients evaluate themselves can be an abstract and difficult concept. To help patients with this process, lead the group in an engaging exercise to visualize their self-evaluation, by drawing a self-evaluation pie chart.

To help explain this concept, providing an example can be helpful. There are four parts to this example: 1) creating a list of how a fictional person, Ray, judges themselves; 2) ranking the items on Ray's list in order of importance; 3) drawing out Ray's pie chart with slices to indicate percentage of evaluation devoted to each slice; and 4) discussing impressions about Ray's self-evaluation pie chart.

Today we will be focusing on ways in which you evaluate yourself, or judge your self-worth. This can be challenging to identify, so to help, let's start by thinking about someone else first, using an example. Ray is a made-up person who does not have an eating disorder. They are an elementary school teacher who performs with an improv group on the weekend, enjoys playing basketball, and makes content for their social media channel. Fashion is important to Ray, especially their sneaker choice and how muscular they think their shape is. Ray has one sister whom they are very close to. Based on this brief vignette, what are the ways you imagine that Ray might evaluate their self-worth? [List the group's ideas on a whiteboard. See Table 12.1.] *I'll now share the order of importance Ray places on each of these items.* [Numbers listed on Table 12.1 are Ray's order of importance.]

Table 12.1 Sample Whiteboard – Ray's Self-evaluation List and Ratings

1	How well I think I am doing as a teacher
5	Relationship with my sister
3	How well I do at improv
4	How well I play basketball
2	Number of new subscribers, likes, or positive comments on my channels
6	How I look – outfits, sneakers, my muscle tone

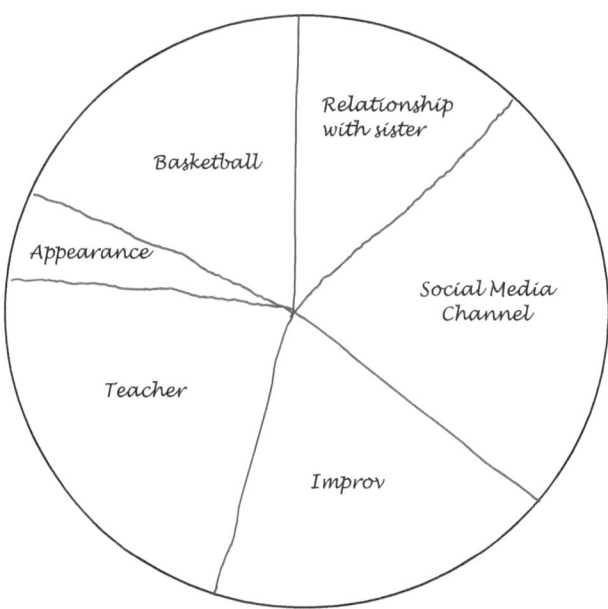

Figure 12.1 Ray's pie chart.

Now, I'd like to share with you how Ray's list looks if we put it into a pie chart. [Draw out Figure 12.1.] *Any overall impressions or thoughts looking at this pie chart? On the chart, you can see 6 slices with the most important being largest (social media channel and being a teacher) and the least important being smallest (appearance).*

After providing the example, each patient will create their own pie chart using the *Self-evaluation* handout. Encourage the group to follow the steps closely on the handout while also reviewing the creation of the pie chart together in the session.

Step 1: Create the list

Ask patients to think of the ways they judge/ evaluate their self-worth. Encourage them to share ideas aloud and to record them on the handout. Sharing areas together is often helpful in generating items that may have been missed or forgotten. Use the example list in Table 12.2 to guide patients if they struggle to come up with items. Most patients will likely have weight, shape, body, and/or appearance included on their list. If

> **Therapist Insight**
>
> Avoid perfection – Some patients can feel that they need to include every single way they judge themselves. Encourage patients to aim to list the main areas and that it is OK to not have every last item. The list can always be updated.

they do not include these, be sure to ask them if they believe these are areas they use to judge themselves. For some patients, these are such obvious items that they do not think to include them.

Table 12.2 Examples of Ways that Patients May Evaluate their Self-worth

How satisfied they are with their body, appearance, shape, or weight	How well they exercise (e.g., following through with an established exercise schedule, exercising at a particular speed or rate)
How they see themselves in a particular role (e.g., parent, partner, child, friend, pet owner)	How well they are performing at work (e.g., praise, reviews, promotions)
How well they are performing at school (e.g., grades, teacher feedback)	How well they perform a certain hobby-related skill (e.g., sports, art)
How spiritually connected they are (e.g., engaging in spiritual rituals and practices)	How knowledgeable they are about a particular interest (e.g., politics, gardening)

Step 2: Rank the items

After creating their individual lists on the *Self-evaluation* handout, ask patients to rank their items in order of importance just as was shown in Ray's example.

Step 3: Create the pie chart

Once patients have identified areas in which they evaluate their self-worth and ranked them, the next step is for them to draw out their pie chart. Ask the patients to use the circle on the *Self-evaluation* handout as a pie chart to divide up how much emphasis they place in each area they have listed. See Figure 12.2 of an example of a sample patient (Ada)'s pie chart.

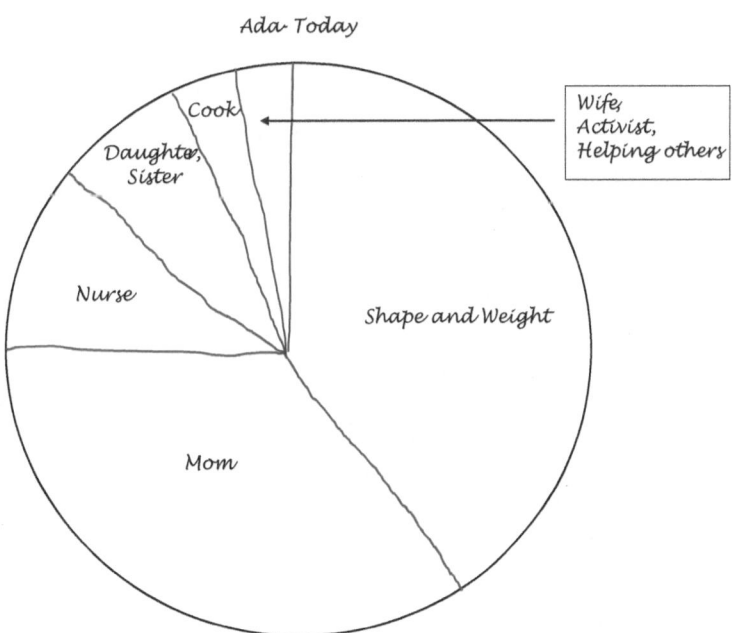

Figure 12.2 Ada's pie chart – Today.

Now we are going to use the circle on your Self-evaluation handout and create your pie chart. Look at your list and estimate how much importance you place on each item as a way to evaluate yourself. This is not meant be exact, so just do the best you can at estimating how much emphasis you put in each area, knowing that you are limited to fit everything into the circle.

Once these individual pie charts are complete, ask patients to estimate what the percentage is of all pie pieces that relate to their shape, weight, and appearance.

What percentage of your pie chart do you estimate is focused on your shape and weight, including anything related to appearance, body, driven exercise, dieting, etc.? Take your best guess as to what that amount is and I am going to go around to collect these numbers, if you feel comfortable sharing. Who would like to start?

Therapist Insight

Judging oneself based on exercise performance or amount is often related to shape and weight for patients. This should be included in the over-evaluation of shape and weight pie piece in these instances.

Going around the group, ask each patient to provide their individual estimation. Once all percentages have been collected, you will share an estimate of the average of all group member percentages and start to create a group pie chart using a whiteboard.

So roughly for our group, the average focus on shape and weight is about ___% [insert estimated amount here]. I am going to create a group pie chart on the whiteboard. Now I want to hear from everyone, what else did you have on your pie chart? What other ways, apart from shape, weight, appearance, exercise, do you evaluate yourself? Just say them aloud and I will include them here on the whiteboard.

Create this group pie chart on a whiteboard (see Figure 12.3). As you can see in the sample, and likely will experience in the session, a large section of the pie chart is taken up by shape and weight, while all of the other areas are squished into the rest of the chart. This is an observation that will be discussed later in the session.

4. Assessing the Impact of the Over-evaluation of Shape and Weight

Next, identify observations and concerns about what the pie chart reveals about self-worth.
   Once the group pie chart visual is completed, start a group discussion to assess patients' reactions and observations related to the group pie chart and their own.

I have illustrated our group self-evaluation. I want to take some time to discuss thoughts, feelings, and reactions you are having to seeing this visual and your own individualized pie chart. Please use your Self-evaluation handout to list observations/concerns as we discuss. What do you notice?

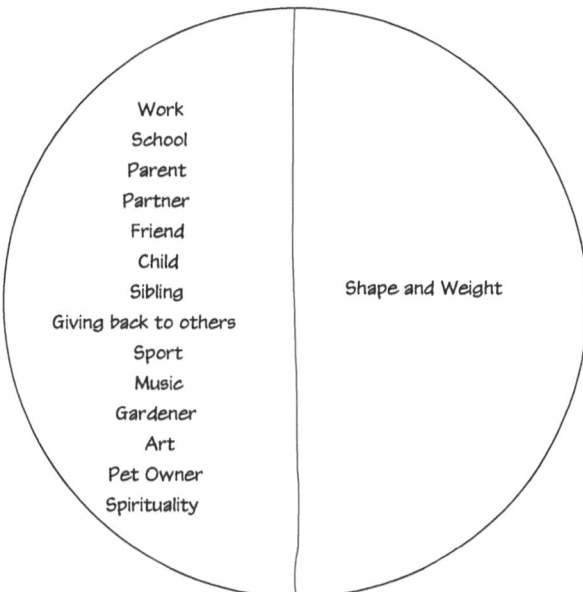

Figure 12.3 Sample whiteboard – Group pie chart.

Depending on patient engagement, typically, the following patient reactions, and discussions, will ensue. If group members are not naturally engaging in all these discussion points, be sure to introduce them yourself. Share your own observations about patterns or concerns that you notice related to the group pie chart. Some sample reactions and responses, adapted from Fairburn (2008), that are important to discuss are:

- *This is depressing. I can't believe that this is my life*. Oftentimes, this exercise can induce negative emotions for patients. In

> **Social Media Alert**
>
> When engaging the group in a discussion reflecting on their responses to their pie charts, ask how social media behaviors impact their self-evaluation. Is their self-judgment informed by how many people like a post where their body is on display? Or perhaps they mostly look at content about dieting and exercise and this keeps them thinking that shape and weight is the most important part of oneself?

many cases, these emotions are sparked from the realization that the way that they are judging themselves is primarily on aspects of life that they do not actually highly value based on their morals (e.g., appearance, body weight). This leads to two important conversational topics:

1. **Values**. *Does this pie chart represent your value system? When you look back at life when you are in old age, is this what you want to look back on?*
2. **Motivation**. Many patients find creating the pie chart (and especially the future-focused pie chart described below) highly motivating. Encourage patients to explore with the group what they find motivating about viewing their pie chart. A common reflection is, "Seeing my life like this makes me really want to be free from this illness." Ask patients to keep track of this motivational insight by writing it on their *Self-evaluation*

handout, sharing their pie charts after the session with a support person, and/or posting their pie charts (particularly the future pie chart which is introduced next) somewhere in their home.

- *All the things that I actually care about are squished into a very small pie piece without much room.* Because there is such a large emphasis placed on one area, other aspects of life become limited, as there is only so much time and energy that one has available. Inevitably, having such a large focus on shape and weight leads to minimization of other areas of life. At times, these are areas of life that were previously (pre-eating disorder) enjoyable to the patient. Therapists should engage the group in a discussion about how they notice this impacting them on a daily basis.

> *It is such a good point that because the shape and weight piece is so large, you have minimal room for everything else in life. I notice this very clearly on our group pie chart. There are so many aspects of life that are squished into one pie piece. I wonder how that impacts your life day to day? I also wonder what areas of life are missing because there isn't room to fit them in? Does anyone have in mind something that didn't make it onto their pie chart that they wish had?*

- *The shape/weight piece is very big.* Having any one piece of self-evaluation significantly dominate can be risky, especially if things aren't going well in that area. The risk lies in overly relying on that one area of life without investing in others, leading to several concerns:
  - One is left with a significant gap in how to define/judge/evaluate oneself. Here it can be useful to include a non-shape and weight example:

> *I wonder if it might be helpful for me to provide an example here of how someone can be impacted when they rely so heavily on evaluating themselves in one area. Consider Che. Che is an executive at a technology company. For their pie chart, there is a dominant slice (70%) of the pie that focuses on work and the rest of their evaluation (e.g., spirituality, partner, friend, musician, sibling, reader) is squeezed into the remaining 30%. What will happen when Che receives negative feedback at work? Is let go because of restructuring? Retires one day? Their "work" pie chart slice will significantly decrease and they will be left with a giant gap to fill. What impact will this have on*

Therapist Insight

This discussion is usually fairly engaging as it is rare to work with a patient who believes that focusing so much on appearance aligns well with their wider value system. Oftentimes, patients find this conversation to be quite obvious in nature and it is not uncommon to hear, "OF COURSE this is not how I want my life to be." Working together as a group can be helpful to decrease shame related to the discrepancy between current self-evaluation and value system.

Che when there is such a big gap in their pie chart? They may feel empty or left without purpose and low in mood. Just like for over-evaluation of shape and weight, Che's over-evaluation of work performance impacts their life significantly. For example, they find that this causes poorer relationships with others; increased anxiety and stress; lack of sleep; and minimal ability to engage with hobbies and other life interests. Even evaluating work performance, a fairly customary/acceptable self-evaluation measure, when done to the extreme, can lead to dysfunction. Do these consequences sound familiar to anyone?

- *If one area of life had to dominate self-evaluation, having that be shape/weight is concerning since this is an aspect of life that is not possible to fully control.* As discussed in Session 6, much of our body size is predetermined by genetics. For many individuals, attempting to influence body size is typically ineffective in the long term, and/or may require engaging in eating disorder behaviors.
- *For individuals with eating disorders, the over-evaluation of shape and weight tends to be a negative evaluation (e.g., "I hate my body," "My shape is gross").* This negative evaluation is maintained by numerous body shape and weight checking behaviors, and avoidance behaviors. These behaviors will be the focus of Sessions 8–10.

It is important to summarize these impressions from the group and also check that all members agree, at least to some extent, that this evaluation is faulty/harmful and something they would like to change.

Reflecting back on this important discussion, it sounds like in drawing out your self-evaluation pie chart, you've noticed that the slices related to body shape, weight, and appearance are large. You've shared that you do not like the way in which areas of life are imbalanced; find this imbalance depressing; believe that it does not align with your values; notice the imbalance squishes out other areas of life that are important; and recognize this pattern can lead to negative feelings about yourself. Does this give some motivation to want to change how you judge yourself?

5. Identifying a Strategy to Address the Over-evaluation of Shape and Weight

Handout: *Over-evaluation of Shape and Weight Extended Formulation*

Next, create a second pie chart to reflect how patients would like their self-evaluation to be in one year.

Ask the group to use the second circle on the *Self-evaluation* handout to create a pie chart reflecting what they would like their self-evaluation to be one year from now. See

Therapist Insight

Sometimes patients will report that they evaluate themselves negatively in all areas identified. Oftentimes in these situations, it is common to hear that a patient's negative view of their body impacts how they see

Figure 12.4 for an example of the sample patient (Ada)'s pie chart one year from now.

I'd like everyone to create a second pie chart reflecting how you would like your self-evaluation to be a year from now. When creating this, consider adding aspects of life that used to be a part of how you judged your self-worth, prior to your eating disorder, that are missing now. Think about areas of life that you are curious about (i.e., activities you have seen others engage in) and ways to evaluate yourself based on that. Think about how much emphasis you are placing on particular areas and how you would like that to look different. Make sure to continue to have shape and weight included on your pie chart as it would be unrealistic to think that you would have none of your self-worth impacted by this. Most people, including those without eating disorders, place some importance on shape, weight, and/or appearance to evaluate themselves.

the rest of life (e.g., "I am unhappy with my relationships but can't start dating because I hate the way I look."). Other times, we hear patients share that evaluating themselves based on shape and weight distracts them from feeling like they don't measure up in other areas of life (e.g., "In some ways, it is easier to try to feel good about how I look than to face how terrible I feel about who I am when I am around others – which feels impossible to work on."). This often highlights the vicious cycle between self-esteem and body image. In these instances, it can be useful to ask patients to consider how this overall perspective about themselves is impacting them, if they may be missing opportunities for other ways to evaluate themselves that they feel good or neutral about, or if they may be evaluating themselves through a particularly harsh, unreasonable lens. Group support can be particularly helpful during these conversations.

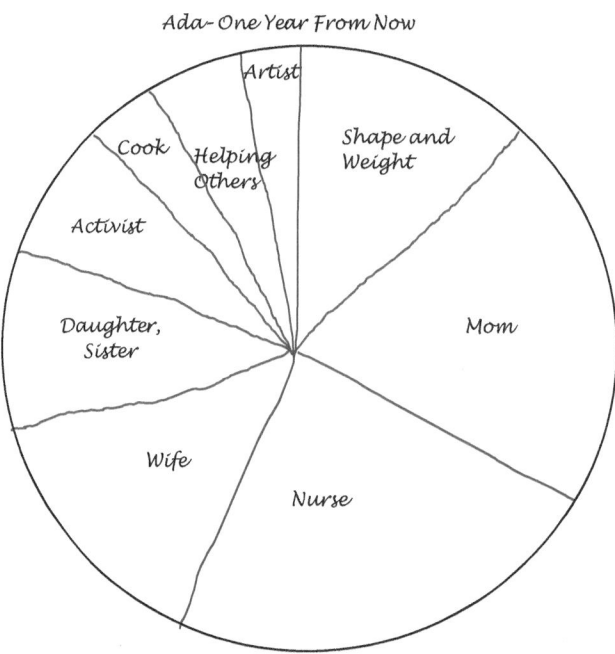

Figure 12.4 Ada's pie chart – One year from now.

After patients have completed a new pie chart highlighting how they would like their self-evaluation to be in one year, the final component of this session is to outline the strategy to reduce the difference between patients' current pie charts and their future pie charts. There are two ways of doing this:

1. Actively *decrease* the over-focus on shape and weight by reducing or stopping the behaviors that keep these slices of the pie chart so large.
2. Actively *increase* focus on, and engagement with, other aspects of life.

> *It is great to think about how you want to see yourself in a year, with less focus on your shape and weight. Now we have to think about how to get there. There are two ways to do this: 1) Shrinking down/reducing the size of the shape and weight pie piece to decrease your focus on evaluating yourselves in this area. This is achieved by decreasing the behaviors and thoughts that keep it so large. 2) Increasing the size of the rest of the pie pieces, as these are areas of life that have been more likely disregarded, or less focused on, because of your focus on shape and weight.*

Decreasing Over-focus on Shape and Weight

To decrease the size of the slices, the behaviors that maintain them need to be stopped or reduced. Figure 12.5 and the *Over-evaluation of Shape and Weight Extended Formulation* handout detail the behaviors and cognitions that are a result of the over-evaluation of shape and weight, as well as how these behaviors and thoughts ultimately maintain this over-evaluation. Additionally, these behaviors and cognitions maintain one another (e.g., shape/weight checking can lead to body dissatisfaction spikes which can cause dieting behaviors,

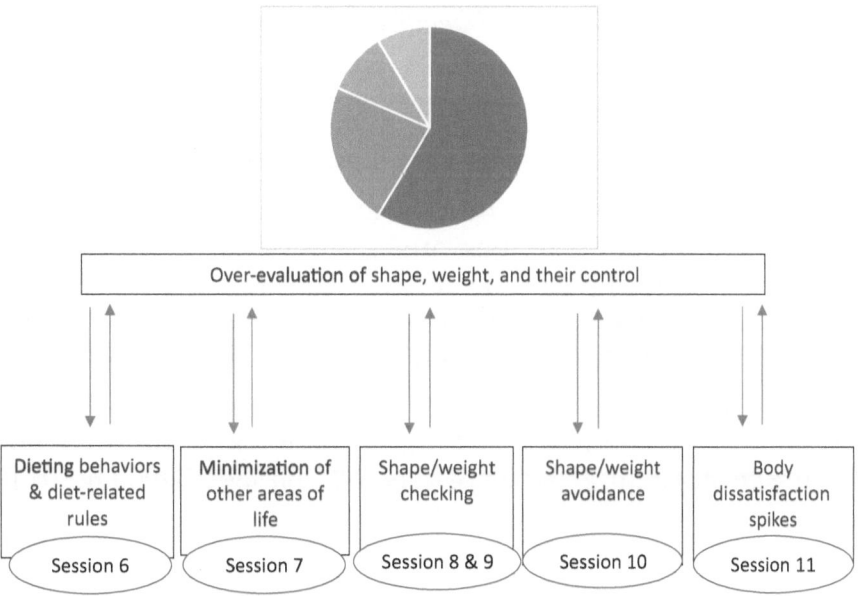

Figure 12.5 Over-evaluation of shape and weight extended formulation.

which can lead back to shape/weight checking). Encourage patients to view the extended formulation as a blueprint or map showing what will be addressed in treatment to reduce the over-evaluation.

> *Your Over-evaluation of Shape and Weight Extended Formulation handout shows the many behaviors and thoughts that maintain, and are maintained by, the over-evaluation, including: dieting behaviors and diet-related rules (which we talked about last session); shape/weight checking and avoidance; and body dissatisfaction spikes. We want to work together to stop or reduce all of the behaviors that keep this aspect of the eating disorder going. Over the next few sessions, we will target each of these behaviors and provide strategies for tackling them. We already started to consider decreasing dieting behaviors and diet-related rules last session. For now, let's focus on the box labeled "minimization of other areas of life" and think about how to increase your focus on other aspects of life.*

Increasing Focus and Engagement With Other Areas of Life

Handout: *Other Areas of Life*

To increase or add areas of life that have been pushed out by the eating disorder, patients will complete the steps on the *Other Areas of Life* handout.

> *Next, let's look at the Other Areas of Life handout. To decrease the size of the shape and weight pie piece, we need to start increasing the importance of, and your engagement with, other areas of life. Increasing these slices, and adding new ones, will help to decrease the focus on some of the eating disordered behaviors and thoughts. Create a list of other areas of life that you would like to start focusing on. These may be activities that you used to enjoy that the eating disorder pushed out, they may be activities that are new to you, or may be areas of life that are currently neglected because of your focus on shape and weight. Let's brainstorm a list of ideas together.*

While patients complete the *Other Areas of Life* handout, encourage them to share their ideas aloud. Oftentimes, this will spark an idea-generating process between group members, and it allows group members to support one another, which is helpful for group cohesion.

After they have created a list of activities, or areas to focus on, ask patients to share their goals related to activities for the coming week. Invite the rest of the group to provide encouragement and praise when patients share the activities they want to work on. For some patients coming up with these ideas may be very difficult. They may not know what to try or add as the eating disorder has been dominant for a long time. Others may feel scared or overwhelmed to try to add new things. These reactions are understandable and make sense. Be sure to normalize this experience. If patients struggle to identify how to start working on their goals, the examples in Table 12.3, and ideas from others in the group, can be helpful.

Table 12.3 Examples of Initial Steps for Working on Goals to Increase Focus and Engagement in Other Areas of Life

Goal	Initial steps for working toward this goal
Increasing social focus	• Text one new friend. • Call one old friend. • Make one social plan this week.
Increasing hobbies/ interests focus (for a patient who struggles to identify hobbies/ interests)	• Make a list this week of all of the interests and hobbies that you have had in the past and that you have been curious about. • Survey others about what interests they have. • Do a quick internet search of lists of hobby ideas and see if any are interesting to you. Rank items on the list based on what sounds most reasonable to start pursuing. Choose the top item on the list and identify the first step in working on this goal.
Increasing work focus	• Create a personal list of strengths and weaknesses in your occupation. • Schedule a meeting with your boss to discuss how to get more involved and identify at least one way to build on strengths and improve weaknesses.
Increasing focus on self-care	• Take a few minutes each day to do a guided meditation. • Buy a scented candle or new body lotion.

For between-session work, ask patients to record on their self-monitoring forms when they have worked on these goals and any barriers that occurred.

6. Preparation for Session 8: Body Shape and Weight Checking

Handouts: *Body Shape and Weight Checking Self-monitoring, Body Shape and Weight Checking Self-monitoring Example*

Before the end of group, let patients know that there will be an additional item of between-session work that needs to be completed prior to the next group: the *Body Shape and Weight Checking Self-monitoring* handout. It is important to look at this handout and the *Body Shape and Weight Checking Self-monitoring Example* handout together and review the following steps for monitoring:

• Begin by defining "body checking" as shape and weight checking and provide some examples listed on the *Body Shape and Weight Checking Self-monitoring* handout. Be sure to introduce the purpose behind addressing body checking.

As you can see on the Over-evaluation of Shape and Weight – Extended Formulation handout, body checking is a behavior that contributes to, and maintains, the over-evaluation of shape and weight. Almost everyone, with or without an eating disorder, checks and compares their body/appearance in some way or another but it is less extreme than the body checking someone with an eating disorder does. For individuals with eating disorders, this checking tends to be frequent and can negatively impact mood and functioning. Oftentimes, body checking becomes a habit. Some people experience both body checking and body avoidance (i.e., behaviors to avoid the discomfort of seeing, or having others see, your body, for example not looking in a mirror). For now, I will ask you to monitor body checking. Later on, we will talk about body avoidance.

- Ask the patients to complete the *Body Shape and Weight Checking Self-monitoring* handouts (instead of their typical self-monitoring forms) over two days in the upcoming week. The days should be chosen based on obtaining data in two different environments (e.g., school/work, home) or schedules (e.g., weekday, weekend).

- Ask the patients to include every time they engage in body checking and complete information in the corresponding columns (time taken, type of body checking, context, etc.).

- Review with the patients the list of body checking examples included on the handout and be sure to be clear that patients may have other body checking behaviors that are not listed.

- Let patients know that they may not be aware of their checking or may not recognize the checking until after it has started. At other times, they may be very aware of their body checking behaviors.

- Stress the importance of completing the monitoring prior to the next group as the main content of the group is guided by the information gathered on these sheets.

- *Most importantly*: Share with patients that completing this handout may cause a certain amount of distress. It is not uncommon for patients to report becoming upset with heightened awareness of the checking they engage in. This distress will pass and the information gathered is vital to reducing checking. Advise patients that they should stop recording if they become overly distressed or dysregulated.

7. Group Wrap-up

Session Summary

Today is our first session focusing on body image. We thought about how you judge yourself and how shape and weight are a significant part of your evaluation. We talked about the consequences of this for you and discovered that many consequences are detrimental. We identified a plan for how to address the over-evaluation of shape and weight. This plan includes both decreasing focus on shape and weight by making behavior changes (which we will actively start working on next session) and increasing the focus and engagement with other areas of life. Everyone has identified one or two new activities to work on this week related to increasing this focus and engagement. Finally, we talked about body checking self-monitoring and set you up to start that over two days this week.

Between-session Work

Remember to encourage patients to write the between-session work on their *Between-session Work Log* handout. The between-session work for Session 7 is:

- Continue work from previous sessions:
  - *Self-monitoring* – to be completed daily, in the moment.
  - *Regular Eating* – continue to prioritize regular eating using *Planning Ahead, Alternative Activities, Urge Tolerating*, and *Feelings of Fullness* to support this work.
  - *My Breaking Food Rules Plan* – continue to plan in avoided foods and break dietary rules.
  - Follow through with any Action Plans identified during the session.
- New work from Session 7:
  - *Self-evaluation* – share with your support person and/or post the future version in your home for motivation.
  - *Other Areas of Life* – take the first steps in adding one or two new/expanded areas over the coming week and add this to your self-monitoring form.
  - *Body Shape and Weight Checking Self-monitoring* – record your body checking on two days.

Higher Level of Care Adaptations: Modular Implementation

When this session is used modularly, the following adaptations are suggested.

Identifying the over-evaluation of shape and weight and its consequences: All elements of this session can be implemented at HLOCs as described. With patients who are significantly underweight, make sure to add in underweight/underfat as an additional – and very powerful – factor that maintains the over-evaluation of shape and weight to the extended formulation. Due to the severity of a patient's disorder in HLOCs, as well as the significant focus on the eating disorder while in an intensive treatment, you may see that the focus of self-evaluation placed on shape and weight is quite significant (i.e., for some patients, it can be close to the entire pie chart). It can be a useful tool to have patients recomplete this pie chart at different time points during their HLOC treatment to show progress and change as they progress through these intensive programs. At times, seeing this change can be motivating and hopeful for patients.

Increasing focus and engagement with other areas of life: When increasing focus and engagement with other areas of life with patients at inpatient or residential settings, focusing on the future after discharge can be helpful since adding in new areas can be difficult, depending on the settings. For these patients who are away from their home environment, find creative opportunities to take initial steps toward addressing minimization of others areas of life. Here are some examples of ways to work on other areas of life when in these more restricted settings:

- *Role as a friend*: Write a letter to, create a piece of artwork for, or make a phone call to a friend; create a hierarchy of social goals to work on once discharged; work on displaying empathy, kindness, and assertiveness to peers in treatment; and/or ask peers ways that they are familiar with how to make new friends in their communities.
- *Hobby of reading*: Ask a support person to bring in a book or borrow a book from the unit library; start reading while in treatment each day if energy allows; make a list of books that peers in treatment recommend; and/or make a list of potential book clubs or libraries to join once discharged.
- *Role as an employee*: Make a list of areas of work that are going well and areas for improvement, and identify Action Plans for each; engage with peers regarding work challenges to solicit their support; start to prioritize a regular schedule of eating and begin to plan when lunch breaks will occur at work; and/or engage a support person during visiting hours to talk through plans related to increasing focus in this area.

Preparation for Session 8 – Body shape and weight checking: In settings where the majority of patients will return the next session, implement as described. If there is likely to be a lot of patient turnover, consider modifying this preparatory work and prepare to review material in the subsequent session with the new patients. If at a residential or inpatient level of care, consider asking patients to engage in body checking monitoring for one day only (as opposed to two days), as this typically offers enough information for patients that are usually quite preoccupied with their bodies.

Group Sesstion 7

Handout 7.1   *Between-session Work Self-review – Session 7*

BETWEEN-SESSION WORK SELF-REVIEW – SESSION 7

Skill/Goal	THIS IS GOING...			MY PLAN		
	Well	OK	Not Well	Make an Action Plan to address	Share with my support person for accountability	Praise myself for working hard on this!
Self-monitoring	☐	☐	☐	☐	☐	☐
Regular eating	☐	☐	☐	☐	☐	☐
Alternative activities	☐	☐	☐	☐	☐	☐
Urge tolerating	☐	☐	☐	☐	☐	☐
Addressing feelings of fullness	☐	☐	☐	☐	☐	☐
Challenging diet-related rules	☐	☐	☐	☐	☐	☐
Eating avoided foods	☐	☐	☐	☐	☐	☐
Additional Items						
	☐	☐	☐	☐	☐	☐
	☐	☐	☐	☐	☐	☐

Which skills are going well? Great work, keep practicing them! Which skills am I struggling to use and need to prioritize? Plan to take action this week – write an **Action Plan** to address these.

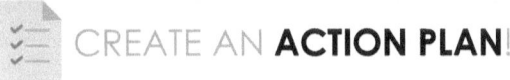

CREATE AN **ACTION PLAN**!

Handout 7.2   *Self-evaluation*

SELF-EVALUATION

Over-evaluation of shape and weight is the over-focus/over-emphasis on shape, weight, and/or your ability to control shape/weight as a means to judge your self-worth. Your group therapist will guide you through an activity to better understand how you tend to evaluate yourself, any thoughts/concerns related to your self-evaluation, and how you would like to evaluate yourself in the future.

Step 1: Create the list: List all of the ways in which you evaluate or judge yourself.

Rank	Item	Rank	Item

Step 2: Rank the items in order of importance to you.

Step 3: Create the pie chart: Reflect how much focus you put in each area.

SELF-EVALUATION

List observations/concerns that you have about your pie chart and what it reveals about self-worth.

Use this circle to create a pie chart to represent what you would like your self-evaluation to be one year from now.

This activity gets me motivated! To help stay on track, I will remember:

____

Handout 7.3   *Over-evaluation of Shape and Weight – Extended Formulation*

OVER-EVALUATION OF SHAPE & WEIGHT
– EXTENDED FORMULATION

The over-evaluation of shape and weight makes it likely that an individual will engage in a number of eating disorder behaviors. And engaging in eating disorder behaviors will strengthen the over-evaluation (see image below). This image shows which behaviors will be targeted, and when, in Group CBT-E. By making changes to these behaviors, we can reduce the importance of the over-evaluation and move more toward recovery goals.

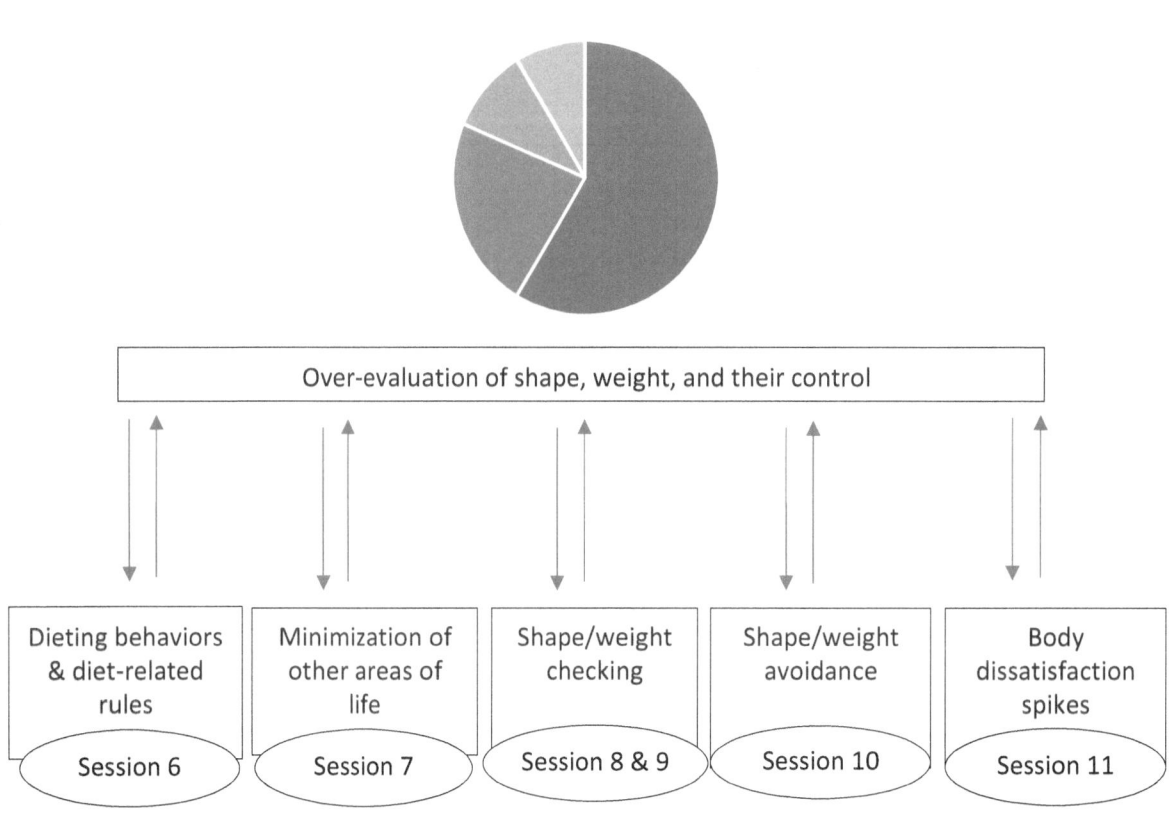

OTHER AREAS OF LIFE

To decrease the amount of focus placed on your shape, weight, and their control, it is very helpful to start engaging in other areas of life that have been minimized by the eating disorder. These are the smaller slices on your pie chart. Spending more time and focus in these areas, and adding new areas, will help these areas to become more important to how you evaluate yourself as a person and reduce the amount of time focused on shape and weight.

Step #1: Make a list of **new** activities that you would like to become involved in and/or **current** activities that you would like to have more focus on.

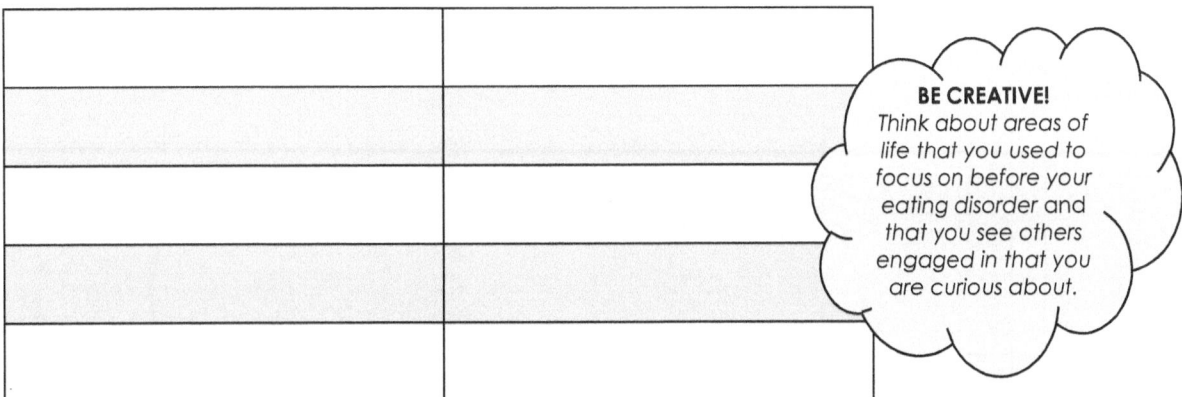

BE CREATIVE!
Think about areas of life that you used to focus on before your eating disorder and that you see others engaged in that you are curious about.

Step #2: Make a plan to try **1–2** of these activities starting this coming week and continuing throughout the rest of group!

Activity	First step for this week	Potential Barriers: Make a plan for these

Step #3: Add this activity to your self-monitoring forms, and any difficulty following through with your plans.

Handout 7.5 *Body Shape and Weight Checking Self-monitoring*

Name: _____   Date: _____   Day of the Week: _____

BODY SHAPE AND WEIGHT CHECKING SELF-MONITORING

Time	Food and Drink	Place	*	v/l/d	e	Body Checking Behaviors & Time Taken	Place	Context and comments

Body Checking Examples: Reflection checking (mirror, selfies, video in virtual meetings); pinching/touching body; weighing; assessing tightness of clothes/accessories; looking down at body; comparing to others; checking photographs; measuring body; using social media to check my body

Handout 7.6 *Body Shape and Wight Checking Self-monitoring Example*

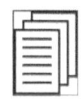

BODY SHAPE AND WEIGHT CHECKING SELF-MONITORING EXAMPLE

Name: Emily Date: 08/27 Day of the Week: Tuesday

Time	Food and Drink	Place	*	v/l/d	e	Body Checking Behaviors & Time Taken	Place	Context and comments
6:45 AM						Checking my face in the mirror while brushing teeth (5 mins)	Bathroom	Ugh – yuck – so puffy and gross.
7:00 AM	Oatmeal, milk, peanut butter, raisins, banana; coffee; piece of toast	Kitchen				Hopped on the scale after going to the bathroom (1min)	Bathroom	Same as yesterday – good – but could be better.
9:00 AM						Took my morning selfie (1min for pic, 10 mins to compare to yesterday's photo)	Bedroom	I look bigger than yesterday.
9:30 AM						Self-view mode – virtual class (3 mins x 5 times)	Class	Readjusting the angle.
10:00 AM	Yogurt, nuts, granola	Desk				Looking down at my body, rubbing my thighs and comparing to my friend (15 mins)	Class	Feels mindless – hate my thighs.
11:00 AM						Scrolling through social media (15 mins)	Class	Checking pictures from this weekend – ugh!
12:00 PM	Sandwich (cheese, turkey, mayo, veggies, bread); chips; apple; water	Cafeteria				Mirror (2 mins)	School bathroom	Checking my hair and thinking about putting on a sweater to cover my stomach.
						Scrolling through social media (10 mins) while waiting for friend		Saw an old friend on social media who has lost a lot of weight. I don't want to eat!
2:00 PM						Weighed myself when I got home (1 min)	Bathroom	Weight is up – I knew I ate too much.

Copyright material from Suzanne Bailey-Straebler and Laura Sproch, *Group Cognitive Behavior Therapy for Eating Disorders* (2025), Routledge

Chapter 13

Group Session 8

Body Shape and Weight Checking –
Part I: Education, Evaluation, and Behavior Change

Overview

Continuing to address the over-evaluation of shape and weight, Sessions 8 and 9 focus on shape, weight, body, and/or appearance checking (see Figure 13.1). We will refer to this as "body checking" throughout the chapter. Reducing body checking behaviors decreases the focus and preoccupation on shape and weight as a means to define self-worth. It also helps to reduce eating disorder behaviors, thoughts, and feelings. As an example, if Ilhan decides to decrease her mirror checking, this will help to reduce thoughts, feelings, and behaviors that are associated with scrutinizing her body in the mirror (e.g., dieting at her next meal, telling herself that she has to start losing weight for her partner to be attracted to her, and increased feelings of anxiety and shame).

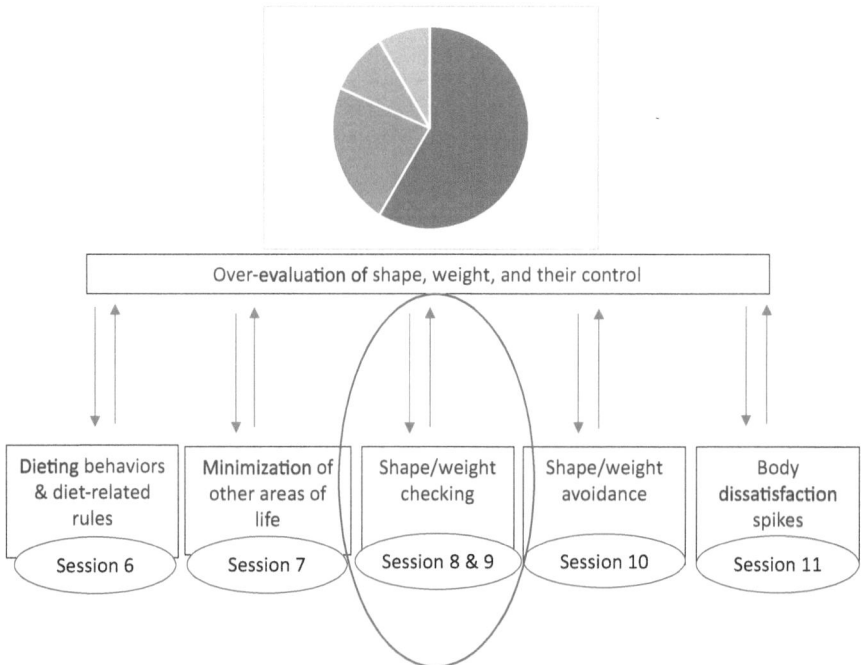

Figure 13.1 Extended formulation – Shape and weight checking.

DOI: 10.4324/9781003450849-17

Body checking is a common practice for many individuals. This often involves a quick glance in the mirror to assess one's appearance (e.g., checking an outfit before going to work, making sure that teeth are clean after a meal, checking a hairdo before a social event). However, for those with an eating disorder, body checking usually takes on a markedly different form, characterized by repetitive and excessive behaviors; regular monitoring; and frequently fixating on perceived flaws, often in areas that are disliked the most. This hyperfocus not only keeps these perceived imperfections at the forefront of one's mind, but also magnifies their perceived severity. This heightened level of scrutiny significantly increases feelings of dissatisfaction with one's body.

Consider a non-eating disordered hyperfocus scenario related to spider phobia. Many people are afraid of spiders or find them "disgusting." We know from phobia research that individuals with phobias scan their environment repeatedly for the feared stimulus (the spider). This scanning or checking has the effect of distracting the person from the environment around them. If they spot a spider while scanning, they are likely to then keep a close watch on the spider – monitoring it for movements and focusing especially on certain aspects they are afraid of (e.g., their legs, their speed, the way they crawl). They become more and more engrossed in monitoring certain parts of the spider, and because of this focus, those feared parts become amplified and highly important. The checking inflates the perceived size of the spider and heightens worries about the spider (e.g., anxiety that the spider might jump and bite). If, however, the person were to instead acknowledge the spider's presence in the room and then move on to something else without constant monitoring, the spider would likely fade into insignificance over time, causing far less distress. We recognize that shape and weight is a more intimate aspect of life than spiders, impacted by weight bias and diet culture. The example can, however, provide a useful illustration of how scrutiny can increase distress and of the importance of modifying checking behaviors.

To minimize the importance of shape and weight, body checking is addressed by guiding patients to stop or reduce checking behaviors. After providing education about body-checking behaviors and how they keep the eating disorder going, Group CBT-E motivates patients to change their checking behaviors using three steps:

1. Increase patient **A**wareness of their own body checking behaviors.
2. Evaluate the **I**mpact of body checking.
3. Encourage patients to **M**ake change to their body checking behaviors.

As you will see in Sessions 8, 9, and 10, these same steps or principles are repeatedly used in the group to bring change to body image behaviors that maintain the over-evaluation of shape and weight. To simplify the steps and to highlight their purpose to patients, we will use the acronym AIM for Change (Figure 13.2).

Because body checking behaviors tend to be quite prevalent and sometimes difficult to change, there are two sessions dedicated to body checking in Group CBT-E. This session, Session 8, focuses more generally on all body checking behaviors and introduces the AIM for Change steps to start addressing body checking. The next session, Session 9, will continue to apply the AIM for Change intervention to three common body checking behaviors: reflection checking, body comparisons, and social media body checking.

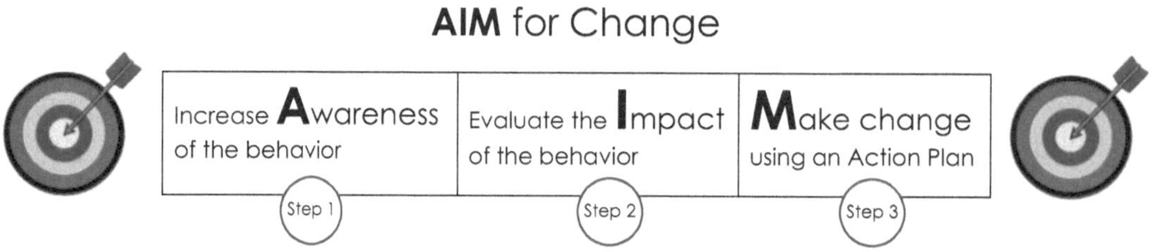

AIM for Change

Increase **A**wareness of the behavior	Evaluate the **I**mpact of the behavior	**M**ake change using an Action Plan
Step 1	Step 2	Step 3

Figure 13.2 AIM for change.

Therapist Preparation

☐ Review this chapter in advance.
☐ Review accompanying handouts and have copies available for patients.

Handouts

- Standard Weekly Handouts
  - *1.3 Self-monitoring form*
  - *1.6 Between-session Work Log*
  - *8.1 Between-session Work Self-review – Session 8*

- Session-specific Handouts
  - *7.3 Over-evaluation of Shape and Weight Extended Formulation*
  - *7.5 Body Shape and Weight Checking Self-monitoring*
  - *8.2 Body Checking*

- Optional
  - *8.3 Weighing*

Group Session Agenda

1. Setting the agenda and orienting to the session (2 minutes)
2. Between-session work self-review (5 minutes)
3. Educating about body checking (5 minutes)
4. Increasing awareness of body checking behaviors (15 minutes)
5. Evaluating the impact of body checking behaviors (15 minutes)
6. Making change using an Action Plan (15 minutes)
7. Group wrap-up (3 minutes)

1. Setting the Agenda and Orienting to the Session

Begin with a positive, encouraging welcome. Share that this is Session 8 of Stage 3 with 6 sessions remaining. Clearly list the session agenda.

2. Between-session Work Self-review

Handout: *Between-session Work Self-review – Session 8*

Ask patients to complete their *Between-session Work Self-review – Session 8* handout. This review continues to check in on the Stage 1 elements and additional Stage 3 interventions (i.e., dieting behaviors, diet-related rules, and enhancing other areas of life). Ask the group to review their ongoing progress with items like self-monitoring, regular eating, and breaking food rules. Breaking food rules will likely continue to be scary, and will continue to need to be worked on, for some weeks. It is important to encourage patients to continue to practice and apply skills to protect themselves from using other eating disorder behaviors in response to breaking rules (e.g., restriction, driven exercise). Additionally, ask patients if they were able to add one or two new activities as a way to enhance other life areas. As always, praise patients for the things that are going well; identify barriers and how to address such obstacles; and build on the existing interventions by identifying increasingly challenging ways to tackle eating disorder symptoms. At the end of the review, encourage patients to create updated Action Plans to reflect goals for the week, and include these on their *Between-session Work Log*.

3. Educating about Body Checking

Handout: *Over-evaluation of Shape and Weight Extended Formulation*

Body checking includes shape and weight checking, which fall into roughly four main categories:

1. Checking with hands (e.g., pinching stomach flesh, rubbing one's collarbone), measurement tools (e.g., scale, measuring tape, fingers around the wrist, rings on fingers, trying on clothes of different sizes), and/or other people (e.g., reassurance seeking about one's shape/weight); and/or looking down at one's body (e.g., looking down at thighs when seated).
2. Reflection checking – repeatedly checking one's image in a mirror, looking at reflective surfaces (e.g., building windows, reflective surfaces), repeatedly taking photographs of oneself, repeatedly checking self-view during virtual meetings.
3. Comparison making – comparing one's shape, weight, or specific body parts to others', comparing to pictures of oneself from different points in life.
4. Social media body checking – comparing one's shape to others' (e.g., various content creators), checking for comments about one's appearance, looking at photos on social media.

Start by reminding patients about body checking, introduced in Session 7, by providing psychoeducation.

Today we are going to talk more about body checking (i.e., shape and weight checking). Remember, body checking is a behavior that contributes to, and is maintained by, the over-evaluation of shape and weight. For individuals with eating disorders, the checking tends to be frequent and extreme, often impacting mood and overall functioning. Let's look together at your Over-evaluation of Shape and Weight Extended Formulation handout to see how these are related. Does anyone relate to this vicious cycle between body checking and over-evaluation of shape and weight?

The four checking behaviors we will explore are: 1.) checking with hands, measurement tools, reassurance seeking from other people, and looking down at your body; 2.) reflection checking; 3.) comparison making; and 4.) social media body checking. Does anyone relate or recognize these various types of body checking behaviors?

Therapist Insight

Some patients may share that they only engage in body avoidance behaviors and do not relate to body checking. While this can happen, it will still be helpful to do a thorough review of body checking behaviors as sometimes people are surprised to learn that they may have body checking behaviors that they just weren't aware of initially. Taking the time to slow down and observe for potential checking behaviors (e.g., body comparisons, looking down at one's body) can be helpful.

Introducing the AIM for Change Strategy

Provide brief education to the group about how body checking will be addressed using a standardized AIM for Change strategy (Figure 13.2). Write out the AIM for Change steps on a whiteboard and remind patients of the steps as you address body checking in the current session and the following sessions.

4. Increasing Awareness of Body Checking Behaviors

To increase patients' awareness of their body checking behaviors we use the following techniques: self-monitoring the behaviors; identifying the specific body checking a patient engages in; and assessing the function, frequency, and focus of the specific form of checking. Doing so provides a comprehensive view of the intensity and severity of the checking. As patients become aware of the extent of their checking and begin to question why they do it, if it is useful, and how it makes them feel, they become ready to make changes to these behaviors.

Identifying Specific Body Checking Behaviors

Handouts: *Body Shape and Weight Checking Self-monitoring; Body Checking*

Explore with patients the specific examples of checking they engage in. Using their *Body Shape and Weight Checking Self-monitoring* handouts completed for between-session work, ask patients to share body checking behaviors they noticed and write these on a whiteboard, as well as ask patients to list these on their *Body Checking* handout. Some patients will feel highly distressed and shameful about some of the behaviors they engage in. Be sure to forewarn patients of this and remind them that the group is a safe space where this information can be shared. It is often helpful to start the list with a few examples before opening it up to the group for their input. Providing examples normalizes these behaviors as a part of having

Table 13.1 Sample Whiteboard – Body Checking Behaviors

Checking with hands, measuring tools, other people, or looking down
Weighing myself 3 times a day
Looking at my step counter on my phone
Looking down at my stomach and thighs when I am sitting in meetings
Trying on my "thin clothes" to see if they still fit
Pinching my stomach and "love handles"
Asking my partner if my stomach looks big every day before work
Checking my calorie counter app

Reflection checking
Scrutinizing my self-view on virtual meetings
Looking at my reflection in car windows and storefronts when I walk to work
Checking my legs in my mirror in my room

Body comparisons
Comparing to everyone I see
Being distracted by comparing my legs to my sister's legs when I am with her

Social media checking
Scrolling through pictures on socials from when I was smaller and weighed less – comparing
  me to me
Looking at dieting and clean eating pages
Following a body builder on social media and comparing their measurements to mine

---

an eating disorder and may reduce the shame of sharing. To help prepare for eventually identifying specific strategies to change these behaviors, list the different checking behaviors under the four main checking behavior headings: checking with hands/measuring tools/ other people and looking down; reflection checking; body comparisons, and social media body checking. [See Table 13.1 for ideas of how this may look].

Assessing the Function of Body Checking Behaviors

Next, support patients to consider why they check their bodies. This allows patients to start looking critically at their body checking which can lead to reducing and/or stopping the behaviors.

> *Why do you think you check your body in so many different ways throughout the day? What information are you trying to find out from checking? Do you think checking provides accurate information about what it is that you are looking for? Remember to continue to complete the Body Checking handout as we go along.*

Often patients report that the reason they body check is to determine how they look, if their weight has changed, or to determine how other people see their bodies. Encourage the group to consider if body checking is a helpful means to find out this information. Create a list of all the reasons patients body check and the groups' view on whether or not the checking provides useful information (see Columns 1 and 2 on Table 13.2. It is intended that this whiteboard will be completed in steps throughout this part of the session and Table 13.2 presents the completed example.)

Table 13.2 Sample Whiteboard – Assessing the Function and Consequences of Body Checking Behaviors

1	2	3	4
Reasons for checking	Does checking provide accurate information?	How long do I spend checking?	Consequences (how checking makes me feel)
To see if I have gained weight	I think I can see small changes – but I know my body doesn't change so drastically over the course of a couple of hours.	Many times during the day	Sometimes I feel relieved when my weight has not changed, but mostly I just feel really depressed.
To see how fat my legs are	They look bigger than I want them to.	Probably over an hour or two in total	I feel horrible.
To encourage me to diet harder	Yes I hate what I see so diet or plan to diet harder. But that doesn't help me with what I am doing here and stresses me out.	All day long	I feel really badly about myself.
So that I know how other people see me	I know my view may be distorted by the eating disorder.	Every time I go near a mirror or a reflective surface, virtual calls are the worst – constantly then.	I feel terrible.
To see how I look compared to others	Maybe? I am not sure.	Every meeting, whenever I see other people	I get so down on myself.

Assessing the Frequency and Duration of Body Checking Behaviors

Many patients check their bodies repeatedly throughout the day and some of them do so for extended periods of time. It is helpful for patients to become aware of the amount of time they spend engaging in checking behaviors. Return to the whiteboard (Table 13.2) and complete Column 3 related to time taken to body check. Then, consider more broadly the following questions to help guide the discussion and exploration.

Let's go back to our whiteboard and think about the examples that we have listed of reasons to body check. Now, we'll consider

- *How many times a day are you body checking?*
- *How long do you take to check? For example, how many minutes do you think you spend body checking on average each day?*
- *What do you think about spending that amount of time body checking?*

- *Do you need to do this behavior so frequently to collect the information that you need? Are there actual changes with your shape/weight that occur so frequently throughout the day? For example, if the function of looking down at your body is to determine if you have gained weight, do you think that looking down at your body all throughout the day helps you to determine if weight gain has occurred? Likewise, if the function of checking your weight so frequently is to assess if your weight is changing throughout the day, is it possible that the changes you are picking up on are related to changes in hydration and not actual weight changes?*

the following questions together as a group, while also adding your personalized information to the *Body Checking* handout.

Typically, patients can see quickly that obtaining such information so frequently and taking a great amount of time to do it does not provide new data that is reliable and useful (and some begin to see that they do not need to check their bodies at all in this way). At this point in treatment, patients usually understand that there are no significant body changes that can occur over the course of a day. If group members are still wondering about this, we have found that using the support of other group members can be very helpful.

Assessing the Focus of One's Body Checking

Next, assess with patients which parts of their bodies they focus on when body checking. The goal is to highlight that often patients focus most on the parts that they like least or are most concerned with. Focusing more on parts of the body that are disliked causes patients to lose perspective and leads to magnification of perceived defects (see spider example in the Overview section). This creates a biased view of one's body that ultimately reinforces body dissatisfaction. Questions to guide this process include:

- *Which parts of your body do you tend to focus most on?*
- *Is it the parts you are most dissatisfied with?*
- *Do you ever check parts of your body that you like or feel neutrally about?*
- *Might you be obtaining biased information if you are only checking parts of your body that you don't like, and potentially missing other aspects of your body, which impacts your overall perspective on your body?*
- *When you weigh yourself, do you tend to focus on the change in weight?*
- *Do you focus more/weigh more often when the change is not in the direction that you would like? Is this biased in any way?*

Therapist Insight

Sometimes to help engage the patients, we will say to a group that is primarily scrutinizing one area, for example the abdominal area, "*I am hearing that many people are zooming in on their stomachs, is this biased in any way? Are we all just stomachs walking around or what else might you be missing?*" Often patients will chuckle thinking about this question, but inevitably it leads to some critical thinking about this bias.

In some ways, it makes sense for someone to repeatedly check something they are highly concerned about; however, checking is problematic for several reasons. This includes magnification of perceived defects and keeping concerns about the body and weight at the forefront of the patient's mind, contributing to preoccupation with shape and weight.

5. 🎯 Evaluating the Impact of Body Checking Behaviors

Handout: *Body Checking*

Therapist Insight

Sometimes patients will quickly report that there are no areas of their body that they like, or even feel neutrally about. In these cases, it can be useful to ask patients to reconsider and reassess if there might just be areas they are not considering – other parts of their body that they are missing entirely. Commonly overlooked areas that can serve as examples are elbows, pinky fingers/toes, feet, and ears.

Next, assess with patients the consequences of body checking. The aim is to build up to the idea of changing these behaviors by highlighting to patients that these behaviors take up time, keep the eating disorder going, do not provide much, if any, useful information, and cause them to feel bad. As you create the group's list on a whiteboard, ask patients to complete Step 2 on their *Body Checking* handout, listing the consequences of body checking that they experience.

Let's start by returning to our list on the whiteboard. What are the consequences of your body checking? [complete Column 4 of Table 13.2]. Now let's think about what we see here. When you engage in body checking, how does it make you feel about yourself? What percentage of the time do you feel good about yourself and/or your body and what percentage of the time do you feel bad?

You can then estimate the average of the group's shared percentage of how often body checking makes them feel bad about themselves. Ask the group what their reaction is to that number. It can be helpful to ask the group to reflect on their reactions to engaging in behaviors that most often make them feel bad about themselves.

What do you think about engaging in a behavior so often that makes you feel bad about yourself? Let's take this outside of your eating disorder for a moment. We have determined as a group that most of the time you feel worse about yourself when you body check. What do you think about this? What would it be like to be in a friendship with someone who made you feel worse about yourself most of the time? Would this be a friendship worth continuing? We can think of body checking in a similar way. Is it worth it to engage in a behavior that makes you feel bad about yourself so often?

At this point, most patients have likely determined that body checking is a flawed means to evaluate what it is that they are looking for (e.g., knowing if their body has changed, determining if they have gained weight). Despite this, it can still be helpful to ask the group to evaluate if what they are looking for when they body check is information that they need in their lives, and if so, if it is needed so frequently.

Through these exercises we have increased your awareness that body checking is something that you do frequently throughout the day. How do you think that impacts your focus on other areas of life? Do you need to know throughout the day if your weight has changed, how other people may see your body, or if your shape has changed? Is this data – which we have just decided is likely quite unreliable – something that you need to collect so frequently and keep at the forefront of your mind, at the risk of taking away from other priorities in life?

While patients continue to add to their *Body Checking* handout, ask the group to summarize the consequences of body checking and record on a whiteboard [see Table 13.3]. The group will likely be able to generate multiple consequences of body checking from the detailed examination of these behaviors.

Sometimes this conversation will lead to discussion about what triggers body checking, such as boredom, anxiety, or loneliness, and some of the emotional outcomes of body checking, such as increased anxiety, shame, or sadness. Highlighting the reciprocal cycle between checking and emotional states can be helpful for patients in understanding the impact of these behaviors.

We have identified several negative consequences of body checking so far in group. I am going to list them on the whiteboard. What can you think of that we have identified so far and what do you want to add?

Table 13.3 Sample Whiteboard – Consequences of Body Checking Behaviors

- I am tired of doing this so much – it takes up so much time!
- It makes me feel bad!
- It stresses me out..
- I don't feel like it is helping me at all.
- I end up feeling bad about myself a lot.
- Whenever I am grumpy, I check more and then I feel worse.
- I am not just a stomach walking around.
- It keeps my eating disorder going!
- It makes me want to diet harder.
- I constantly need to check my weight and obsess about the number.
- I spend so much time doing it all day and it isn't giving me the information I want (i.e., if my partner is still attracted to me).
- I do think that I can see shape changes, but I don't think that there is a purpose for me to be trying to find these out while I am at school or out with friends.
- I can't focus on work – I am so distracted by this!

6. 🎯 Making Change Using an Action Plan

Handouts: *Body Checking,* Optional: *Weighing*

After patients have identified the consequences of body checking and have considered reasons to change, they are now well set up to make Action Plans. Ask patients to use the *Body Checking* handout to create an Action Plan. There are two strategies, adapted from Fairburn (2008) for change: stopping behaviors that likely exclusively serve the eating disorder and reducing, or modifying, behaviors that have additional non-eating disordered purposes. Some behaviors may naturally fall into both categories and require thoughtful assessment to individualize for each patient.

Stopping behaviors, or aspects of behaviors, that exclusively serve the eating disorder

Examples include:

- measuring one's body with a measuring tape, hands, etc.
- using a step counter, exercise tracker, or other methods of movement and/or calorie burning apps from devices (Though this is an indirect form of body checking, it can reinforce dieting behaviors and contribute to the maintenance of the eating disorder, making it important to address in this session.)
- trying on clothes that don't fit to measure body size
- checking one's body naked in the mirror
- checking to see if there is a "thigh gap" (i.e., a gap between the patient's legs when standing with ankles together)
- repeatedly touching or pinching body parts
- looking down when sitting to assess the width of one's thighs
- posting images online to get "roasted" (i.e., posting on social media sites for the specific purpose of having others comment on your appearance negatively)

Stopping these behaviors can be done by stopping immediately (i.e., immediate extinction) or by phasing out the behavior.

Immediate extinction. Depending on the patient's motivation, some of these behaviors can be stopped immediately. Removing access to various checking methods, such as removing measuring tapes and clothes that no longer fit, can be useful to help stop these behaviors.

Phasing out. Other behaviors may require a phasing out approach. For behaviors that seem to be more habit driven, a two-part process can be helpful. First, encourage patients to more closely monitor the behavior on their self-monitoring forms. Then, suggest that they question themselves before engaging in the behavior (e.g., "Do I want to engage in this behavior?", "Will it tell me anything helpful?", "Could it possibly harm me, by making me feel bad or cause me to engage in eating disorder behaviors?"). This process will bring the behavior into the patient's awareness allowing them to make a decision about whether to engage in the checking. In the short term, it can also be helpful to utilize competing response techniques such as tying a reminder string around wrists or carrying around a stress ball to use hands in a new way.

For the final section on the handout, we will think about what action you can take to begin to reduce your checking and create your Action Plans. Some behaviors are best stopped completely. These are behaviors that serve the eating disorder only. Posting images online to get "roasted" would be an example of this. These behaviors can be stopped immediately, often by removing access to the checking tool, or by phasing them out. If you can stop immediately based on what you now know about the consequences of these checking behaviors, go for it! If you need to take a slower approach and phase it out, one way to start doing this is by monitoring each time this behavior occurs on your self-monitoring forms. Recording the behavior on your forms will make you more aware of it and give you the opportunity to decide if you wish to continue it. Then, if you would like to try to stop, perhaps question yourself about the function and consequences of your behavior, engage in a competing response (e.g., squeezing a stress ball), and/or practice other strategies (e.g., alternative activities, urge tolerating) to help with the desire to check. After monitoring, consider setting goals using your Action Plans to gradually make change to these behaviors.

Modify Aspects of Behaviors That Have Other Non-eating Disorder Purposes

Some body checking behaviors serve other functions in addition to serving the eating disorder; it is the frequency and extent of them that is problematic. Rather than identifying a strategy to eliminate such behaviors, the focus is on finding more balanced approaches to these behaviors.

One common body checking behavior that requires modification is weight checking. While we want patients to stop repeated weight checking (multiple times per day or week), we do not aim for patients to completely avoid knowing their weight, as there can be non-eating-disorder purposes of knowing one's weight (e.g., weight-dependent medications; fitted sports equipment). Therefore, this is a behavior that requires modification. Table 13.4 has information about modifying weight checking. For patients who need to address weight

Tips for phasing out checking behaviors

1. Record the behaviors on the self-monitoring forms, especially during times when the behaviors are likely to be more apparent and frequent (e.g., at the office, at night, on a date).
2. Consider the consequence(s) of engaging in the checking behavior.
3. Use specific tools to support making changes:

   a. specific environmental cues to increase awareness (e.g., cover mirrors used when getting in and out of the shower to resist checking one's body naked; get rid of clothes that no longer fit).
   b. competing response to urges to check (e.g., put hands by one's sides and make a fist for one minute each time one has touched their clavicle).
   c. stimulus control techniques (e.g., avoid going into the bathroom/bedroom after dinner as that triggers reflection checking or weighing at a difficult time).

Table 13.4 Modifying Weight Checking

Depending on the extent, checking weight often requires specific attention and time. For many, weight changes on a scale are viewed as fully objective data that can be relied upon. In these situations, weight movement that is higher than the last reading is interpreted as weight gain, and weight movement that is lower is interpreted as weight loss. While this may be the case, comparing data points that are taken so closely together (e.g., gathered on the same day or multiple times per week) is far more likely to be capturing changes in one's hydration levels rather than actual changes in body weight. Because these hydration level changes or fluctuations are viewed by patients as accurate indicators of weight change, frequent weighing keeps the eating disorder going by: 1) making particular numbers highly significant (e.g., "I must not go over xyz pounds"); 2) encouraging dieting (e.g., "my weight has gone up – I must diet more until my weight has gone down," "I must keep dieting, it is working"); and 3) greatly influencing one's overall emotional state (e.g., "My weight is down, I feel good and it's a good day," "My weight is up, I feel bad and it is a bad day"). For patients who report engaging in weight checking, provide them with the Weight Checking handout. This handout provides more in-depth information about weight, weight checking, and a method for decreasing the behavior.

checking, provide them with the *Weighing* handout. This handout provides psychoeducation about weight checking and avoidance behaviors and ways to address this, including a weekly weighing intervention. If time allows and this behavior is relevant for many patients in the group, review this handout as a group.

Other behaviors that require modification are reflection checking, body comparisons, and social media body checking. Reducing these behaviors will be the focus of the next session.

If there is time, prior to ending the session, ask patients to share aloud their body checking Action Plans that they have identified for the week ahead.

7. Group Wrap-up

Session Summary

Today we continued working on reducing the over-evaluation of shape and weight by focusing on body checking. We walked through the AIM for Change steps to 1) increase Awareness of body checking behaviors by identifying what types of body checking behaviors you have, thinking about the function of these behaviors, as well as the frequency, duration, and focus of these behaviors; 2) evaluate the Impacts of these behaviors, including how they make you feel and how they impact your eating disorder; and 3) Make plans to engage in change by identifying individual Action Plans to eliminate, reduce, and/or modify body checking behaviors.

Between-session Work

Remember to encourage patients to write the between-session work on their *Between-session Work Log* handout. The between-session work for Session 8 is:

- Continue work from previous sessions:
    - *Self-monitoring* – to be completed daily, in the moment.
    - *Regular Eating* – continue to prioritize regular eating using *Planning Ahead, Alternative Activities, Urge Tolerating*, and *Feelings of Fullness* to support this work.
    - *My Breaking Food Rules Plan* – continue to plan in avoided foods and break dietary rules.
    - *Other Areas of Life* – continue to work on adding in one or two new/expanded areas over the coming week and record this on the self-monitoring form.
    - Follow through with any Action Plans identified during the session.

- New work from Session 8:
    - *Body Checking* – create and implement Action Plans to reduce body checking, focusing on stopping behaviors that only serve the eating disorder and modifying behaviors that have additional purposes.
    - *Weighing* – if using this handout, review the material and put a plan in place to start the weekly weighing intervention this week.

Higher Level of Care Adaptations: Modular Implementation

When this session is used modularly, the following adaptations are suggested.

Body shape and weight checking: This session can be implemented as described at HLOCs. Patients knowing, or not knowing, their weight is likely decided by the program and setting. Be sure to acknowledge this with patients when reviewing the material about weight checking so that it is relevant to your patients' experience.

HLOC environments often provide opportunities for eliminating body checking behaviors due to limited access to checking tools. For example, patients typically do not have access to measuring tape, old clothing, and calorie/exercise trackers while in treatment. This creates a natural opportunity for elimination of these behaviors. Additional planning related to generalizing that elimination when a patient returns home can be useful. An additional benefit of HLOC is the opportunity to utilize patient monitoring by staff members to help support elimination of more habit-driven behaviors. For example, nursing staff (or any staff equipped to monitor behaviors) can be incredibly useful in helping to redirect a patient away from touching their clavicle, pinching parts of their body, measuring their wrists, or looking down at their body.

In other situations, particularly in inpatient or residential programs, body checking behaviors that require modification may or may not be able to be practiced in balanced ways. For example, many HLOC programs do not have mirrors in the therapeutic space, have limits on using technology (e.g., social media), and do not allow patients to see their weight. In these situations, you will need to be thoughtful about how to address body checking behaviors that require modifications. At times, these modifications will need to be planned for future lower levels of care.

Finally, it is not uncommon in HLOCs that patients who are undergoing the weight regain process may believe strongly that they need to engage in body checking in order to determine what their body looks like as they gain weight. They may believe that frequent checking does help them to see the rapid ways that their body is changing. We recommend validating this experience. In these conversations, it can be useful to consider if there is anything other than weight change that may impact their impression of their shape and weight, as well as identify consequences of the body checking behavior.

Group Session 8

Handout 8.1 *Between-session Work Self-review – Session 8*

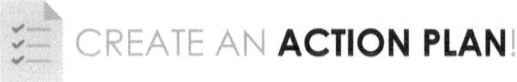

BETWEEN-SESSION WORK SELF-REVIEW – SESSION 8

Skill/Goal	THIS IS GOING...			MY PLAN		
	Well	OK	Not Well	Make an Action Plan to address	Share with my support person for accountability	Praise myself for working hard on this!
Self-monitoring	☐	☐	☐	☐	☐	☐
Regular eating	☐	☐	☐	☐	☐	☐
Alternative activities	☐	☐	☐	☐	☐	☐
Urge tolerating	☐	☐	☐	☐	☐	☐
Addressing feelings of fullness	☐	☐	☐	☐	☐	☐
Challenging diet-related rules	☐	☐	☐	☐	☐	☐
Eating avoided foods	☐	☐	☐	☐	☐	☐
Engaging in 1–2 other areas of life activities	☐	☐	☐	☐	☐	☐
Additional Items						
	☐	☐	☐	☐	☐	☐
	☐	☐	☐	☐	☐	☐

Which skills are going well? Great work, keep practicing them! Which skills am I struggling to use and need to prioritize? Plan to take action this week – write an **Action Plan** to address these.

CREATE AN **ACTION PLAN**!

Handout 8.2   *Body Checking*

BODY CHECKING

Body checking is a behavior that contributes to, and maintains, over-evaluation of shape and weight.

MY BODY CHECKING			
Checking with hands, measurement tools, and/or other people; looking down at my body			
☐	Weighing myself frequently	☐	Looking down at my body
☐	Measuring my body	☐	Pinching/touching my body
☐	Assessing tightness of clothes/accessories	☐	Checking with others for reassurance about my appearance
☐		☐	
Reflection Checking			
☐	Mirror checking	☐	Checking myself in the video during virtual meetings
☐	Taking multiple selfies	☐	Looking at my reflection in windows/ buildings
☐		☐	
Body Comparisons			
☐	Comparing to old photographs of myself	☐	Comparing myself to strangers
☐	Comparing myself to family and friends	☐	
☐		☐	
Social Media Checking			
☐	Looking at social media to compare my body to others	☐	Following eating disorder-focused social media accounts
☐	Following diet culture accounts	☐	
☐		☐	

AIM for Change

Increase **A**wareness of the behavior	Evaluate the **I**mpact of the behavior	**M**ake change using an Action Plan
Step 1	Step 2	Step 3

Step 1: **A**wareness of the behavior

What is the **function** of my body checking? Why am I checking and does checking provide accurate information?

What is the **frequency** and **duration** of my body checking? How long do I spend checking?

What is the **focus** of my body checking? What specific parts am I most concerned with/parts I am most dissatisfied with (e.g., the number on the scale, abdominal area).

Step 2: Evaluate the **I**mpact of the behavior

What are the **consequences** of my body checking? How does it make me feel?

 Step 3: Make change using an Action Plan

IDEAS TO CONSIDER INCORPORATING INTO MY ACTION PLAN

Examples of Behaviors to Eliminate
Repeatedly touching or pinching body parts
Measuring my body with a measuring tape
Trying on clothes that don't fit to measure my size
Checking my body naked in the mirror
Checking to see if there is a "thigh gap" (i.e., a gap between legs when standing with ankles together)
Looking down when sitting to assess the width of my thighs

Examples of Behaviors to Modify *These will continue to be addressed in the next session
Repeatedly weighing myself (see *Weighing* handout for additional guidance)
Reflection checking
Body comparisons
Social media body checking

SAMPLE ACTION PLAN		DATE: 12/2
PROBLEM:	Weighing myself	
CURRENT FREQUENCY (IF APPLICABLE):	1–2 times a day	
GOAL FOR UPCOMING WEEK:	1 time this week	
SPECIFIC PLAN:	**MY PLAN:**	**MY SUPPORT:**
	Decrease access to the scale	Remove the scale from my bathroom and hide it in the closet.
		Tell my roommate my plan.
		Put a positive affirmation in my phone to encourage myself.
	Resist urges to weigh myself	When I have an urge, use an alternative activity or urge toleratingto get through the urge.

ACTION PLAN		DATE:
PROBLEM:		
CURRENT FREQUENCY (IF APPLICABLE):		
GOAL FOR UPCOMING WEEK:		
SPECIFIC PLAN:	MY PLAN:	MY SUPPORT:

WEIGHING

Some individuals with eating disorders engage in frequent self-weighing, while others may completely avoid seeing their weight. When present, these behaviors contribute to your over-evaluation of shape and weight and it is important to address them. This handout outlines a strategy called *weekly weighing* which aims to minimize the consequences of both frequently checking body weight and avoiding weight completely. Weekly weighing can be implemented on your own or it can be part of individual therapy work. **You know yourself best** – so make the best choice for yourself about whether or not to try weekly weighing on your own. If you feel that it would be best to approach this with the support of a professional, talk to your group therapist for recommendations.

WEEKLY WEIGHING

WHAT IS IT?

Weekly weighing is weighing yourself once a week, plotting your weight on a graph, and then reflecting on your experience. With weekly weighing, you will no longer be participating in avoidance of knowing your weight or over-checking your weight, both of which lead to increased focus on weight and keep the eating disorder going.

1. Weigh **once a week**.
2. **Plot weight** using the weight chart.
3. **Avoid any self-weighing** outside of the once weekly weighing.
4. **Record** reflections.
5. Put into place any **environmental strategies** needed to help avoid weighing in-between sessions:
   - Give my scale to a support person after I am done weighing.
   - Hide my scale after weighing.
   - Get rid of my scale and only complete weighing in my provider's office.

Frequently weighing oneself can be a common body checking behavior. Sometimes people weigh themselves multiple times per week or multiple times per day. Some people believe they must get their weight, naked, first thing in the morning after they have moved their bowels and then weigh themselves throughout the day to assess for changes. Some people weigh after eating avoided foods to assess the impact of eating this food on their weight. Some people weigh after engaging in an eating disorder behavior, like self-induced vomiting, to see the effect on their weight. This behavior both maintains, and is maintained by, the over-evaluation of weight. Take a look at your over-evaluation of weight and shape pie chart to remind yourself about how this might be impacting you. Does weight checking cause you to engage in any eating disorder behaviors? (e.g., dieting, vomiting)? Modifying weight checking will likely be very useful to help decrease the emphasis on weight as a way to judge your self-worth and reduce associated eating disorder behaviors.

Weekly weighing allows you to take a scientific approach, not controlled by the eating disorder, to knowing your weight (i.e., you weigh yourself once per week, not when your eating disorder worries or thoughts tell you to). Having a more scientific, controlled approach helps to address unscientific assumptions about weight and instead, helps to think about weight using actual data.

For example, Ari frequently weighs themselves. On Tuesday, they weigh themselves and the number on the scale is higher than Monday (Arrow 1 on chart). They interpret this change to

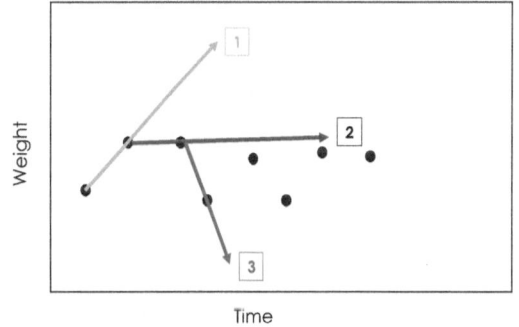

indicate that their weight has increased, and will continue to go up and up. As a result, they feel badly about their weight and decide to diet for the rest of the day to stop further weight gain. On Wednesday, their weight stays the same as Tuesday (Arrow 2) and they tell themselves "Ugh, my dieting didn't work yesterday and now I need to double my efforts to lose this weight." On Thursday, the number on the scale is lower than Tuesday (Arrow 3). They interpret this to indicate that they have lost weight. They think, "Finally I have lost weight. I will keep dieting to lose more." As you can see – no matter what happens with their weight, the outcome is to **keep dieting**.

Although Ari is interpreting these weight changes on the scale as weight loss and weight gain, what Ari is actually experiencing are healthy, typical weight fluctuations (see the dots on the scatterplot above) most often caused by hydration levels (see more information below). All bodies experience weight fluctuations. You can see how these typical fluctuations were interpreted by Arias meaningful, long-term weight change which was very distressing for them and caused them to engage in eating disorder behaviors (dieting). Weekly weighing allows for a more objective, scientific understanding of weight that helps to decrease false assumptions and takes a longer-term view of weight trends.

Examples of Reasons for Weight Fluctuations
Water (Up to 60% of the human body is water)
Hormones (e.g., various points in the menstrual cycle are associated with water retention)
Periods of sleeping (i.e., due to fluid loss without replacement while asleep)
Salt intake
Bowel movements
Temperature
Alcohol consumption
Sweating

WEEKLY WEIGHING TO DECREASE WEIGHT AVOIDANCE

Avoiding knowing one's weight is a body avoidance behavior. Just like over-checking weight, completely avoiding weight also maintains, and is maintained by, the over-evaluation of weight. Avoiding weight can lead to increased thoughts, assumptions, and worries about weight. Working toward modifying weight avoidance will likely be very useful to help decrease the emphasis on weight as a way to judge your self-worth. Not knowing your weight and being afraid to know what it is can also negatively impact other areas of life, like not attending medical appointments where weight may need to be assessed. If weight avoidance is keeping your eating disorder going and interfering with other areas of your life, addressing it is important.

Exposure to weight in a balanced way over weeks often can have a neutralizing effect similar to other exposure-based interventions. Despite often increased anxiety of looking at weight in this way initially in the short-term, the repeat exposure then often decreases anxiety and discomfort long-term, as you become more acclimated to your feared stimulus (i.e., the number on the scale). Ultimately, the goal is to work closer toward having a more neutral perspective on your weight. Take a look at your Exposure handout to be reminded of how this works! Keep in mind, though, that we live in a weight-biased world. Weight exposures may increase your risk of encountering shame related to your weight. For this reason, it can sometimes be most helpful to do weight exposure work with a trained eating disorder professional who can support you through this work and help you to reach your goals. If you would like to try weight exposures on your own, be kind to yourself, appreciating the fear that weekly weighing may cause. Use the support of the group to discuss challenges.

Step #1	Record the date in Column B of the Weight Reflection Log.
Step #2	Obtain your weight. • Record this in Column C of the Weight Reflection Log. • Use the same scale (placed on a hard surface) each week. 　• If using different scales, be aware they may be calibrated differently and give somewhat different information. This is ok and can help in tolerating slight differences. • Weigh only once.
Step #3	Apply any environmental strategies that are needed if your scale is in your home environment (for example, give to a support person until next week, hide in your car).
Step #4	Plot your weight on your Weight Chart. *To set up your chart for the first time, review the sample weight chart provided to see how the first 4 weeks of weekly weighing was charted. Remember, in order to complete the weight column in the chart, start by placing the number of your first weight in the middle of this column and then have each row represent 2 pounds/1 kilogram.*
Step #5	Complete Columns D and E on the Weight Reflection Log. • Take time to reflect on what you learned as a result of obtaining your weight. Remember Ari's experience and avoid making interpretations about changes from one point to the next. • If you are experiencing an emotional reaction to seeing your weight, what will you plan to put in place to take care of yourself? • Likewise, if seeing your weight is making you want to engage in eating disorder behaviors, what plan can you put in place to prevent this?
Step #6	Recognize the accomplishment of completing this difficult task.
Step #7	Repeat next week (and not before)

Group CBT-E is not a weight loss intervention.

If you are at a weight that is lower than what your body needs or are underfat, a goal of Group CBT-E is to increase weight to get to a healthier weight. If you do not have a weight regain goal, with regular eating patterns, your weight may stay the same, may increase, or may decrease as your body adjusts to regular eating patterns and eating more flexibly.

Wait until you have 4 data points.

Try to avoid making significant interpretations of your weight graph until there are at least 4 data points on the graph. This is because a more reliable trend cannot be determined with minimal data points. For example, having just two data points does not give enough information about a stable pattern as that change could be impacted by typical weight fluctuations (e.g., water consumption). The weight chart is not meant to be used to interpret any one data point, but instead is meant to be a visual of weight trends over time. Remember, an exact stable weight (i.e., weight that is the same at each weighing session) is an impossible goal, as healthy weight fluctuates.

Stop when you are ready.

It is recommended to continue this intervention at least until the end of Group CBT-E and then decide if you would like to continue this intervention and for how long. This decision will be a part of your Staying Well Plan which is created in the final session. Some patients feel that they need much more time with it, while others feel that they need just a short while longer. Some continuation of this intervention following the conclusion of the group will likely be useful.

WEIGHT REFLECTION LOG

A	B	C	D	E
Week	Date	Weight	What is my interpretation of my weight graph?	Ways I will take care of myself (if needed), including using supports
#1				
#2				
#3				
#4				
#5				
#6				
#7				
#8				
#9				
#10				

WEIGHT CHART

WEIGHT											
WEEK	1	2	3	4	5	6	7	8	9	10
DATE										
TIME										

*To complete the weight in the chart, start with your first weight number in the middle of the weight column, then have each row represent 2 pounds/1 kilogram. Each week, record the date and plot your weight.

SAMPLE WEIGHT CHART

WEIGHT										
216										
214										
212										
210										
208										
206										
204										
202										
200										
198										
196										
194										
192										
190										
188										
186										
184										

WEEK	1	2	3	4	5	6	7	8	9	10
DATE	1/2	1/9	1/16	1/23						

TIME

Chapter 14

Group Session 9

Body Shape and Weight Checking – Part II: Reflection Checking, Body Comparisons, and Social Media Body Checking

Overview

Session 9 is the second session focused on body checking. In Session 8, body checking was introduced and strategies to begin to reduce checking described. Patients will have already engaged in initial discussion and evaluation of the ways in which they are checking their bodies and consequences that come from these behaviors. Between sessions, patients will have started to modify, reduce, and/or eliminate some body checking behaviors. Session 9 focuses more extensively on three common body checking behaviors: reflection checking; body shape and size comparisons ("body comparisons"); and social media body checking.

As introduced in Session 8, AIM for Change (see Figure 13.2) will continue to be applied to stop or reduce reflection checking, body comparisons, and social media body checking.

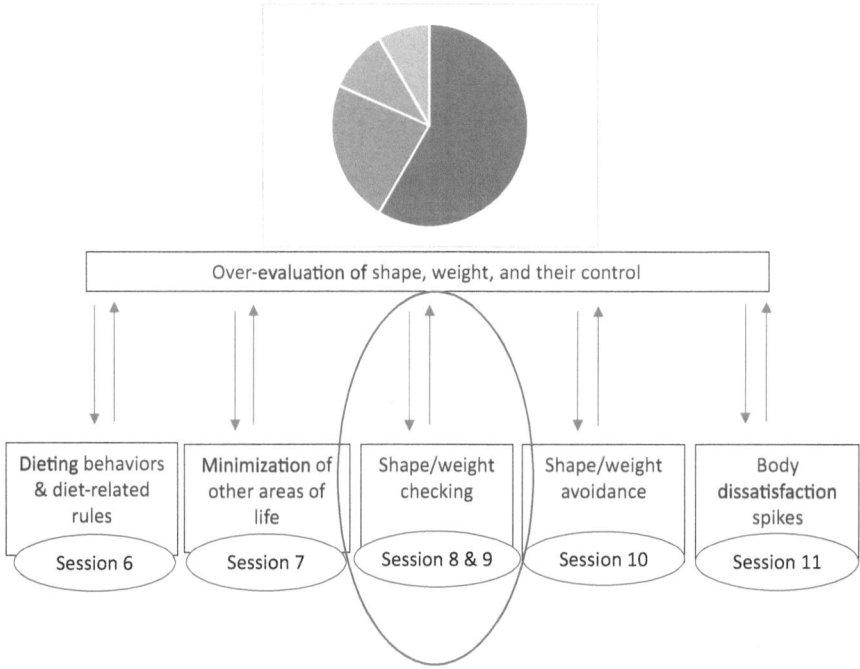

Figure 13.1 Extended formulation – Shape and weight checking.

DOI: 10.4324/9781003450849-18

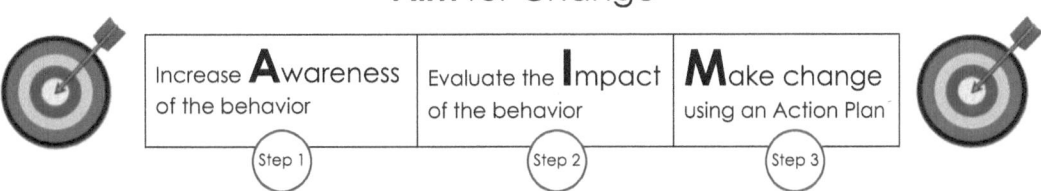

Figure 13.2 AIM for change.

Therapist Preparation

☐ Review this chapter in advance.
☐ Review accompanying handouts and have copies available for patients.

Handouts

- Standard Weekly Handouts
  - *1.3 Self-monitoring*
  - *1.6 Between-session Work Log*
  - *9.1 Between-session Work Self-review – Session 9*

- Session-specific Handouts
  - *7.5 Body Shape and Weight Checking Self-monitoring*
  - *9.2 Reflection Checking*
  - *9.3 Body Comparisons*
  - *9.4 Social Media Body Checking*

Group Session Agenda

1. Setting the agenda and orienting to the session (2 minutes)
2. Between-session work self-review (5 minutes)
3. Addressing reflection checking (20 minutes)
4. Addressing body comparisons (15 minutes)
5. Addressing social media body checking (15 minutes)
6. Group wrap-up (3 minutes)

1. Setting the Agenda and Orienting to the Session

Begin with a positive, encouraging welcome. Share that this is Session 9, Stage 3, and that there are 5 sessions remaining. Clearly list the session agenda.

2. Between-session Work Self-review

Handout: *Between-session Work Self-review – Session 9*

Ask patients to complete their *Between-session Work Self-review – Session 9* handout. This review asks patients to reflect on progress with Stage 3 elements and Stage 3 interventions (dieting behaviors, diet-related rules, enhancing other areas of life, and initial efforts to reduce/eliminate body checking behaviors). As always, the idea is to celebrate the things that are going well, identify barriers and how to address such obstacles, and build on the existing interventions by identifying increasingly challenging ways to tackle eating disorder symptoms. For this session, ask about patients' progress with reducing or eliminating body checking behaviors. Sometimes body checking is so engrained as a habit that patients may not be aware in the moment that they are engaging in these behaviors. If patients report this, use methods to increase their awareness of the behavior. For example, if a patient is uncon-

sciously pinching their body fat, ask them to wear gloves for a short while, which should heighten their awareness of the behavior. If another patient is unable to stop frequently weighing themselves, encourage them to return to the information and intervention described in the *Weighing* handout. For example, removing the scale from easy access when not needed – such as keeping it in the car trunk or on a high closet shelf – can help protect against frequent weighing. Involving a support person in this task is useful to ensure the scale is not easily accessed and to provide additional support. At the end of the review, encourage patients to create updated Action Plans to reflect goals for the week, and include these on their *Between-session Work Log*.

This session has a sizable agenda. Share this with the group and let them know that it will be your job to move things along. Make sure to cover all the components of this session. The AIM for Change strategy is applied repeatedly throughout the session. As the patients get used to practicing these skills, they will likely be able to move quickly through the process. Depending on the size of the group, you may not be able to hear from each patient individually regarding each of their body checking behaviors. Encourage patients to complete their handouts, continue the discussion with a support person (if available), and follow through with Action Plans, to further support this work.

3. Addressing Reflection Checking

Handout: *Reflection Checking*

Session 8 built momentum around changing body checking behaviors and introduced reflection checking as an example of one checking behavior. The start of this group opens with a more detailed exploration of reflection checking. Reflection checking comprises all forms of using a reflective surface to body check, including mirrors, windows, photographs of self (i.e., selfies), and videos of self (e.g., checking the "self-view" during a virtual meeting). We will use "reflection checking" as an abbreviated term to capture all forms of this behavior. Reflection checking is a common and acceptable practice in many cultures. For patients with eating disorders, reflection checking can extend beyond the typical behavior of perhaps using a mirror to check appearance in a functional way, and can become quite dysfunctional. Patients often significantly scrutinize their bodies when looking at their reflection, leading to body dissatisfaction and furthering the over-evaluation of shape and weight.

The AIM for Change strategy will be used again in this session. Write out the three steps of the strategy shown in Figure 13.2 on the whiteboard and review with the group.

> **Therapist Insight**
>
> Check for all forms of reflection checking and ask about specifics of the behavior. A patient once shared that she took hundreds of selfies throughout the day to constantly assess her shape.

 ### Increasing Awareness of Reflection Checking

Assessing the Frequency, Duration, and Focus of Reflection Checking Behaviors

The first step to increasing awareness of reflection checking began in the last session with the review of the body checking monitoring records. The next step is to draw attention to the specific ways group members check their reflection using the *Reflection Checking* handout. This handout will be used throughout the session for patients to complete as they follow along with the discussion. Similarly to the last session, patients are asked to consider the frequency, duration, and focus of the reflection checking. The following questions provide a helpful guide for the conversation (adapted from Fairburn et al., 2008):

- *How often/for how long do you look at your reflection?*
  - *How often do you look in the mirror?*
  - *How often do you take selfies or use your phone camera to check your appearance?*
  - *How often do you use virtual meeting spaces to check your body in self-view?*
  - *Are there other reflective surfaces that you frequently check (e.g., a television that is turned off, glass walls in an office space, a window in a bedroom)?*

- *What exactly do you look at?*
  - *Do you tend to look at your whole body or body parts?*
  - *If you zoom in on body parts, which parts do you tend to look at?*
  - *Do you look at anything other than your body?*

- *Other specific questions to consider:*
  - *How many different mirrors do you use and where are they located (think about mirrors at home and away from home)?*
  - *What types of mirrors and/or reflection tools do you use (e.g., full-length, half-length, face, full wall; self-view; selfies)*
  - *Do you get dressed in front of the mirror or take photos of yourself in different outfits?*
  - *Do you stand naked in front of the mirror or take images of yourself naked to assess your body?*
  - *Do you ever visit the restroom only to check in the mirror?*
  - *Do you ever use your phone to check your appearance in the camera?*
  - *Do you take images of yourself throughout the day to assess your body?*

Unless they are engaging in complete reflection avoidance (Session 10), patients frequently share that they have multiple mirrors they use both inside and outside their homes and that they spend significant time scrutinizing their appearance in the mirror. Some share that they take selfies of themselves throughout the day. Others frequently attend virtual meetings and use this as an opportunity to check themselves on the video, enlarging the self-view image. Many patients report that checking behaviors have increased greatly with the popularity of selfies and virtual meetings. Following this conversation, to increase awareness of reflection checking, provide a summary to patients of what was discussed.

> **Therapist Insight**
>
> If no one mentions standing in front of the mirror naked to check their body – ask! This behavior is so common, and yet there is rarely ever a practical reason to stand in front of the mirror to body check.

> *In this group, and in last week's group, you shared that you check your reflection a lot – multiple times throughout the day and then again at work/school/outside your home. You've also shared that you check in virtual meetings. Some of you shared taking multiple selfies to check. You've mentioned that you mostly look at the parts of your body you like the least or are most concerned about (stomach, thighs), though mentioned that you cannot do this in virtual meetings and instead at these times focus more on your jawline and cheeks.*

Assessing the Function of Reflection Checking Behaviors

Next, explore why patients are checking their reflection in this way and what they hope to find out.

> *Now that we have had a chance to better identify what reflection checking you engage in, let's think together about what you are trying to find out when reflection checking. Do you think you can find it out this way?*

As mentioned in Session 8, patients frequently check their reflection with a goal of determining how they look, if their shape and weight has changed, or how other people see their bodies. As patients start to examine the function of their reflection checking, help them to look critically at this function to determine if they are getting reliable and accurate information, and if this information is needed. Table 14.1 provides examples of therapeutic responses to common reflection checking functions identified by patients.

Avoiding Avoidance

In teaching patients to reduce their reflection checking behaviors, we must be careful to not give the impression that we want them to avoid seeing their reflections. The goal is for them to be able to use reflective surfaces in ways that are useful, view their reflection ideally with

Table 14.1 Examples of the Functions of Reflection Checking and Therapeutic Responses

Function of Checking	Sample Response
To determine how I look	*What one sees in one's reflection can be biased by how one focuses one's attention, is thinking, and is feeling. This can be related to:*
	• *How someone focuses their attention- what someone sees in their reflection typically depends on how they are looking at their reflection. The scrutiny that typically occurs when body checking leads to a faulty understanding about how one's body actually looks. If someone is scrutinizing their body, then the images that they see will be impacted by this scrutiny. For example, if I was to spend 2 hours a day looking really closely at my pinky finger – examining it closely for flaws (e.g., wrinkles, blemishes, crookedness) – over time, I would see my pinky in a negative light. The very same pinky that previously had been a neutral part of my life. Later on, when I look at it, I would be naturally scrutinizing it for these flaws. Imagine how this relates to areas of your body when scrutinizing your reflection.*
	• *Thoughts and feelings. Let's use an example – has anyone ever looked in the mirror/taken a selfie multiple times in a day and had different impressions each time? Was this actually related to a change in your appearance? Might this have been related to your mood and/or negative self-talk at different points during that day?*
To determine how others see me	*What you see in your reflection provides no information about what someone else may think about your body. We have no control or knowledge of someone else's perspective.*
To determine if weight has changed	*There is no scientific way of measuring weight change just by looking at one's reflection. That is not a way to collect reliable data. Looking at your reflection is a very subjective process which can be influenced by mood and thoughts.*

neutrality in the longer term, and, in the shorter term, avoid using their reflection to judge their shape and weight. For example, mirror use is normative to many cultures and there are useful reasons to look in a mirror. It is equally important to support group members in becoming comfortable with, or taking a neutral approach to, seeing their reflection. Create a list together with patients of way that mirrors or other reflective surface can be used in less disordered ways [see Table 14.2].

Table 14.2 Sample Whiteboard – Helpful/Normative Uses of Mirrors and Reflective Surfaces

- general sweep of my appearance
- making sure I do not have seeds in my teeth
- checking my outfit quickly
- shaving
- putting in contact lenses
- doing my hair
- putting on makeup
- taking a selfie on vacation to post to a friend – not to scrutinize myself!
- quickly making sure that I am in the camera frame for a meeting

 Evaluating the Impact of Reflection Checking

Explore with patients the consequences of reflection checking. Reflection checking can lead to negative and uncomfortable thoughts and feelings about oneself.

We have a good idea now that many of you are reflection checking throughout the day, and we've started to consider that not only does the checking not tell you what you want to know, but also causes magnification, scrutiny, and provides biased information. I'd like to better understand the consequences of reflection checking. [Create a whiteboard list using Table 14.3 as a sample.]

The list highlights how reflection checking leads to increased body dissatisfaction as well as other consequences. As with the last session, we want patients to consider if these consequences are worth it.

Now that we have had a chance to look at the consequences of reflection checking, what do you think about engaging in a behavior that leaves you feeling so badly, so often? For those of you that have expressed that reflection checking helps to provide a momentary reduction in worry, but leads to more checking overall, and keeps your eating disorder going, what do you think about that? Do you want to keep engaging in a behavior that makes you feel so badly and keeps the eating disorder going?

Table 14.3 Sample Whiteboard – Consequences of Reflection Checking

- I feel gross.
- I hate myself.
- I feel reassured that my shape is not changing, but worry it could change at any moment.
- I am certain that my cheeks are bigger than before and I need plastic surgery and need to suck my cheeks in.
- I push myself harder on my run.
- I cut back on my food intake.
- It takes up a lot of time and distracts me.

Therapist Insight

Occasionally patients will describe that reflection checking is reassuring as it shows them that their body has not changed. Often this leads to an increased desire to continue to check as this "reassurance" is short-lived. Continually checking ultimately places more focus on shape and weight.

 Making Change Using an Action Plan

As a final step, ask patients to complete Action Plans for reducing, stopping, or modifying their reflection checking using the *Reflection Checking* handout. The group discussion can be used to help support patients in creating individual Action Plans. The same change strategies introduced in Session 8 apply here too:

1. Stopping reflection checking, or aspects of reflection checking, that exclusively serves the eating disorder. Examples of these behaviors include:
    a. Naked mirror/selfie checking
    b. Getting dressed in front of the mirror
    c. Lifting one's shirt in mirrors to assess the size of the abdomen
    d. Taking multiple selfies to assess shape
    e. Frequently viewing self in the camera during a virtual meeting

For patients who struggle exclusively with reflection *avoidance*, making change using an Action Plan is not relevant. Reflection avoidance will be addressed further in the next session, Session 10.

2. Modifying aspects of behaviors that have other non-eating disordered purposes. As described, reflection checking is common in many cultures and can serve useful purposes. For example, while we want to stop mirror checking behaviors like getting dressed in front of a mirror, other useful purposes, like putting in contact lenses, are to be continued. Therefore, modifying some reflection checking is required. See Table 14.4 for examples of strategies to modify reflection checking.

4. Addressing Body Comparisons

Handouts: *Body Shape and Weight Checking Self-monitoring; Body Comparisons*

The next agenda item is addressing body comparisons. Comparing to others is a common behavior – people compare education levels, careers, finances, accomplishments, relationships, houses, or other material goods. Comparing body shape and weight is also a common behavior for people with and without eating disorders. However, the intensity and frequency of comparing bodies is far greater for patients with eating disorders. For patients, these

Table 14.4 Examples of Strategies to Modify Reflection Checking

Reduce the number of mirrors available	Ask patients how many mirrors they have in their homes. Typically, we recommend reducing mirrors to two: one full-length and one facial mirror.
Limit access to reflections	Consider turning some mirrors around, placing tapestry/fabric over mirrors, and covering mirrors with paint or sticky notes with positive messages. Ask patients to consider limiting self to a certain number of selfies per week. Encourage patients to turn off their self-view in virtual meetings after checking the initial camera placement.
Increase awareness of when a patient is going to check their reflection	Reflection checking often goes unnoticed and it may require strategies to bring more awareness to it. For example, anything placed on the mirror (like a sticky note) will be a new stimulus heightening one's awareness. And as awareness increases, behavior changes are more likely.
Determine if the reflection checking actually answers what a patient wants to know	Encourage patients to catch themselves before reflection checking and decide if it is helpful. Suggest that patients ask themselves, "Can I accurately check changes to my body this way?" If the answer is no, then the recommendation is to avoid checking.

comparisons can be very distracting; negatively impact mood and self-esteem; limit social interactions and behaviors; increase preoccupation with weight and shape; decrease the focus on other areas of life; and ultimately maintain the eating disorder. Similar to other body checking behaviors, comparisons often involve scrutiny and selective attention, which puts someone at risk of collecting information that is biased. As with all checking behaviors, Group CBT-E addresses body comparisons using the AIM for Change strategy.

 ### Increasing <u>A</u>wareness of Body Comparisons

The first step to increasing awareness of body comparisons is assessing the frequency and duration of body checking, which was introduced in Session 8.

In the last group, a number of you noted that you compare your body shape and size to others quite frequently. While it is somewhat human nature to compare to others in a variety of areas (e.g., clothes, house, etc.), body comparisons are particularly problematic when trying to overcome an eating disorder. As we have done with other checking behaviors, we will explore your body comparisons and the impact that these have on you. Please take out the Body Comparisons handout, which I am going to ask you to take notes on throughout our discussion. Remember to use your Body Shape and Weight Checking Self-monitoring handout to remind yourself of how often, and how long, you are comparing yourself to others over the course of a day.

Assessing the Focus of one's Body Comparisons

To explore body comparisons, engage patients in a group activity to survey their approach to comparison making.

Therapist Insight

The intention of this activity is to help patients realize (both individually and collectively) the biased nature of their body comparisons. It is also a means to help with group cohesiveness, as body comparisons, and the biases attached, are typically a vulnerable topic. Identifying commonalities can help to reduce shame and guilt related to comparison making.

Let's explore a little more about how you make comparisons. I am going to ask a series of questions related to seven types of body comparisons and also some questions about what you are comparing to. I'd like you to indicate if you do this type of comparison making by giving a thumbs up for yes and down for no [use any rating system that you prefer]. *OK, let's begin.* [Ask patients the questions listed on Table 14.5.]

Table 14.5 Questions to Guide Comparison-making Discussion

Who in the group compares their body/weight to:	
General	*Others' bodies?*
Type of People	*People you know?*
	Strangers?
	Celebrities/Social media influencers?
	People in this group?
Age	*People of your age only?*
	People who are younger than you?
	People who are older than you?
	People of all ages?
Gender	*People of your gender only?*
	People of other genders?
Height	*People who are around your height only?*
	People who are of a different height than you?
Size	*People who are in a smaller body than you?*
	People who are in a larger body than you?
Weight	*Others' weights (number on the scale)?*
Attraction	*People who you believe are more attractive than you?*
	People who you believe are less attractive than you?
Types of Images	*People in real life?*
	Photos of myself from different stages of my life and illness?
	Social media/media images?

(Continued)

Table 14.5 (Continued)

Who in the group compares:	
Subject of Comparison	*Your specific body parts to others' specific body parts?*
	Parts of your body that you dislike to others' same body parts?
	Parts of your body that you like to others' same body parts?
	Your whole body to others' whole body?
	To others with a focus on other aspects of life based on personality, lifestyle, sense of humor, etc.?

In your feedback from this exercise, you want to highlight two things:

1. How much comparison making is occurring:

    Nearly everyone indicated that they are engaging in a great deal of body comparisons.

2. How narrow and biased the comparing is, highlighting the inherent flaws in the approach to comparison:

    It sounds like a lot of you compare almost exclusively to people who you believe to be closer to your view of an ideal shape, your age or younger, your gender, etc. And most of you said that you focus in on comparing to parts of your own body that you are most dissatisfied with. Many of you shared that you are often focusing in on your shape and weight as a way to compare to others, as opposed to other aspects of life. What do you think about this?

In asking patients to consider if their body comparisons are skewed, make sure to ask about specific comparisons and how those may be biased. For example, consider the biased nature of comparing one's body to a younger body. Bodies are meant to age and develop over time. Disregarding this and instead setting an expectation that bodies should be comparable despite age is both a faulty comparison and just nonscientific. As another example, consider the biases in comparing one's body to that of a celebrity, model, or social media influencer. Many of these individuals dedicate a lot of time and resources to their appearance as their livelihood is dependent on it. Professional tools (e.g., photographers, lighting, photoshopping) are often used to display a particular image in a way that will be useful for promotional purposes. Consider the unfair nature of comparing to bodies of different genders, heights, etc.

 ### Evaluating the Impact of Body Comparisons

As with the previous checking interventions, you want to find out how comparison making impacts the group.

We have identified two interlinking problems: 1) you are comparing yourself to others a great deal (multiple times each day); and 2) you mostly compare to others' bodies that you consider "ideal" in some way and/or compare yourself to others more exclusively based on

Table 14.6 Sample Whiteboard – Consequences of Body Comparisons

- I never feel good enough.
- I want to lose weight and diet.
- I want to avoid going outside.
- I want to leave social situations.
- I want to wear baggy clothes.
- I feel anxious and hopeless.
- I may as well binge.

your shape/weight. In general, comparisons to others' body shapes are unhelpful, but they can be especially harmful when the sample is so skewed. [Create a list on the whiteboard and engage in discussion (see Table 14.6 for a sample).] *When you compare your shape/weight so frequently, and to "ideal" shapes and weights, this leads to unhelpful thoughts and feelings about your own shape and weight (e.g., "I am ugly," "My body is so big," "I weigh too much.") and keeps you focused on your body. We know from your formulations that these types of thoughts keep the eating disorder going. They can cause further dieting, driven exercise, or other behaviors. What do you think about this – that body comparisons with others lead you to feel badly and encourage eating disorder behaviors?*

As described, comparison leads to increased body dissatisfaction, with most people reporting that it causes them to think negatively about themselves. This is not unique to patients with eating disorders. If we asked people who do not have struggles with body image to spend large amounts of time comparing their body to other bodies they find "ideal," they too would experience increased levels of body dissatisfaction. Again, the aim is to provide this information to build momentum to change these behaviors.

 ## *Making Change Using an Action Plan*

As detailed earlier, body comparisons are common in our culture. It is likely impossible to fully eliminate comparison making. Therefore, the focus is on eliminating types of comparisons that can be stopped and modifying other types of comparisons. The same change strategies introduced earlier apply here too:

1. Stopping comparison making that exclusively serves the eating disorder. Examples of these include:

   a. Comparing to specific body parts that patients are most dissatisfied with
   b. Comparing to others that patients find "ideal" in some way
   c. Comparing to celebrities, social media content creators, or models

2. Modifying comparison making that has other non-eating disordered purposes. See Table 14.7 for examples of strategies to modify body comparisons in this way.

Table 14.7 Examples of Strategies to Modify Body Comparisons

Plan in advance a competing and/or neutral comparison	Neutral comparisons that patients have come up with include shoes, earrings, hair style, rings, glasses, etc. This can be turned into an information-gathering action plan. For example, a patient may tell themselves, "Ok, let's see how many people I spot wearing flats versus heels." Be careful with comparisons of certain items, such as clothing, which can lead back to body comparisons and can be unhelpful.
	Encourage patients to practice, and plan in advance for, situations where they are likely to engage in comparison making (e.g., virtual meetings, shopping with friends). This technique relies on patients being aware of their comparison making and perhaps using a distraction activity to turn their attention back to the current situation.
Encourage "catching" when a patient is about to engage in, or is engaging in, body comparisons	Ask patients to catch themselves before they start to engage in body comparisons (or even after they have started) and ask themselves, "Do I want to do this behavior that I know will make me feel bad about myself?" If the answer is no, ask patients to consider stopping the comparison and praise themselves for resisting/stopping the urge to compare.

5. Addressing Social Media Body Checking

Handout: *Social Media Body Checking*

Nearly all patients engage in social media body checking, which is another example of reflection checking and comparison making. Social media is extremely pervasive, easy to access, and checking can be done privately, potentially making it far more harmful than other forms of body checking. Though there is overlap between this behavior and those discussed above, there are particular considerations unique to social media use that warrant separate clinical focus.

Certain forms of social media use are correlated with increased mental health symptoms, such as anxiety, depression, and loneliness. While in other instances, social media use has been found to lead to decreased mental health symptoms, for example, decreased loneliness in marginalized groups (e.g., LQBTQ+, neurodivergent) that have access to an online community. Specific to eating disorders, total time on social media is associated with increased eating disorder symptoms, thin ideal internalization, drive for thinness, and body dissatisfaction. In particular, social media use that is focused on appearance and body checking seems to have the most detrimental impacts for patients with eating disorders. How patients use and engage with social media makes a difference. Social media behavior that is primarily appearance related (e.g., viewing, posting, manipulating, emphasizing, tagging, comparing, commenting on photographs of one's own or someone else's body) negatively impacts body satisfaction and can contribute to eating disorder behaviors.

For the purposes of this intervention, it is likely that social media behaviors that are not purely body checking behaviors, and include other forms of social media use that perpetuate the eating disorder, will be addressed (e.g., photoshopping images, watching videos about what others "eat in a day," commenting exclusively on appearance when leaving comments for others, following pro-eating disorder content). We recommend being flexible and including all social media behaviors that patients find could be contributing to their eating disorder. As with the other checking behaviors, social media body checking is addressed using the AIM for Change strategy.

 *Increasing **A**wareness of Social Media Body Checking*

Begin by engaging the group in a discussion about their social media use. You want to know more about the types of social media they follow, how they post their own content (e.g., using filters, using photoshop, posting temporary versus permanent posts), and how long

> **Therapist Insight**
>
> Keep in mind that some social media behaviors have likely become so normative that patients may not even be aware of how their engagement with social media may be related to their eating disorder. In other situations, social media use and its connection to the disorder may be quite obvious- for example, patients may post specific eating disorder content (e.g., goals related to dieting, exercise, and weight loss) on social media.

they spend engaging with social media. Ask patients to use the *Social Media Body Checking* handout to take notes throughout the discussion and create a list with the group of examples of social media body checking behaviors. Table 14.8 offers an example of what this may look like.

In addition to reflection checking and body comparison, did you know that social media use can also be a body checking behavior? And just like the other body checking behaviors, it contributes to the over-evaluation of shape and weight, and body dissatisfaction. It is interesting to think about just how much time you may spend on social media sites engaging with content that will keep your eating disorder going. Have you ever thought about this? Let's make a list of social media behaviors on our whiteboard that you think may be examples of body checking. As we make the list, think about how much time you spend engaging in these behaviors.

Table 14.8 Sample Whiteboard – Examples of Social Media Body Checking

- Looking at hundreds of photos before selecting one to post.
- After posting a photo, scrutinizing comments about my appearance.
- Looking at my photo history to compare my body to old pictures of my body.
- Following certain social media content focused on dieting, exercise, and body building/lifting/sculpting.

Now that the group has generated a list of behaviors, ask the group to reflect on what they think about these behaviors. The following questions can guide the conversation:

Let's look at your social media body checking behaviors. In instances where you are comparing your shape to others, are you comparing in the narrow way we discussed earlier? That is, comparing only to others who have your "ideal" body? Comparing to others who may be unrealistic to compare to – like celebrities or content creators? What about the use of filters, editing, image modification? Do you think that the people you follow use any of these techniques to modify their image or content?

 ### Evaluating the Impact of Social Media Body Checking

As with other forms of body checking, social media checking often has negative consequences. Patients will spend long periods of time body checking and often hyperfocus on content and creators that cover topics that maintain eating disorder symptoms. Using social media in this way causes increased body dissatisfaction and negative thoughts and feelings about oneself. By this point in the group, patients are familiar with the AIM for Change strategy and understand that engaging in behaviors that lead them to feel badly is probably best changed in some way.

Therapist Insight

Often by this point, as there has been so much practice, group members are able to identify the next steps on their own. Acknowledge that they may be finding the repetition a bit boring, but most importantly, they are learning the steps required for change. If useful, involve them in leading various sections of this session.

Now we are at our "I" in our AIM for Change strategy. That means, let's talk about the consequences of using social media in the ways you described. What do you think about the way you use social media and how it is likely keeping your eating disorder going? What thoughts, feelings, and behaviors are consequences of your social media body checking?

 ### Making Change Using an Action Plan

As you did with previous body checking behaviors, support patients in identifying behaviors that are best stopped and those that would benefit from being modified/reduced. Ask patients to complete Action Plans related to these changes. The same change strategies introduced earlier apply here too:

1. Stopping social media behaviors that exclusively serve the eating disorder. Examples of these include:
   a. Following particular people/sites on social media whose content is focused on body shape, weight, and appearance (e.g., fashion influencers, exercise influencers,

pro-eating disorder sites, peers who spend a lot of time posting photoshopped images, dieting sites).
  b. Spending excessive amounts of total time on social media. Spending any time on social media may put patients at increased risk of the usage turning to body checking.
2. Modifying aspects of social media behavior that have other non-eating disordered purposes. There are many different social media body checking behaviors and strategies to address these behaviors. A group brainstorming activity can be useful for identifying the best strategies for individual group members. As members identify strategies, record these on a whiteboard. See Table 14.9 for examples of strategies that may be helpful for patients to consider.

Table 14.9 Examples of Strategies to Modify Social Media Body Checking

- Decrease the number of social media platforms that one engages with.
- Decrease/remove social media apps from one's cell phone to be forced to more thoughtfully interact with a social media platform using a computer.
- Review a list of friends/pages one is following and eliminate following friends/pages that are wrought with body comparisons (e.g., celebrity, athletic build, model sites).
- Add in new sites that cover other areas of interest – using the other areas of life that were identified in Session 7 as a guide.
- Make specific plans to reduce total use (e.g., 1 hour/day).
- Set a timer for the amount of time one is willing to engage with social media.
- Install an app that stops access after a certain amount of overall use.
- Complete self-monitoring before, during, and after social media use.
- Reduce/stop posting pictures seeking reassurance/praise about one's appearance/body.
- Reduce/stop commenting on others' pictures in a way that suggests the focus is on appearance.
- Avoid posting selfies and limit photograph posting to images with environments or situations that are highly valued by the patient and not eating disorder-related.
- If posting a high number of photographs, start to significantly decrease this number.

6. Group Wrap-up

Session Summary

In today's session, we talked about ways to address three types of body checking that maintain body dissatisfaction and keep the eating disorder going: reflection checking, body comparisons, and social media body checking. We thought about the consequences (often negative feelings) of each of these behaviors and made plans to change these behaviors. We talked about behaviors that are best to stop – like taking multiple selfies throughout the day to assess shape. We also talked about behaviors that require modification – like how we compare ourselves to others. The between-session work is to act on the Action Plans you each created.

Between-session Work

Remember to encourage patients to write the between-session work on their *Between-session Work Log* handout. The between-session work for Session 9 is:

- Continue work from previous sessions:
  - *Self-monitoring* – to be completed daily, in the moment.
  - *Regular Eating* – continue to prioritize regular eating using *Planning Ahead, Alternative Activities, Urge Tolerating*, and *Feelings of Fullness* to support this work.
  - *My Breaking Food Rules Plan* – continue to plan in avoided foods and break dietary rules.
  - *Other Areas of Life* – continue to focus on the one or two new/expanded areas.
  - *Body Checking* – create and implement Action Plans to reduce body checking, focusing on stopping behaviors that only serve the eating disorder and modifying behaviors that have additional purposes.
  - Follow through with any Action Plans identified during the session.

- New work from Session 9:
  - *Reflection Checking, Body Comparisons*, and *Social Media Body Checking* – create and implement Action Plans to reduce body checking, focusing on stopping behaviors that only serve the eating disorder and modifying behaviors that have additional purposes.

Higher Level of Care Adaptations: Modular Implementation

When this session is used modularly, the following adaptations are suggested.

Reflection checking, Body comparisons, and Social media body checking: At HLOCs, each of the checking behaviors (reflection checking, body comparisons, and social media body checking) could be separated out into individual complete group sessions. This can be done by introducing the AIM for Change strategy at the start of each session, taking more time to generate checking behavior lists together, and taking more time to process the impact of these behaviors with patients. Really emphasizing the impact often becomes further motivation for these patients to meet their individual treatment goals while at an HLOCs.

As well as the HLOC recommendations outlined in Body Checking – 1 (Session 8), there are some additional considerations for this particular body checking session. For reflection checking and social media body checking, when implemented as one group, Steps 1 and 2 of AIM for Change (i.e., increasing awareness and evaluating the impact of the behavior) can be implemented as described at all levels of care. Step 3 (i.e., making plans to engage in change) may be challenging to implement in inpatient and residential settings. As mentioned in previous sessions, consider whether or not to include this step and if it seems appropriate, consider finding creative solutions for creating Action Plans. For body comparisons, we find that this checking behavior is often quite strong at HLOCs, as patients are frequently preoccupied with comparing their bodies to other patients' bodies, as well as staff's bodies. For example, it is not uncommon for some patients to experience increased eating disorder behaviors, urges, or thoughts as they compare their body to a very low-weight patient newly admitted to the unit. Talking openly to the group about the tendency to compare bodies while in treatment, and making Action Plans for how to address this, can be a useful tool at HLOCs. At partial hospitalization programs and intensive outpatient programs, the complete intervention can be implemented as described.

Group Session 9

Handout 9.1   *Between-session Work Self-review – Session 9*

BETWEEN-SESSION WORK SELF-REVIEW –SESSION 9

Skill/Goal	THIS IS GOING...			MY PLAN		
	Well	OK	Not Well	Make an Action Plan to address	Share with my support person for accountability	Praise myself for working hard on this!
Self-monitoring	☐	☐	☐	☐	☐	☐
Regular eating	☐	☐	☐	☐	☐	☐
Alternative activities	☐	☐	☐	☐	☐	☐
Urge tolerating	☐	☐	☐	☐	☐	☐
Addressing feelings of fullness	☐	☐	☐	☐	☐	☐
Challenging diet-related rules	☐	☐	☐	☐	☐	☐
Eating avoided foods	☐	☐	☐	☐	☐	☐
Engaging in 1-2 other areas of life activities	☐	☐	☐	☐	☐	☐
Reducing body checking	☐	☐	☐	☐	☐	☐
Additional Items						
	☐	☐	☐	☐	☐	☐
	☐	☐	☐	☐	☐	☐

Which skills are going well? Great work, keep practicing them! Which skills am I struggling to use and need to prioritize? Plan to take action this week – write an **Action Plan** to address these.

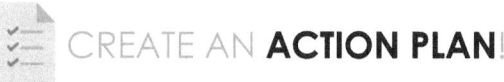

CREATE AN **ACTION PLAN**!

Handout 9.2 *Reflection Checking*

REFLECTION CHECKING

Reflection checking is a common behavior. It is typical in most cultures to use mirrors, take selfies, and check appearance in the camera during virtual meetings. For patients with eating disorders, reflection checking can extend beyond a more functional use of looking at one's reflection and instead, can become quite dysfunctional. Often, individuals with eating disorders significantly scrutinize their bodies when checking, which negatively impacts their over-evaluation of shape and weight and encourages engaging in eating disorder behaviors.

AIM for Change

Step 1: Awareness of the behavior

What is the **nature** of my reflection checking – how often/how long do I look at my reflection? What exactly do I look at?

[ ]

What is the **function** of my reflection checking – why am I checking in this way and what am I hoping to find out?

[ ]

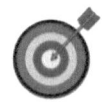 **Step 2:** Evaluate the **I**mpact of the behavior

What are the **consequences** of reflection checking? How does it make me feel? Does it make me want to engage in any eating disorder behaviors?

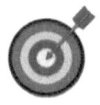 **Step 3:** **M**ake change using an Action Plan

IDEAS TO CONSIDER INCORPORATING INTO MY ACTION PLAN

Examples of Behaviors to Eliminate	
Behavior	Tips
Naked mirror/selfie checking	Place a towel over the mirror in my bathroom to help when taking showers.
Getting dressed in front of the mirror	Place a sticky note on my mirror as a reminder to avoid changing in the mirror. Consider picking out clothes ahead of time.
Lifting one's shirt in mirrors to assess size of stomach	Place a positive affirmation next to the mirror where I typically check.

Examples of Behaviors to Modify	
Behavior	Tips
The number of mirrors available.	Consider one full length and one facial mirror. Turn mirrors around, place tapestries/fabric over mirrors, or cover mirrors with paint or sticky notes with positive messages.
Selfie-taking	Limit myself to a certain number of selfies per week. Identify alternative activities when urges to take more come up. Don't edit selfies.
Looking at myself during virtual meetings	Turn off my self-view in virtual meetings. Apart from checking on the initial camera placement, there is no reason to watch myself in a meeting.

SAMPLE ACTION PLAN		DATE: 4/22
PROBLEM:	Reflection checking in video meetings	
CURRENT FREQUENCY (IF APPLICABLE):	Almost the entire work day – I work remotely!	
GOAL FOR UPCOMING WEEK:	Just a couple of minutes a day	
SPECIFIC PLAN:	MY PLAN: Look at my video for the first 1 minute of each meeting to make sure that the position of my camera is correct and then turn off the self-view video feature.	MY SUPPORT: I will put a reminder in my phone for each day to remember to do this. I will put a sticky note next to my computer to remember. After 2 full days of completing this, I will treat myself to going to the movie theater to reward myself for accomplishing this!

BODY COMPARISONS

Body shape and weight comparisons are common behaviors. For individuals with eating disorders, these comparisons can be very distracting; negatively impact mood and self-esteem; limit social interactions and behaviors; contribute to eating disorder symptoms; increase over-evaluation of shape and weight; and decrease the focus on other areas of life that are more personally valuable. AIM for Change provides a useful strategy for addressing body comparisons.

AIM for Change

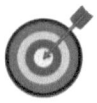

Step 1: Awareness of the behavior

How often, and for **how long**, do I spend engaged in shape/weight comparisons? What is the **focus** of my comparison making? Who am I comparing to? What part of their body am I comparing to? Do I compare to others' weights?

| |
| |
| |
| |

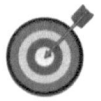

Step 2: Evaluate the Impact of the behavior

What are the **consequences** of comparing my shape and/or weight to others' in this way? How does it make me feel? Does it make me want to engage in eating disorder behaviors?

| |
| |
| |
| |

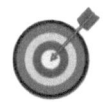 Step 3: Make change using an Action Plan

Overall Tips
When you catch yourself about to engage in body comparisons, or when you notice body comparisons: 1. Ask, "Do I want to do this behavior that I know will make me feel bad about myself?" 2. Stop engaging in the comparison-making (move your eyes to something else). 3. Praise yourself for resisting/stopping the urge to compare.

Examples of Behaviors to Eliminate	Tips
Comparing specific body parts that I am most dissatisfied with	When noticing myself comparing a specific body part to someone else, shift my attention away from that body part and compare to a body part that I am more satisfied with, or to my whole body.
Comparing to others that I find "ideal" in some way	When possible, eliminate situations where this behavior would occur (e.g., particular social media, television, or magazine use); plan a distractor in situations that are unavoidable; and complete a self-check about whether I am engaged in a biased comparison and how this may impact me.
Comparing my weight to other people's weights	Consider putting in place goals to eliminate this behavior (e.g., stop looking up celebrity weights online, stop following influencers who share their weight openly, and get rid of the notebook I keep of my daily weights).

Examples of Behaviors to Modify	Tips
Biased body comparisons	Plan in advance to compare to someone else in a less biased and shape/weight-focused way: • Consider comparing something that may seem more neutral (e.g., shoes, earrings, hair style, color, rings, glasses). Consider this an information-gathering Action Plan (e.g., how many folks can you spot wearing flats versus heels?). • Identify specific situations that are coming up and may trigger body comparisons (e.g., virtual meeting, going shopping with friends) and plan tools to implement to stay focused and present on the activity.

SAMPLE ACTION PLAN			DATE: 7/19
PROBLEM:	Comparing my body negatively and in a shape/weight-focusedway as I walk to and from work.		
CURRENT FREQUENCY (IF APPLICABLE):	About 40 minutes, 5 times a week.		
GOAL FOR UPCOMING WEEK:	20 minutes, 5 times a week.		
SPECIFIC PLAN:	MY PLAN:	MY SUPPORT:	
	To compare something more neutral when I find myself comparing.	I will set a timer and in the course of 3 minutes, I will survey how many folksare wearing jewelry compared to folksnot wearing jewelry.	
		I will take 3 minutes to compare my eyes to others' eyes.	
	To distract myself when walking.	I will download that new podcast I have been wanting to listen to and play that while walking.	
		I will try calling my friend while walking, who I have been meaning to catch up with.	

SOCIAL MEDIA BODY CHECKING

Particular forms of social media use are correlated with mental health symptoms, such as anxiety, depression, and loneliness. Social media use also impacts eating disorder symptoms. There is a correlation between total time on social media and eating disorder symptoms, body ideal internalization, and body dissatisfaction. Social media use that is focused on appearance and body checking seems to have the most detrimental impacts on patients with eating disorders. How you use social media makes a difference.

AIM for Change

Step 1: Awareness of the behavior

What are my social media body checking behaviors? How long do I spend using social media this way?

```
┌─────────────────────────────────────────────────────────┐
│                                                         │
│                                                         │
│                                                         │
│                                                         │
│                                                         │
│                                                         │
└─────────────────────────────────────────────────────────┘
```

Step 2: Evaluate the Impact of the behavior

What are the **consequences** of social media body checking? How does checking in this way make me feel? Does it make me want to engage in eating disorder behaviors?

```
┌─────────────────────────────────────────────────────────┐
│                                                         │
│                                                         │
│                                                         │
│                                                         │
│                                                         │
│                                                         │
└─────────────────────────────────────────────────────────┘
```

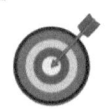

Step 3: Make change using an Action Plan

IDEAS TO CONSIDER INCORPORATING INTO MY ACTION PLAN

Examples of Behaviors to Eliminate
Following accounts/sites that focus on shape, weight, and appearance (e.g., fashion influencers, exercise influencers, pro-eating disorder sites, weight loss sites, peers who spend a lot of time posting photoshopped images).
Spending excessive amounts of total time on social media sites.

Tips to Modify Behaviors
Decrease the number of social media platforms that you engage with.
Review a list of friends/pages that you are following and eliminate following friends/pages that are wrought with comparisons (e.g., dieting, exercise, food, pro-eating disorder, cooking, clean eating, celebrity sites).
Make specific plans to reduce total use (e.g., 1 hour/day).
Install an app that stops access after a certain amount of overall use.
Reduce/stop posting pictures seeking reassurance/praise about your appearance/body.
Decrease/remove social media apps from your cell phone to be forced to more thoughtfully interact with a social media platform using a computer.
Follow new sites/accounts that cover other areas of interest – explored when identifying the other areas of life to focus on (Session 7).
Set a timer for the amount of time you are willing to engage with social media.
Complete self-monitoring before, during, and after social media use.
Reduce/stop commenting on others' pictures in a way that suggests the focus is on appearance.
Avoid posting selfies and limit photograph posting to images with environments or situations that are highly valued by you and not eating disorder related.
If posting a high number of photographs, start to significantly decrease this number.

SAMPLE ACTION PLAN		DATE: **9/12**
PROBLEM:	Spending a long time scrolling on social media looking at photosand videos	
CURRENT FREQUENCY (IF APPLICABLE):	About 3 hours a day	
GOAL FOR UPCOMING WEEK:	Decrease to 1 hour a day	
	MY PLAN:	MY SUPPORT:
SPECIFIC PLAN:	Delete Instagram from my phone so it is just on my tablet.	I will do this right now in group and will commit to not redownloading it for an entire week.
	Before I go to sleep, instead of scrolling, I will plan a different activity.	Tomorrow, I will get a book from the library to read. I will plug in my phone across the room when I get into bed.
	When I first wake up in the morning, instead of scrolling, I will plan a different activity.	I will plan to set my alarm for 20 minutes later so that I don't have time to scroll, but instead will need to get up and in the shower to get to work on time.

ACTION PLAN		DATE:
PROBLEM:		
CURRENT FREQUENCY (IF APPLICABLE):		
GOAL FOR UPCOMING WEEK:		
	MY PLAN:	MY SUPPORT:
SPECIFIC PLAN:		

Chapter 15

Group Session 10
Body Shape and Weight Avoidance

Overview

This session introduces body avoidance. Body avoidance is another set of behaviors that maintains, and is maintained by, the over-evaluation of shape, weight, and their control (see Figure 15.1). There are two main forms of body avoidance: shape-related avoidance and weight-related avoidance. In this chapter we will refer to both using the term body avoidance.

In contrast to Sessions 8 and 9, which covered checking behaviors, avoidance behaviors exist on the other end of the behavior continuum. Body avoidance can be significantly distressing and dysfunctional for patients with eating disorders. It can limit participation in activities that are highly valued and keep thoughts about one's shape and weight at the forefront of one's mind. This ultimately increases preoccupation with shape and weight,

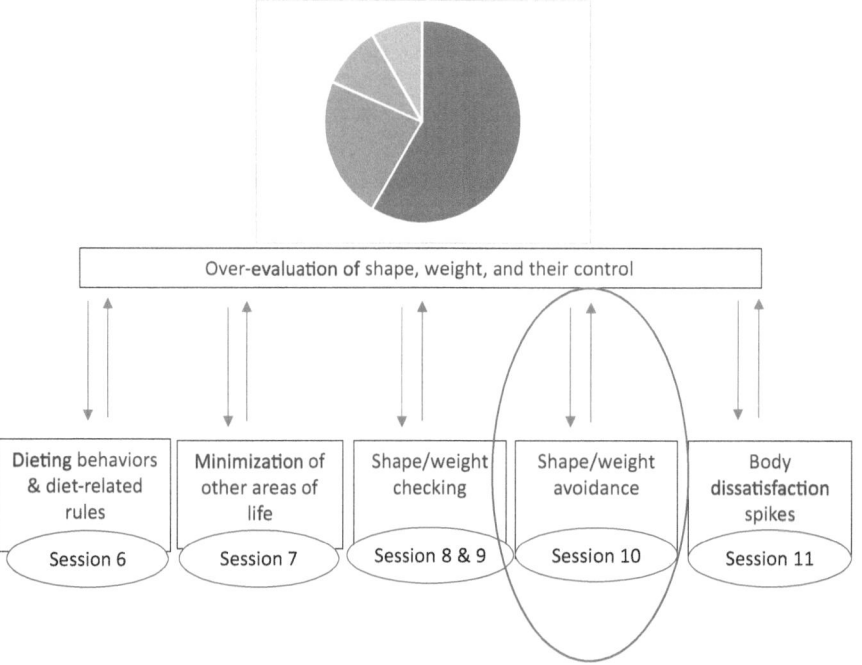

Figure 15.1 Extended formulation – Shape and weight avoidance.

DOI: 10.4324/9781003450849-19

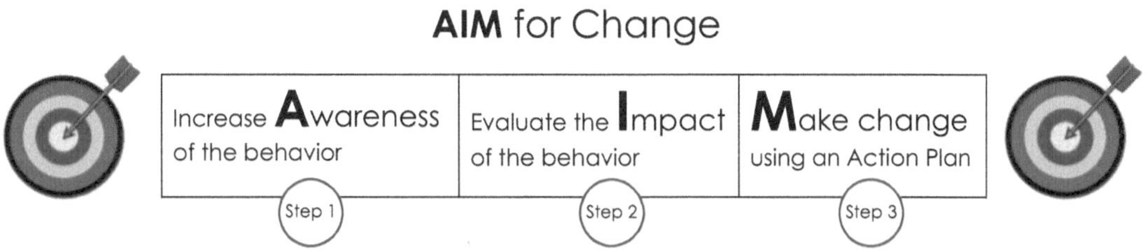

AIM for Change

Figure 13.2 AIM for change.

contributes to the over-evaluation of shape and weight, and decreases involvement in joyful aspects of life, negatively impacting self-esteem and mood.

Avoidance behaviors are addressed using the AIM for Change strategy (see Figure 13.2).

Therapist Preparation

☐ Review this chapter in advance.
☐ Review accompanying handouts and have copies available for patients.
☐ Familiarize yourself with the use of exposure hierarchies regarding avoidance behaviors.
☐ At the end of this session, specific between-session work needed for Session 11 (recording body dissatisfaction spikes) is described. Be sure to have familiarity with this content to adequately explain the between-session work.

Handouts

- Standard Weekly Handouts
    - *1.3 Self-monitoring Form*
    - *1.6 Between-session Work Log*
    - *10.1 Between-session Work Self-review – Session 10*
- Session-specific Handouts
    - *7.3 Over-evaluation of Shape and Weight – Extended Formulation*
    - *10.2 Body Avoidance*
    - *6.5 Exposure*
    - *10.3 Body Dissatisfaction Spikes Self-monitoring*
- Optional: *Weighing*

Group Session Agenda

1. Setting the agenda and orienting to the session (2 minutes)
2. Between-session work self-review (5 minutes)
3. Increasing awareness of body shape and weight avoidance (10 minutes)
4. Evaluating the impact of body shape and weight avoidance (15 minutes)
5. Making change using an Action Plan (20 minutes)
6. Preparing for Session 11 (5 minutes)
7. Group wrap-up (3 minutes)

1. Setting the Agenda and Orienting to the Session

Begin with a positive, encouraging welcome; share that this is Session 10, Stage 3 with 4 sessions remaining. Clearly list the session agenda.

2. Between-session Work Self-review

Handout: *Between-session Work Self-review – Session 10*

Ask patients to complete their *Between-session Work Self-review – Session 10* handout. This review asks patients to reflect on progress with Stage 1 elements and Stage 3 interventions (dieting behaviors, diet-related rules, enhancing other areas of life, and reducing or eliminating all body checking behaviors). As always, the idea is to celebrate the things that are going well; identify barriers and how to address such obstacles; and build on the existing interventions by identifying increasingly challenging ways to tackle eating disorder symptoms. For this session, continue to support patients to reduce their body checking behaviors. Check that they have removed/altered mirrors, stopped taking a large number of selfies, and continued to reduce weighing, if needed. Support patients in making meaningful Action Plans and involving their support people for help. Have group members remind each other why they are reducing these behaviors (e.g., checking makes you feel bad and takes up a lot of brain space) and the importance of sticking with their goals. At the end of the review, encourage patients to create updated Action Plans to reflect goals for the week, and include these on their *Between-session Work Log*.

3. Increasing <u>A</u>wareness of Body Shape and Weight Avoidance

Handouts: *Over-evaluation of Shape and Weight Extended Formulation*; *Body Avoidance*

Start by providing brief psychoeducation about body avoidance and the content for the group. Share Figure 15.1 with the group and read aloud, or have a volunteer read aloud, the three AIM for Change steps.

> *In the last couple of sessions, we have discussed body checking in all of its different forms. Today we are going to think about the other side of the spectrum, which is body avoidance behaviors. The avoidance behaviors we will consider are to do with shape avoidance and weight avoidance. Looking at the extended formulation (on your Over-evaluation of Shape and Weight – Extended Formulation handout), we can see how avoidance like this keeps the over-evaluation of shape and weight going. Now, let's think about how avoidance does this. Many people believe that avoidance is a helpful tool in reducing distress or anxiety. While it often is in the short term, it frequently causes heightened distress or anxiety in the long term. In the case of body avoidance, it may also lead to missing out on important or fun experiences. Today, we will take time to consider any avoidance behaviors you engage in and the consequences of doing so. We will use the AIM for Change strategy to guide us. [Elicit group feedback about the plan to discuss body avoidance and ask if anyone is aware of how avoidance can worsen things in the long term, before moving on to the next part of group.]*

Table 15.1 Sample Whiteboard – Consequences of Body Avoidance

Avoidance	Short-term consequences	Long-term consequences
Avoid medical appointments where my weight/shape will be discussed and/or I might be weighed.	Feel less anxious and also feel better knowing I won't be judged by doctors for my current weight.	I twisted my ankle and it still hurts a couple of months later – it is possibly fractured. I have a mole on my arm that looks suspicious and could do with being examined.
Never weigh myself – I am scared that it is shooting up out of control.	Feel better.	Even more worried about what I weigh now – It must be the highest it has ever been – so I need to diet to lose weight.
I won't be naked around my partner.	Feel better. I don't want to see my body. But it is awkward sometimes with my partner.	Miss feeling close to them; miss intimacy; they are upset too.
No bathing suits.	Happy to not see my thighs and stomach so exposed.	I love swimming and have missed out on two family beach holidays.
Avoid having sex.	I feel relieved.	I enjoy sex and would like this back in my life.
Avoid being in photographs.	I am glad to not have to see myself in a picture – I'll just obsess about it over and over but it can be awkward when I am with groups that want to take pictures with me.	I have no pictures of my life – and none with my partner or children. I am really sad about this.
No shorts or short-sleeved tops.	Feel better about not seeing my upper arms or legs. But I can get sweaty which makes me uncomfortable.	I'm uncomfortably hot in the summer. And missing out on wearing cute clothes!
I always wear a baggy sweatshirt.	Don't have to see my body.	Feel sloppy, overly hot sometimes which makes me even more aware of my body. Sometimes I feel unprofessional at work.
Shower in the dark.	Don't see my body.	I've slipped before from not being able to see. I feel really badly about myself for showering in the dark.

Following the AIM for Change strategy, the first step to addressing body avoidance is to first increase awareness of the various types of avoidance that patients are engaging in. Some patients are highly aware of their body avoidance; many are less aware. In either case, focused exploration is useful to uncover the behavior.

Using Step 1 of the *Body Avoidance* handout, engage the group in considering what they avoid and if they can relate to one another's avoidance. Brainstorm places, people, poses, etc. that are avoided in an effort to avoid seeing one's body or knowing one's weight. Ask patients to share aloud any behaviors they engage in and create a shared list on a whiteboard. The first column of Table 15.1 provides an example of a shared list. The second and third columns will be completed as a group activity as a part of the next agenda item. Consider building onto this whiteboard as you proceed through this piece of the agenda.

For some individuals, body avoidance can be a response to past trauma, serving as a coping mechanism to distance themselves from feelings or memories associated with their body. As with all Group CBT-E interventions, it's essential to carefully consider the patient's unique experiences and work collaboratively to determine whether a particular session or intervention is appropriate, ensuring that it aligns with their needs and comfort level.

On your Body Avoidance handout, place a checkmark next to any behaviors you are avoiding and add other behaviors that are not listed. You don't need to fill out the "Stop Now" or "Rank" columns just yet, we will return to these later. We will talk together as a group and I will list ideas on the whiteboard. Make sure to check off the relevant boxes on your handout as we go along.

4. Evaluating the Impact of Body Shape and Weight Avoidance

Next, explore with patients the consequences of their body avoidance. In some cases, body avoidance can lead to short-term reductions in shape- or weight-related anxiety. However, the long-term impacts can be profoundly impairing. Patients will likely identify some positive consequences. Normalize these experiences, while also helping patients to consider any possible longer-term harms.

*We've created quite an extensive list of different body avoidance behaviors the group engages in. And I imagine there are even more that you did not think of since it can be challenging to be aware of something that you are **not** doing. I'd like to now think about the consequences of body avoidance. Some of the consequences may be seen as positive, which they very well may be; however, some of these consequences may also have longer-term negative impacts. I'd like us to think about both the immediate and long-term consequences. Take a few moments to write some ideas you have about the consequences of your body avoidance in the Step 2 box on your Body Avoidance handout.*

Engage the group in a discussion about how their body avoidance has impacted their lives, both in the short and long term. For example, it is common to hear from some patients that they haven't worn a bathing suit in years. Patients will describe that the anxiety of even thinking about purchasing a bathing suit is so high that they can't even imagine ever wearing one again. This short-term anxiety is often quite strong and leads to total avoidance. Avoidance decreases/eliminates their significant anxiety and fear. The same patients may also share that since their avoidance and fear prevent them from going swimming, they miss out on an activity that they greatly enjoy. Their avoidance may have caused further avoidance of activities, such as going to the beach or on a vacation where swimming might be involved. They feel that ever going swimming again is impossible due to their current avoidance, their body dissatisfaction, and societal pressures. This is one example, of many, of how body avoidance can negatively impact engagement in life activities (e.g., avoiding dating, missing out on opportunities to see old friends due to fears of them noticing body changes, avoiding taking a dance class because others will see one's body in tight clothes). Engage patients in a discussion about how their body avoidance has caused a lack of participation in valued life activities.

As patients identify consequences, add two further columns to the whiteboard list of avoidance behaviors to include the long- and short-term consequences patients described. See Table 15.1 whiteboard sample for ideas.

Ask group members for their views on the consequences of body avoidance and provide a summary of the findings:

Therapist Insight

Body avoidance is impacted by cultural messages about body ideals. If group members share that their avoidance is related to society's message that certain behaviors should be avoided because of body size, meet this with active listening and compassion. Some patients may be interested in considering shifting their perspective on whether their beliefs and behaviors need to align with society's messaging. When this occurs, discussion questions to challenge societal norms may be useful. For example, in a discussion about wearing a bathing suit/going to the beach, you may ask patients to consider:

- Should our society be judging people on the beach in this way?
- Should people of all shapes and sizes be able to enjoy swimming?
- Should going to the beach be about what people look like in bathing suits?
- Do we make choices to go against societal expectations because we disagree with them?

Considering challenging societal norms can be intensely difficult. However, in having this conversation, some patients may begin to think more about self-acceptance for who they are (regardless of their body size) and some initial ideas about how they want to react against, or respond to, societal standards.

It sounds like many of you engage in some form of body avoidance, which is expected given how everyone in the group reports high levels of body dissatisfaction. For most of you, there is a positive benefit, at least initially. You all did a great job thinking about the longer-term impacts of your body avoidance. What do you think about this? Does it make sense to consider changing some of your body avoidance in an effort to reduce some of those longer-term impacts?

5. Making Change using an Action Plan

Handouts: *Exposure**, Optional: *Weighing**

The final step is to support patients in creating Action Plans for reducing, stopping, or modifying their body avoidance using the *Body Avoidance* handout. The group discussion is used to help support patients in creating individual Action Plans. The main change strategy for reducing most body avoidance is through gradual exposure.

Gradual Exposure

As reviewed in Session 6, exposure therapy is the most effective treatment for anxiety and has been shown to be highly effective in addressing fears for patients with eating disorders. It is a psychological tool used in many behavior therapies. Exposure is the opposite of avoidance and ultimately means "facing fears." When someone avoids something that is anxiety provoking, the fear strengthens and the avoidance does not allow for learning about the ability to cope with, habituate to, or tolerate distress. Exposure is used to change the way someone responds to feared stimuli. If fears are faced and distress tolerated, learning occurs that allows one to be better able to manage similar situations in the future. Consider reviewing the *Exposure* handout again with the patients if a refresher related to this concept would be useful to the group. It is important to highlight that most exposure treatments assume that the feared stimuli are neutral and the fear exaggerated, which is not the case regarding some shape and weight avoidance behaviors. Table 15.2 describes this issue in more depth.

Body Avoidance Exposure

Ask patients to return to Step 1 of their *Body Avoidance* handout and indicate, using the columns on the handout, any behaviors they believe they can stop now and to rank the others in order of easy to most difficult to change.

Returning to the avoidance behaviors you identified on Step 1 of the Body Avoidance handout, I want you to first identify any avoidance that you can stop immediately. Then, rank the remaining behaviors in order from easiest to change to most difficult to change. You can use numbers (e.g., 0 = no problem at all changing, 100 = seems impossible to change) or you can categorize them into groups (e.g., easy, kind of tough, difficult), whatever works best for you.

You may be familiar with the Subjective Units of Distress Scale (SUDS). SUDS is a tool used to measure the intensity of emotions or physical sensations, with a "0" indicating no intensity (i.e., completely relaxed) and "100" indicating extremely high intensity (i.e., the highest amount of anxiety ever experienced defined by the individual). If interested in using SUDS to aid in helping to identify initial exposure goals, consider identifying exposures that place patients' anxiety and discomfort around a SUDS score of 50.

Table 15.2 Weight Stigma and Body Avoidance

As described, exposure therapy aims to support patients in confronting anxiety-inducing situations in an effort to reduce fear and improve their quality of life. Exposure therapy is most effective when anxiety arises from an exaggerated fear. For instance, an individual with snake phobia will often describe worry that encountering a snake will lead to them being bitten and killed. In many parts of the world snake bites are uncommon and death from a snake bite is even more unlikely. Exposure therapy would expose this individual to a snake and support them in tolerating their distress while not engaging in safety behaviors (e.g., scanning the room for an escape route, closing their eyes when looking at a snake). This would allow them to confront their fear and observe their distress naturally reduce over time. Now imagine an environment where death from a venomous snake bite was an everyday experience. Exposure strategies here would require modification. In this case, the identified exposure exercise would need to consider the very real danger, while still including some gradual exposure to improve quality of life. Some safety behaviors and avoidance tactics might be appropriate and even encouraged (e.g., carrying snake repellant spray at times of a likely encounter with a snake, but not at all times).

In our diet-positive culture, which promotes an idealized body shape, weight stigma is a reality. It is therefore crucial to approach body shape and weight exposure work with sensitivity. When considering exposure work for patients encountering weight-related stigma and shame, consider these societal factors. Openly discussing these challenges and aligning exposure goals with the patient's needs and treatment objectives is key. For example, if a patient avoids medical appointments due to fear of weight-related stigma, exposure therapy may involve gradually confronting this fear while also acknowledging the potential for stigmatizing treatment and supporting behaviors that might otherwise be seen as "safety behaviors" (e.g., letting their PCP know they do not wish to be weighed). Table 15.3 offers guidance on navigating such exposures. In fostering a supportive environment for patients' recovery journey, exposures should be tailored to each patient's unique experiences, treatment goals, and the societal pressures they encounter.

Once the group has an idea of behaviors they can stop immediately, as well as has ranked the rest of the behaviors based on how difficult it would be to change, ask patients to make two Action Plans: 1) commit to stopping all (or most) of the behaviors they believe can be stopped now and 2) engage in gradual exposure to one of their avoidance behaviors. For this second Action Plan, encourage patients to review the gradual exposure examples on the *Body Avoidance* handout. The patient needs to experience heightened anxiety and tolerate that feeling, without avoiding, to learn that they can accomplish this task, experience fear, and move closer to their goals. Over time, the patient's anxiety may reduce when confronted with the feared experience. The intention is that patients start by exposing themselves to an item that is quite anxiety provoking, but not so fear inducing that they will not be able to follow through with their goal. Remind patients to use graded steps that increase in difficulty when creating their Action Plans. See Table 15.3 for examples of gradual exposure steps.

Now that you have identified behaviors you feel you can stop, please make an Action Plan to commit to this for the next week. After you have done that, we will create Action Plans for engaging in a gradual exposure. Choose an avoidance behavior that you feel would be difficult to change, but is doable if you push yourself, and most importantly, is something that you want to change. When creating the exposure steps, review the examples on the Body Avoidance handout. It provides guidance on setting graded steps. You will know where is best to start on the steps that you outline – something that is challenging, but manageable – trust yourself! And if it ends up being too easy, quickly move to the next step, or of it feels too hard, go back a step, or add in an earlier step. Remember, it will feel uncomfortable, but your end goal is important and tolerating the distress caused by the anxiety will help the distress to reduce and stop these behaviors from interfering with your life in time.

Support the patients in identifying specifics about when, how often, and how their exposure tasks will be completed. The more specifications identified (i.e., what day, what time, what event), the more likely the exposure will occur. The more frequently the patient is willing to practice the exposures, the more quickly the work will be accomplished. Encourage patients to engage in some type of exposure task at least four times over the course of the week. Daily exposure will likely have the best effect. At times, introducing body avoidance exposures in such a brief format (i.e., one group therapy session) may not be adequate for patients who struggle with particularly significant body avoidance behaviors or intense anxiety related to exposure. These individuals may require short-term, brief exposure-based individual sessions to help them meet their goals.

Weight avoidance may require special attention to modify. Avoiding knowing one's weight can be problematic in that it not only contributes to the over-evaluation of shape and weight, but has other negative consequences as well (e.g., preventing attending medical appointments, increased worrying about what might be happening to one's weight without knowing). It is important to understand if a patient's desire to not know their weight is truly avoidant and leading to distress or not. For example, Patient A may not have a scale in their home and are only weighed annually at medical appointments. Not knowing their weight is not distressing, nor does it cause them to avoid activities where they would be told/need to know their weight. They are not preoccupied with their weight or potential weight changes. Patient B may also not have a scale in the home but is highly preoccupied with their weight and possible weight changes, which is very distressing. When they see their weight annually at medical appointments, they experience significant anxiety before, during, and after the appointment. They also no longer engage in a once greatly enjoyed sport which would require them to know and share their weight to obtain the correct gear. Each individual patient should consider if their current relationship with seeing their weight reflects avoidance and if it is contributing to their eating disorder.

Table 15.3 Gradual Exposure Step Examples

Avoidance Behavior	Exposure Steps
Avoid medical appointments where my weight/shape will be discussed and/or I might be weighed	1. Find weight-inclusive PCP where possible. 2. Schedule an appointment. 3. Attend appointment, bring a support person, and let PCP know my wishes about knowing my weight and being weighed, as well as about my eating disorder treatment. 4. Attend a future appointment alone.
Avoid weighing myself for fear that it is shooting up out of control	1. Talk to my support person about how weight exposure may be useful for me. 2. Decide to weigh once weekly for the rest of CBT-E group using the guidance on the *Weighing* handout. 3. Make a plan with my support person to be with me to obtain my first weight directly before the next CBT-E group and give the scale to my support person after. 4. Do weekly weighing without my support person. 5. Plan to find out my weight in my next PCP appointment.
Avoid being naked around my partner	1. Wear short-sleeved shirt around them. 2. Wear tank top around them. 3. Wear underpants and swimming top around them. 4. And so on...
Avoid wearing a bathing suit	1. Purchase a new bathing suit. 2. Wear a bathing suit around at home (with or without someone else present). 3. Go to the beach and spend x minutes without a cover-up. 4. Go to a pool and engage in lap swim. 5. Walk along the beach in a bathing suit. 6. Wear a two-piece bathing suit.
Avoid having sex	1. Hold hands. 2. Hug. 3. Wear a more revealing outfit at home with partner present. 4. Allow a partner to touch/kiss one's body with clothing on and eventually with more revealing clothing on. 5. Be physically intimate with increasing levels of lighting.
Avoid being in photographs	1. Take a selfie, do not edit. 2. Ask a trusted support to take a photograph, do not edit. 3. Include self in a group photograph, do not edit. 4. Post an unedited photo on social media. 5. Tag self in an unedited photo on a friend's social media page. 6. Post an unedited close-up photo on social media. 7. Text an unpreferred photo to someone else, commenting only on the image's representation of the experience, not on physical appearance. 8. Post an unpreferred photo on social media, commenting only on the image's representation of the experience, not on physical appearance.

For patients who identify this avoidance behavior and want to change it, gradual exposure can be applied. Recommend implementing the weekly weighing intervention outlined in the *Weighing* handout. As described in Table 15.2, addressing weight avoidance is often complicated by weight stigma. For some patients, consider recommending a short course of individual therapy focusing on weight avoidance, using a CBT-E approach.

6. Preparing for Session 11: Body Dissatisfaction Spikes

Handout: *Body Dissatisfaction Spikes Self-monitoring*

In the next session, patients will work on exploring body dissatisfaction spikes. These are feelings of intense body dissatisfaction that can occur at various times throughout the week or day. Provide the *Body Dissatisfaction Spikes Self-monitoring* handout to the patients and ask them to complete this form twice this week instead of their typical self-monitoring forms. As with body checking, patients will be asked to complete this form over two different days (e.g., once on a work/school day and the other during a home day). Ask patients to focus on moments when they experience *particularly strong* body dissatisfaction, as some patients will report a consistent level of body dissatisfaction throughout the day, and it is the fluctuations within this experience that will provide useful data. Ask patients to use the form to also ask themselves what else might be going on in the moments when they are experiencing these body dissatisfaction spikes. Let patients know that the next session relies on having this important information prepared.

Social Media Alert

Some patients, despite regularly using social media, will completely avoid posting images of themselves. Or they will spend an exceedingly long time selecting an image that allows them to avoid displaying an aspect of their body that they are dissatisfied with. This contributes to shape and weight preoccupation and takes time and focus away from other areas of life. It is important to ensure that these social media behaviors are captured on a patient's fear hierarchy. Some examples of strategies include:

- When taking photographs, resist using photoshop or filtering tools.
- Instead of taking many selfies to choose which to post, set a specific expectation of a limited number of selfies to take, with a limited timeframe to choose, before posting a selfie.
- Reduce hiding or adjusting the body in photographs to avoid unflattering angles (e.g., only taking profile views, standing behind others).
- Post an image of oneself (perhaps with gradual exposure) if images of oneself have not been posted in a while.
- Post an image that shows a particular aspect of one's body that is disliked (i.e., a full body image, a warm weather image when wearing summer clothes, a face close-up).

For the coming week, I am going to give you a new self-monitoring form to complete twice this week on two different days (e.g., work/home, weekday/weekend, day with others/day alone). This form will ask you to record all the same information as your typical form and will also ask you to record times when you experience particularly strong increases in your body dissatisfaction, which we call body dissatisfaction spikes. These are times when you feel particularly uncomfortable in your body and may believe that there may have been body changes. If you are finding that you have too many instances to record, please focus on the most significant instances that occur. As always, the intention of self-monitoring is to better understand the function and nature of the experience. Start thinking about what else might be triggering these experiences other than changes to your body. We will start the next session by exploring what you have learned from monitoring.

7. Group Wrap-up

Session Review

In today's session, we explored the topic of body shape and weight avoidance. We explored how avoidance keeps the eating disorder going. Although it can feel like a helpful method to decrease body awareness and dissatisfaction, it often has the opposite effect over time. We talked about ways to decrease avoidance when it is interfering with your life and keeping the eating disorder going. We also considered doing shape/weight exposures, given our knowledge of the reality of weight stigma. When a body avoidance behavior is interfering with enjoyment of your life, but engaging in an exposure activity may make you more vulnerable to experiencing weight stigma, choose your exposures thoughtfully in a way that helps you achieve your goals, while also recognizing potential stigma.

Between-session Work

Remember to encourage patients to write the between-session work on their *Between-session Work Log* handout. The between-session work for Session 10 is:

- Continue work from previous sessions:
  - *Self-monitoring* – to be completed daily, in the moment.
  - *Regular Eating* – continue to prioritize regular eating using *Planning Ahead, Alternative Activities, Urge Tolerating*, and *Feelings of Fullness* to support this work.
  - *My Breaking Food Rules Plan* – continue to plan in avoided foods and break dietary rules.
  - *Other Areas of Life* – continue to focus on the one or two new/expanded areas.
  - *Body Checking* – create and implement Action Plans to reduce body checking in all its forms, focusing on stopping behaviors that only serve the eating disorder and modifying behaviors that have additional purposes.
  - Follow through with any Action Plans identified during the session.

- New work from Session 10:
  - *Body Avoidance* – create and implement Action Plans related to body exposures.
  - *Exposure* – review this handout again, if needed.
  - *Weighing* – if a patient is using this handout for the first time, review the material and put a plan in place to start the weekly weighing intervention.
  - *Body Dissatisfaction Spikes Self-monitoring* – record any experiences of intense body dissatisfaction and what else is occurring at the time.

Higher Level of Care Adaptations: Modular Implementation

When this session is used modularly, the following adaptations are suggested.

Body shape and weight avoidance: Steps 1 and 2 of AIM for Change (i.e., increasing awareness and evaluating the impact of the behavior) can be implemented as described at all levels of care. Step 3 (i.e., making plans to engage in change) may be challenging to implement at inpatient and residential settings due to patients' high severity of illness, likely high levels of anxiety related to their shape and weight, and lack of engagement with typical life activities. For example, patients who are struggling with a significantly high intensity of symptoms, and who are working on facing fears related to reducing these symptoms, may not yet be well set up to start also taking on the significant challenge of facing body avoidance fears. For patients at significantly low weights for their body, the work of engaging in body avoidance exposures when significantly underweight may not lead to translatable changes when the patient is at a higher, safer weight. Once weight is gained, new avoidance behaviors may arise or avoidance behaviors may return. Additionally, in residential and inpatient levels of care, many exposures are often not possible (e.g. wearing a bathing suit, going to a dressing room, having sex) due to the fact that patients are not in their home environments. Some creativity could be used to consider exposure work at these settings (e.g., avoiding wearing makeup, using a mirror, wearing colorful clothing), if this seems clinically appropriate. Depending on your program, consider whether or not to include Step 3. At partial hospitalization programs and intensive outpatient programs, the complete intervention can be implemented as described. Finally, as with HLOC recommendations in Session 8, weight avoidance goals may or may not be able to be addressed at HLOCs, depending on whether or not weights are shared openly with patients.

Preparation for Session 11: body dissatisfaction spikes: In settings where the same patients will return the next session, implement as described. If there is likely to be a lot of patient turnover, this preparatory work may not work well for the flow of the group. Consider how your program/service handles follow-up work in this way given patient turnover. Additionally, for the highest levels of care, consider decreasing the body dissatisfaction spikes self-monitoring from two days of monitoring to one day or one part of a day. Typically, patients struggle with high levels of body dissatisfaction in HLOC and will be able to collect sufficient data even in a short period of time. Be sure to be very clear that if patients are experiencing high levels of body dissatisfaction distress fairly constantly throughout the day, they can record just the highest intensity spikes in this dissatisfaction.

Group Session 10

Handout 10.1   *Between-session Work Self-review – Session 10*

BETWEEN-SESSION WORK SELF-REVIEW – SESSION 10

Skill/Goal	THIS IS GOING...			MY PLAN		
	Well	OK	Not Well	Make an Action Plan to address	Share with my support person for accountability	Praise myself for working hard on this!
Self-monitoring	☐	☐	☐	☐	☐	☐
Regular eating	☐	☐	☐	☐	☐	☐
Alternative activities	☐	☐	☐	☐	☐	☐
Urge tolerating	☐	☐	☐	☐	☐	☐
Addressing feelings of fullness	☐	☐	☐	☐	☐	☐
Challenging diet-related rules	☐	☐	☐	☐	☐	☐
Eating avoided foods	☐	☐	☐	☐	☐	☐
Engaging in 1–2 other areas of life activities	☐	☐	☐	☐	☐	☐
Reducing body checking overall	☐	☐	☐	☐	☐	☐
Reducing reflection checking	☐	☐	☐	☐	☐	☐
Reducing body comparisons	☐	☐	☐	☐	☐	☐
Reducing social media body checking	☐	☐	☐	☐	☐	☐

Which skills are going well? Great work, keep practicing them! Which skills am I struggling to use and need to prioritize? Plan to take action this week – write an **Action Plan** to address these.

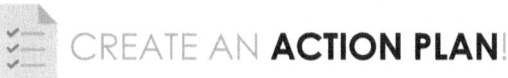

CREATE AN **ACTION PLAN**!

Handout 10.2   *Body Avoidance*

BODY AVOIDANCE

Body shape and weight avoidance, or *body avoidance* for short, can greatly limit participation in activities that are highly valued. Although avoidance behaviors can sometimes feel helpful in the moment in reducing anxiety, engaging in avoidance can often lead to more intense feelings of anxiety in the future. Body avoidance increases preoccupation with weight and shape and decreases involvement in joyful aspects of life, impacting self-esteem and mood.

AIM for Change

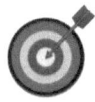

Step 1: Awareness of the behavior

Do you engage in any of the avoidance behaviors below? Add a check mark for any that you recognize. Add in any additional behaviors in the space provided.

I avoid....	√	Stop now	Rank
Medical appointments due to reasons related to weight and shape?	☐		
Situations where I may need to be weighed?	☐		
Knowing my weight?	☐		
Buying new clothes?	☐		
Posting my image on social media, despite a desire to want to share updates?	☐		
Wearing clothes of a particular style or color?	☐		
Physical activity that might draw attention to my appearance or body (e.g., dancing, exercising)?	☐		
Being seen by others when I am not "made up" in some way (make-up, hair)?	☐		
Seeing my body (e.g., looking in the mirror, looking at photographs)?	☐		
Activities that might "mess up" my appearance (sweating, swimming)?	☐		

My partner(s) seeing me naked?	☐		
Physical touch in which others would be able to feel my body (hug, massage, sex)?	☐		
Taking photographs and/or videos?	☐		
Certain places or events where my body might be on display (beach, dressing room, gym, fancy occasion)?	☐		
Certain people who talk a lot about physical appearance and/or do a lot of things to "look good"?	☐		
Certain people who I tend to compare to?	☐		
People who may make comments about my appearance?	☐		
People who I think are good looking?	☐		
Certain poses that I think are not flattering (profile, head-on, smiling, hand gestures)?	☐		
Certain sexual positions due to having my partner(s) see body parts that I dislike?	☐		
Other body avoidance behaviors:			

Step 2: Evaluate the Impact of the behavior

What are the **consequences** of body avoidance (e.g., missing important medical appointments, not going to the beach, not being in photographs)?

Short-term consequences	Long-term consequences

 Step 3: Make change using an Action Plan

IDEAS TO CONSIDER INCORPORATING INTO MY ACTION PLAN

Overall Tips
Remember to start small and slowly build up to what you can safely tolerate. Use urge tolerating to support staying with the exposure.

Examples of Gradual Exposures

Avoidance behavior	Exposure strategy
Avoiding wearing a bathing suit	1) Purchase a new bathing suit 2) Wear a bathing suit around at home (with or without someone else present) 3) Go to the beach and spend x minutes without a cover-up 4) Go to a pool and engage in lap swim 5) Walk along the beach in a bathing suit 6) Wear a two-piece bathing suit
Avoid being in photographs	1) Take a selfie, do not edit 2) Ask a trusted support to take a photograph, do not edit 3) Include self in a group photograph, do not edit 4) Post an unedited photo on social media 5) Tag self in an unedited photo on a friend's social media 6) Post an unedited close-up photo on social media 7) Text an unpreferred photo to someone else, commenting only on the image's representation of the experience, not on physical appearance 8) Post an unpreferred photo on social media, commenting only on the image's representation of the experience, not on physical appearance

SAMPLE ACTION PLAN		DATE: 3/19
PROBLEM:	Not wearing a bathing suit	
CURRENT FREQUENCY (IF APPLICABLE):	Most days in the summer and vacation days in winter	
GOAL FOR UPCOMING WEEK:	Start working on gradual exposure by following steps that are doable for me. This Sample Action Plan is Step One. I will also use urge tolerating to support myself in sitting with the anxiety.	
SPECIFIC PLAN:	MY PLAN: Buy 4 new (returnable) bathing suitsonline tonight. I will try them on (2 at a time) on Saturday and Sunday without engaging in body checking.	MY SUPPORT: I will tell my partner I am going to buy one and ask that they check in with me about this. I will try them on in the morning after I take a shower and will plan urge tolerating after. I will plan to watch my favorite movie Sunday night as a reward for completing this task.

Handout 10.3 *Body Dissatisfaction Spikes Self-monitoring*

Name: _____ Date: _____ Day of the Week: _____

BODY DISSATISF ACTION SPIKES SELF-MONITORING

Time	Food and Drink	Place	*	v/l/d	e	Spike?	What else is happening that might be causing the spike?	Context and comments

Chapter 16

Group Session 11

Stage Three Check-in and Body Dissatisfaction Spikes

Overview

Session 11 offers an opportunity to review all Stage 3 interventions covered thus far, including reducing dieting behaviors, body checking and avoidance, and increasing minimized areas of life. Session 11 also introduces the concept of body dissatisfaction spikes as another factor maintaining the over-evaluation of shape and weight.

Stage 3 contains numerous interventions that are introduced in the sessions and then worked on by the patients at home (e.g., eating avoided foods, reducing frequent weighing). Throughout the sessions, review of this material is primarily patient led, through between-session work self-reviews. Patients typically are making many difficult changes over this time in areas of life that are significant for them (e.g., dieting, body image). These changes are critical for recovery. Additional review of the patient's progress with these changes is beneficial, with the hope that this supports patients with their momentum in treatment. Session 11 provides more in-depth group time to review engagement with the material and follow through on Action Plans.

The second part of the session explores body dissatisfaction spikes (see Figure 16.1). Body dissatisfaction spikes are common occurrences experienced by most people. These experiences are often transient – they come and go and usually do not have a significant impact on daily life experiences and goals. They are often triggered by physical sensations, thoughts, emotions, or behaviors. For individuals with eating disorders, these spikes can be more intense, longer lasting, significantly impact quality of daily living, and lead to eating disorder behaviors.

During this session, you will review and implement Group CBT-E's RAD Approach, used here to address body dissatisfaction spikes (see Figure 16.2).

Therapist Preparation

☐ Review this chapter in advance.
☐ Review accompanying handouts and have copies available for patients.
☐ Have access to each patient's *My Formulation* handout as this will be used in part of the session to highlight how body dissatisfaction spikes maintain their eating disorder.

DOI: 10.4324/9781003450849-20

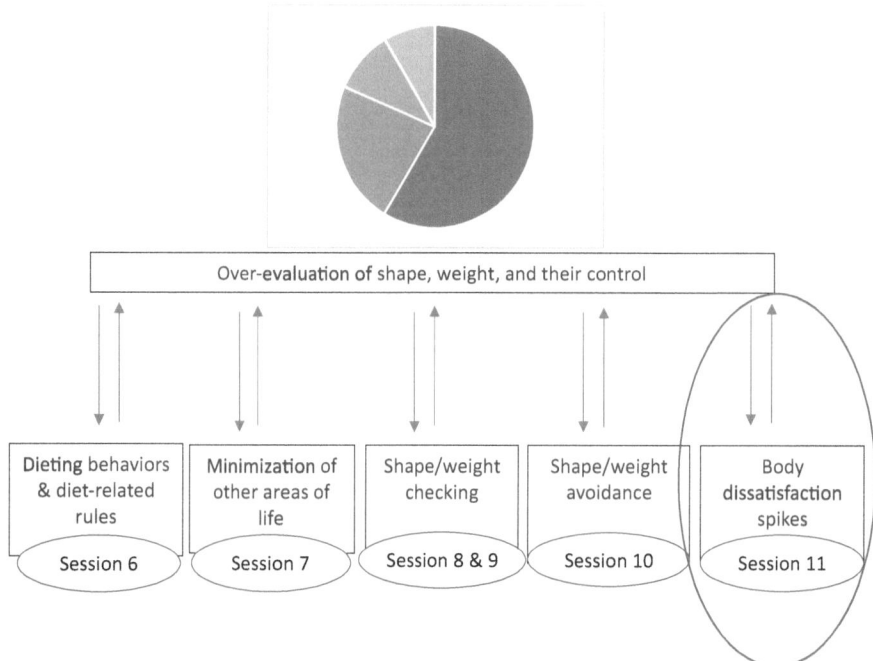

Figure 16.1 Extended formulation – Body dissatisfaction spikes.

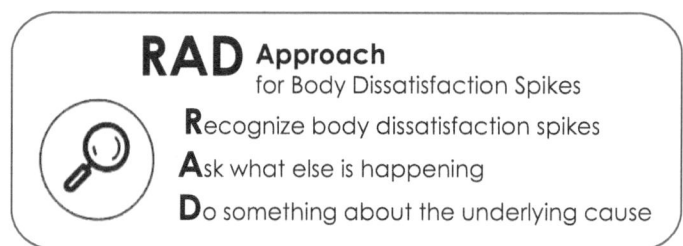

Figure 16.2 RAD Approach for body dissatisfaction spikes.

Handouts

- Standard Weekly Handouts
  - *1.1 My Formulation*
  - *1.3 Self-monitoring Form*
  - *1.6 Between-session Work Log*
  - *11.1 Between-session Work Self-review – Session 11*

- Session-specific Handouts
  - *11.2 Stage three Check-in*
  - *10.3 Body Dissatisfaction Spikes Self-monitoring*
  - *11.3 Body Dissatisfaction Spikes*

Group Session Agenda

1. Setting the agenda and orienting to the session (2 minutes)
2. Between-session work self-review (5 minutes)
3. Reviewing Stage 3 interventions (20 minutes)
4. Identifying body dissatisfaction spikes (10 minutes)
5. Identifying the triggers for body dissatisfaction spikes (10 minutes)
6. Addressing body dissatisfaction spikes (10 minutes)
7. Group wrap-up (3 minutes)

1. Setting the Agenda and Orienting to the Session

Begin with a positive, encouraging welcome; share that this is Session 11, Stage 3 with 3 sessions remaining. Clearly list the session agenda.

2. Between-session Work Self-review

Handout: *Between-session Work Self-review – Session 11*

Before handing out the between-session work self-review, let patients know that it is shorter than previous weeks. It only contains Stage 1 skills, as the group will be reviewing Stage 3 skills more in depth this session. Since the handout only contains Stage 1 skills, ask patients to pay close attention to how they are progressing with these items. As you have been, ask group members to share their progress and to specify what their Action Plans are. Encourage them to write the Action Plan on their *Between-session Work Log*.

3. Reviewing Stage Three Interventions

Handout: *Stage 3 Check-in*

At this point in the sequential format, the group has been putting in great effort to reduce the over-evaluation of shape and weight by removing or reducing its maintaining mechanisms. These include dieting behaviors and diet-related rules (Session 6), body checking (Sessions 8 and 9), and body avoidance (Session 10). The group has also been increasing minimized other areas of life (Session 7). Support the group in reviewing their progress in implementing related Action Plans and update any plans as needed. This session also serves as a time to check in with the patients about their treatment momentum – how much energy, commitment, and motivation they have at this point and how they can maintain or bolster this for the final sessions.

Before we move on to new content in group today, I wanted to take some time to check in on how you are doing with implementing your Action Plans and update these plans together if needed. I also wanted to check in on energy levels regarding the group and treatment. It is common to start to feel tired out by working so hard on challenging the eating disorder. First, we will go around to share how we are currently feeling about group and our ability to keep going for the final important weeks.

As patients share their thoughts and feelings about treatment and continuing for the final sessions, validate feelings of "treatment fatigue,'" praise their commitment so far, and emphasize the importance of finishing strong. Normalize any expressions of anxiety about the group coming to an end.

> *Some of you mentioned feeling a bit anxious about group coming to an end. This is under-standable and a common feeling about group ending. We have been together as a group for 11 weeks and during this time you have made tremendous changes. It makes sense that you may be nervous about losing the support of the group and worry about being able to continue to make progress after group is over. Let's take a moment to share these concerns together.*

Next, ask the group to take out their *Stage 3 Check-in* handout and complete Step 1 on the handout. Step 1 asks patients to consider each treatment intervention they have learned about in Stage 3. They are asked to consider a plan for addressing areas that would benefit from further improvement. Next ask patients to turn to Step 2 which provides space to consider which areas are "going well" and should be continued, and which areas are "not going well," or are "going ok." These areas are highlighted as opportunities to set new Action Plans and update existing Action Plans. Have the group share aloud with each other about their positive progress, as well as their plans for ways to improve areas they may be strug-gling with. One helpful Action Plan is to review relevant treatment materials from previous sessions in areas requiring more focused work.

> *Let's summarize some of what you have learned from Step 1 and now work to complete Step 2 on your Stage 3 Check-in handout. I will give you a minute to complete this step individu-ally and then we will discuss as a group. Please share what you have learned about things that are going well and why, as well as areas where you are struggling and thoughts you have about how to make change. Please use one another for support in identifying barriers and opportu-nities to try new strategies.*

Along with addressing all Stage 3 interventions, spend specific time exploring progress in reducing body avoidance introduced in the previous session. Check in on the exposures com-pleted between sessions, and how the exposure may have impacted feelings, behaviors, and thoughts. Praise patients for following through with avoidance exercises as these are often highly anxiety provoking to complete. Encourage the group to support and acknowledge each other's successes in tolerating anxiety and continuing with the exposure activity. Support patients in committing to the next step on their exposure hierarchy or working on a new exposure goal. This will be a between-session work item for the rest of the treatment. Patients will be expected to independently identify an exposure task that is progressively higher up on their hierarchy as they experience success with lower rated items.

After the check-in, give the group a moment to transition to the next agenda item focusing on new material related to identifying body dissatisfaction spikes.

4. Identifying Body Dissatisfaction Spikes

 Recognize Body Dissatisfaction Spikes

Handouts: *Body Dissatisfaction Spikes Self-monitoring; Body Dissatisfaction Spikes*

Briefly introduced in the last session, body dissatisfaction spikes are feelings of intense body dissatisfaction. They are often experienced as highly distressing and are associated with engaging in eating disorder behaviors. Many times, body dissatisfaction spikes occur as a result of behavior (e.g., body checking) or negative feelings (e.g., loneliness). Often when a patient experiences a spike, they believe the associated negative thoughts are true and may react with eating disorder behaviors to reduce the uncomfortable feelings and thoughts. For example, Alexis has the spike/thought: "Ugh, my thighs are disgusting," which she takes as fact and responds by increasing the number of lifting sessions she does at the gym and cutting back on her eating. The *cause* of the spike was the trigger of scrutinizing images of herself from a recent vacation. Stopping that body checking behavior could have prevented the spike and resulting eating disorder behaviors. Learning that feelings/thoughts are not facts; recognizing when these spikes happen and what they are related to/what triggers them; and identifying ways to address the underlying cause is essential to removing this maintaining mechanism.

> **Therapist Insight**
>
> We use the term *body dissatisfaction spikes* to capture all types of intensifications of body dissatisfaction. Patients will have their own term for this phenomenon. Be sure to use the language that best describes their experience. For some patients this may be "feeling gross," while for others, it may be "hating my body" and so on.

Begin by reviewing what body dissatisfaction spikes are and the three steps of the RAD Approach for addressing these spikes (share Figure 16.2 on the whiteboard). Remind patients that they used the RAD Approach as a tool to better understand *feelings of fullness* in Session 4. For the purposes of body dissatisfaction spikes, the language attached to the RAD Approach is slightly modified from feelings of fullness but maintains the same principles. To start, engage in the first step, **R**ecognize body dissatisfaction spikes. Ask patients to take out both their *Body Dissatisfaction Spikes Self-monitoring* and *Body Dissatisfaction Spikes* handouts.

Body dissatisfaction spikes are common for most people whether they have an eating disorder or not. They come and go and can often be related to thoughts, feelings, behaviors, and physical sensations. For people with eating disorders, body dissatisfaction spikes can have particularly unwanted long-term consequences, including keeping the eating disorder going. Take a look at your Body Dissatisfaction Spikes Self-monitoring handout that you completed this week. Let's start a list of body dissatisfaction spikes that you noticed [start creating a list like Column A in Table 16.1]. As we write these on the whiteboard, make sure to also include those that are relevant to you on your Body Dissatisfaction Spikes handout.

Table 16.1 Sample Whiteboard – RAD Approach for Addressing Body Dissatisfaction Spikes

A	B	C
Body dissatisfaction spike	Anything else happening?	Do something about the underlying cause
Feeling really gross at around 3pm Monday.	My period was just about to start and I always feel extra dissatisfied with my shape then – really bloated too.	Recognized my hormones are causing all the feels. Be gentle with myself and use some pampering or self-care that I like – taking a hot bath, drinking extra water, getting to bed early.
Hate my body 12pm Saturday.	Was walking with a friend and noticed I am not as built as he is.	Recognize our bodies are different. He spends a lot of time at the gym and in the end, that is not an important long-term value for me. I want to spend more time getting out and spending time with friends. Review comparison-making materials.
My stomach is just ick 11pm Friday.	Squeezing my belly.	Review body checking materials. Stop checking my body this way!
No part of my body looks good right now Sunday 2pm.	Preparing for a date and feeling nervous. Trying on lots of outfits, scrutinizing in the mirror.	Give myself grace – dating is anxiety provoking. Stop the checking behaviors. Call a friend for a pep talk session.
Nope, nope, nope! All parts of me. Yuck. 5:30pm Tuesday.	Fighting with my mom.	Review my formulation – no wonder I am obsessing about my body when I am fighting with mom, I have a really strong arrow there. Limiting what I eat is not going to solve the fight with my mom. In fact, it hurts me in the long run because I end up bingeing. Instead, distract myself for a little while and speak with mom when I feel calmer.
Feeling depressed about the way I look – for hours all day Wednesday.	Tons of scrolling on social media – comparison making.	Of course this is happening! Stop comparison making and stop social media time for now – change my environment, turn off my phone, and review related treatment material.

5. Identifying Triggers for Body Dissatisfaction Spikes

 <u>A</u>sk What Else is Happening

Handout: *My Formulation*

Next, ask patients to consider what may have triggered the spike in their body dissatisfaction. Frequently these spikes indicate that something else is happening (often unrelated to one's body or body changes) and instead are due to the over-evaluation of shape and weight. At times, these spikes may be viewed as evidence of actual body, shape, and/or weight changes. Support patients to challenge themselves to go beyond their assumption that body dissatisfaction spikes are a sign of a problem with their body or that their body has changed, to find the underlying cause of the increased dissatisfaction.

As an example, Devin is on his way to his office. He gets into the elevator on the way to the 10th floor. When he steps into the elevator, he is feeling pretty good. It is a beautiful spring day, he has a meeting at work that he is well prepared for, and thinks he has an innovative idea to share. He has planned an exciting date with his girlfriend after work. During the course of the elevator ride, Devin's mood becomes more negative, and he starts to feel disappointed in his body shape. By the time he gets off at the 10th floor, he is feeling horrible about his body. He has lots of thoughts about the parts he hates the most, and is having a hard time remembering why he was so excited about the day. Over the course of 10 floors, his view on the day and his body changed rapidly. Devin is not sure why he feels so badly about his body shape now.

In exploring what else was going on at the time when Devin was in the elevator, the following was uncovered: He walked into the elevator and, out of habit, immediately compared his body to others. He initially assessed that his muscular build and body size was about average compared to the other men in the elevator and felt OK about this. At the 5th floor, two more men got into the elevator and Devin compared his shape to theirs and determined that he was one of the least attractive men in the elevator. His body dissatisfaction started to spike. On the 7th floor, another man got into the elevator whom Devin saw as very fit and muscular. He started to feel that he was the least attractive person in the elevator and his body dissatisfaction really intensified.

In Devin's situation, it is the trigger of comparing his body to other men's bodies that caused this body dissatisfaction spike. Sometimes it can be difficult to identify the triggers for body dissatisfaction spikes, especially if the trigger occurred the previous evening, or earlier in the day. Encourage the group to go slowly back through a recent time when a spike occured to consider if there were any events, changes in emotional state, or thoughts that may have ultimately led to the spike. See Table 16.2 for examples of common triggers for body dissatisfaction spikes. Group members are particularly helpful in supporting one another to find triggers. If there does not seem to be a cause, that is OK too.

Now, let's move on to the next part of our RAD Approach. The A – asking yourself what else might be happening when you experience an increase in body dissatisfaction. Like we just did, use your Body Dissatisfaction Spikes handout and Body Dissatisfaction Spikes

Table 16.2 Common Triggers for Body Dissatisfaction Spikes

Shift in mood state (e.g., sad, guilty, anxious, bored, embarrassed)
Eating differently than intended (e.g., breaking a diet rule, eating more food, eating a challenging food)
Body checking behaviors (e.g., comparing to others, scrutinizing one's body in the mirror, looking down at one's body, scrolling on social media)
Sensations related to feeling clothes on one's body (e.g., wearing form-fitting clothes, wearing ill-fitting clothes, wearing more revealing clothes)
Seeing one's weight
Physical sensations (e.g., feelings of fullness, bloating, gastrointestinal upset, feeling hot/ sweaty)
Hearing someone else comment on their body size or diet plan
Social media use
Not sleeping well

Self-monitoring handout to help with this next step. Looking at our list on the whiteboard, let's think about the instances when you recorded a body dissatisfaction spike. Let's consider what else might have been happening? Make sure to pay particular attention to the thought itself, as well as any other behaviors, emotions, or situations that were going on. [Add another column, using Column B in Table 16.1 as an example.]

Next, ask patients how they would typically respond to experiencing a spike. Many patients react by engaging in eating disorder behaviors in an attempt to address the unpleasant feeling or thought.

It sounds like everyone in the group noticed that at some point in the last week, they experienced a body dissatisfaction spike. When this occurred, how did you respond? Did the intensity of this feeling make you engage in, or have the urge to engage in, eating disorder behaviors? Were there other consequences related to other feelings, behaviors, or thoughts?

For patients that do experience eating disorder behaviors/urges, validate that it is understandable that one would experience such behaviors/urges. Boxes A and F on the personalized formulations highlight the mechanism that eating disorder behaviors can be a response to the intensification of body dissatisfaction. For example, many patients share that they try to "diet harder"/restrict their intake when they experience a spike, or that these spikes cause feelings of being a failure, which can lead to other eating disorder symptoms (e.g., binge eating). The thoughts associated with body dissatisfaction spikes are frequently intensifications of the cognitions that drive the eating disorder (Box F). Have patients review their *My Formulation* handout to help visually explain this.

It makes sense that you would react to a spike by using an eating disorder behavior. If we look at your personalized formulations, you can see how many of the body dissatisfaction spikes are intensifications of what you put in this top box here, Box F. And we can see how these thoughts already drive the rest of the eating disorder. So it is understandable, if you felt a spike in one of these thoughts, that you would react by using the behaviors listed.

Therapist Insight

Encourage patients to view body dissatisfaction spikes as alarms signaling them to check in with themselves to see if some other matter or issue needs resolving.

6. Addressing Body Dissatisfaction Spikes

 ### Do Something about the Underlying Cause

Next, support patients in addressing body dissatisfaction spikes by recommending that they respond to what is causing the spikes (i.e., addressing the trigger directly), rather than the spike itself. This is not only helpful for decreasing the over-evaluation of shape and weight, but can also be helpful for making effective change to life problems (e.g., having an assertive conversation with a triggering father could potentially have much more positive benefits to the relationship than binge eating). Brainstorm together ways of responding to the underlying cause of the spike once it is identified and record these on the whiteboard (see Column C in Table 16.1). Patients can sometimes struggle with this last step. Encourage them to remember the strategies learned thus far related to addressing triggers to engaging in eating disorder behaviors, such as alternative activities, urge tolerating, and reducing or eliminating body checking and avoidance behaviors. Group members are often extremely helpful in providing each other with ideas on targeting the underlying issue(s).

7. Group Wrap-up

Session Review

In today's session, we reviewed all the different skills you have been working on in Stage 3.

Social Media Alert

Social media is a common trigger for body dissatisfaction spikes. It is important to assess for this and to discuss this openly in the group. If this is not brought up as an example of a trigger in the session, make sure to ask patients to consider this common trigger. Engage the patients in a discussion to apply the RAD Approach to social media behavior. For example:

- **R**ecognize body dissatisfaction spikes
  - I am at the train station and suddenly feel more depressed about my body.
- **A**sk what else is happening
  - I've been scrolling on social media while I wait for my train. While scrolling, I looked at dieting information and compared myself to a person I used to go to school with.
  - I am bored and have nothing else to do.
- **D**o something about the underlying cause
  - Stop using social media in this way (review Session 9). Occupy my brain with other things like math and word puzzles.

In the example above, this patient may consider using the information from the RAD Approach to also plan for the future. Perhaps they will realize that mindless social media scrolling when bored is a particularly

We considered how you are doing with sticking to Action Plans, updated plans, and made new Action Plans. We also explored body dissatisfaction spikes. We talked about how common they are, how they keep the eating disorder going, and how to address them when they occur. Over the next week and weeks to come, look out for these spikes and work to address the underlying cause as described in group today. Doing so will help protect you against feeling negatively about your body shape and weight, and also prevent engaging in eating disorder behaviors.

common personal trigger for body dissatisfaction spikes (as it is with many patients) and they will decide to plan ahead alternative activities during their commute. It may also benefit the patient to remember that starting to scroll through social media is a signal that they are at risk of body dissatisfaction spikes. The patient may need to identify common situations when this scrolling typically occurs and a plan for how to distract from this activity (e.g., if interested in current events, downloading a news app to occupy time instead).

Between-session Work

Remember to encourage patients to write the between-session work on their *Between-session Work Log* handout. The between-session work for Session 11 is:

- Continue work from previous sessions:
  - *Self-monitoring* – to be completed daily, in the moment.
  - *Regular Eating* – continue to prioritize regular eating using *Planning Ahead, Alternative Activities, Urge Tolerating*, and *Feelings of Fullness* to support this work.
  - *My Breaking Food Rules Plan*– continue to plan in avoided foods and break dietary rules.
  - *Other Areas of Life* – continue to focus on the one or two new/expanded areas.
  - *Body Checking* and *Body Avoidance* – create and implement Action Plans to reduce body checking and avoidance in all its forms.
  - Follow through with any Action Plans identified during the session.

- New work from Session 11:
  - *Body Dissatisfaction Spikes* – create and implement Action Plans to address body dissatisfaction spikes using the RAD Approach.

Higher Level of Care Adaptations: Modular Implementation

When this session is used modularly, the following adaptations are suggested.

Stage 3 check-in: Check-ins are an important part of HLOC treatment. Depending on the level of care, assessing treatment progress, skill implementation, and symptom change could happen on a daily or weekly basis, as this information is a useful part of a treatment plan to inform treatment needs both for the patient and the treatment team. These types of reviews can occur in a variety of different formats (e.g., group therapy, individual meetings, family therapy, community meetings) and with different providers (e.g., therapists, nurses, psychiatrists). We recommend that there are opportunities to have these check-ins in the format that works for your service and program to best support the patient in getting the full benefit of treatment. These types of reviews can occur as a piece of a session (as presented here) or can be an entire session, based on the needs of the group and the time resources available.

Body dissatisfaction spikes: This topic could be a standalone topic at HLOCs, or could be applied in conjunction with a review, depending on the needs of the group and the level of care. Addressing body dissatisfaction spikes can be implemented at all levels of care. However, for patients actively working on treatment goals to regain weight, these spikes can be difficult to differentiate. These patients often share that they are in a constant heightened state of body dissatisfaction as their body is actively changing. The process of regaining weight, a common and significant fear, often leads to intense body dissatisfaction. In these cases, it is crucial to support patients in tolerating the body dissatisfaction in order to return to health. It is important to validate this experience and help patients to identify particularly strong body dissatisfaction spikes that may occur during a treatment day. Apply the RAD Approach in these situations. Helping patients to view times when dissatisfaction spikes are even higher in a day can provide useful information about what else may be going on other than just dissatisfaction related to body changes, such as anxiety, body comparisons, guilt, breaking a diet rule, and feelings of fullness. Help to identify plans for addressing those triggers directly. Also, be aware of triggers that patients will identify related to body dissatisfaction spikes that are specific to HLOC treatment, for example, being asked to drink (or not to drink) a nutritional supplement, being told to prepare for discharge to a lower level of care, body comparisons with patients arriving to treatment that are in need of significant weight gain, and eating with new patients who are refusing their meals. In these situations, it can be useful to both plan for how to address these treatment-specific triggers, and explain how these concerns are generalizable to life outside the program (e.g., learning to complete your meal around another patient who is restricting will help to be able to eat at school one day even though friends may not be eating).

Group Session 11

Handout 11.1 *Between-session Work Self-review – Session 11*

BETWEEN-SESSION WORK SELF-REVIEW – SESSION 11

Skill/Goal	THIS IS GOING...			MY PLAN		
	Well	OK	Not Well	Make an Action Plan to address	Share with my support person for accountability	Praise myself for working hard on this!
Self-monitoring	☐	☐	☐	☐	☐	☐
Regular eating	☐	☐	☐	☐	☐	☐
Alternative activities	☐	☐	☐	☐	☐	☐
Urge tolerating	☐	☐	☐	☐	☐	☐
Addressing feelings of fullness	☐	☐	☐	☐	☐	☐
Additional Items						
	☐	☐	☐	☐	☐	☐
	☐	☐	☐	☐	☐	☐

The between-session self-review for Session 11 only contains Stage 1 interventions. This is because the first part of Session 11 is an in-depth, shared exploration of progress with Stage 3 interventions.

Which skills are going well? Great work, keep practicing them! Which skills am I struggling to use and need to prioritize? Plan to take action this week – write an **Action Plan** to address these.

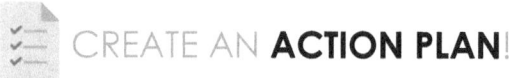

CREATE AN **ACTION PLAN**!

Handout 11.2   *Stage Three Check-in*

STAGE THREE CHECK-IN

You have been working on many different skills to reduce the over-evaluation of shape and weight that keeps the eating disorder going.

As a reminder, here are the Stage 3 topics you have covered so far:

- Session 6 – Reducing dieting behaviors and diet-related rules
- Session 7 – Increasing focus on other areas of life
- Session 8 & 9 – Reducing shape and weight checking behaviors
- Session 10 – Reducing shape and weight avoidance behaviors

Changing each of these takes time and lots of practice. Checking in to see how you are doing and sharing this with the group and your therapist will help you continue to make progress towards your recovery goals.

Step 1: Consider each element of treatment.

Skill/Goal	THIS IS GOING...			MY PLAN		
	Well	OK	Not Well	Make an Action Plan to address	Share with my support person for accountability	Praise myself for working hard on this!
Challenging diet-related rules	☐	☐	☐	☐	☐	☐
Eating avoided foods	☐	☐	☐	☐	☐	☐
Engaging in other areas of life activities	☐	☐	☐	☐	☐	☐
Reducing body checking with hands, measuring tools, and/or other people; and/or looking down at my body	☐	☐	☐	☐	☐	☐
Reducing reflection checking	☐	☐	☐	☐	☐	☐
Reducing body comparisons	☐	☐	☐	☐	☐	☐
Reducing social media body checking	☐	☐	☐	☐	☐	☐
Reducing body avoidance	☐	☐	☐	☐	☐	☐

Step 2: Reflect on the following questions. Be as specific as possible in identifying ways to continue practicing.

Which areas are going well?

What will help me to keep working on areas that are going well?

Which areas are going ok?

How might I continue to improve them?

Which areas are not going well?

What action can I take to improve them?

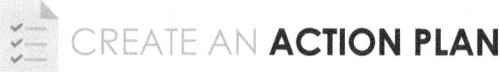 CREATE AN **ACTION PLAN**!

Handout 11.3   *Body Dissatisfaction Spikes*

BODY DISSATISFACTION SPIKES

Body dissatisfaction spikes are increases in body dissatisfaction. These occur for everyone; however, they tend to have increased severity and frequency for individuals with eating disorders. Oftentimes, these spikes are triggered by thoughts, feelings, behaviors, and/or events that may not be related to shape and weight changes, but are experienced as if they are **facts**.

See the example below of how body dissatisfaction spikes can occur throughout the day and examples of events, behaviors, feelings, and thoughts that can trigger the body dissatisfaction.

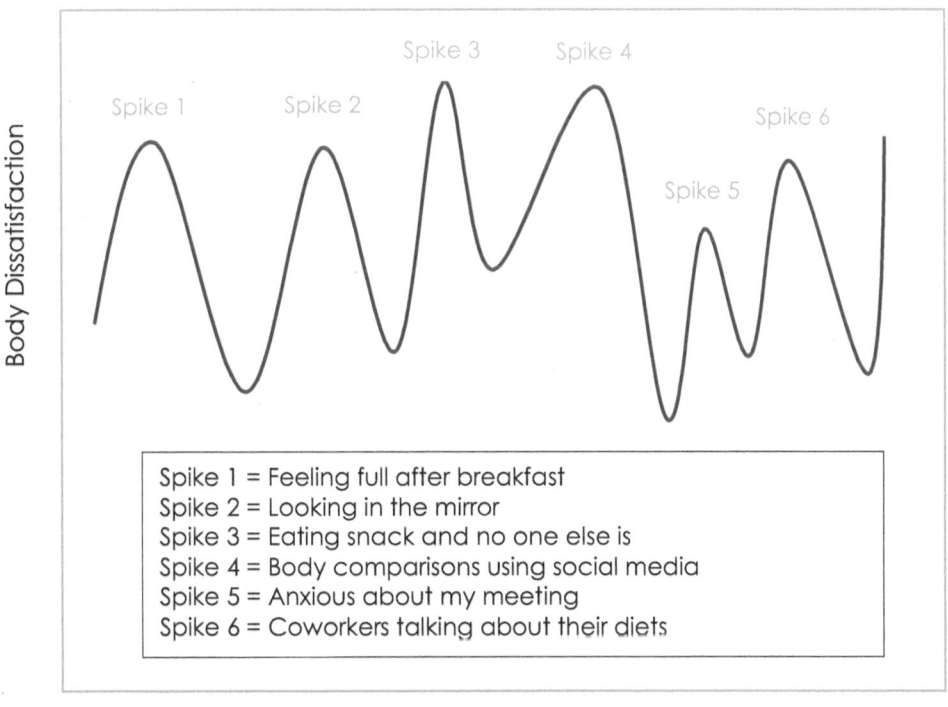

Spike 1 = Feeling full after breakfast
Spike 2 = Looking in the mirror
Spike 3 = Eating snack and no one else is
Spike 4 = Body comparisons using social media
Spike 5 = Anxious about my meeting
Spike 6 = Coworkers talking about their diets

In order to address body dissatisfaction spikes, try using the RAD Approach.

RAD **Approach**
for Body Dissatisfaction Spikes
Recognize body dissatisfaction spikes
Ask what is happening
Do something about the underlying cause

R: Recognize body dissatisfaction spikes	A: Ask what else is happening?	D: Do something about the underlying causes
Examples of my spikes	*Trigger(s)*	*How else could I address the trigger(s)?*

Overall Tips
Remember that addressing body dissatisfaction spikes means addressing the actual trigger directly.
Sometimes the best way to address body dissatisfaction spikes may be to reframe your thought. For example, as opposed to "I feel gross right now," relabel what is actually going on, for example, "I am tired and want to relax right now."
Sometimes, using the skills that you have already learned of alternative activities and urge tolerating can be very helpful with body dissatisfaction spikes.

SAMPLE ACTION PLAN		DATE: 11/9
PROBLEM:	Body dissatisfaction spikes	
CURRENT FREQUENCY (IF APPLICABLE):	Throughout the day	
GOAL FOR UPCOMING WEEK:	Use RAD each time I have a spike in body dissatisfaction.	
SPECIFIC PLAN:	MY PLAN:	MY SUPPORT:
	When body dissatisfaction spikesare related to my mood, use supports.	Call my sibling and vent. Send a text to a friend. Distract myself by looking up a fun community activity to do in my town.
	When body dissatisfaction spikes are related to my thoughts, reframe thoughts.	Write down my thoughts and write out the RAD Approach.

Chapter 17

Group Session 12
Events, Emotions, and Eating

Overview

Life events and changes in one's emotional state can greatly impact eating behavior. This is not only true for individuals with eating disorders, but is also typical for most people without eating disorders. It is common for media to portray food or eating as a soothing strategy after a difficult day. Think of the many gifs and memes featuring someone looking stressed eating a pint of ice cream with the aim of feeling better. In fact, this particular food has become so synonymous as a way to reduce stress or relax that it has its own term: "an ice-cream binge." While this misuse of the term "binge" here is problematic as it diminishes the seriousness of binge eating for those with eating disorders, the common use of the term highlights that food can, and often does, settle our emotions.

This group focuses on the impact that life events and emotions have on eating. As highlighted on the formulation, both life events and various emotional states can keep the eating disorder going. Expanding on the original Individual CBT-E formulation which has life events and emotions leading to binge eating, we have added bidirectional arrows to indicate that binge eating also impacts life events and emotions (described in Session 1). We have also added other bidirectional arrows indicating that for many people, events and emotions have an impact on all aspects of the eating disorder and vice versa. Figure 17.1 shows that events/emotions not only impact binge eating in this example, but likely also dieting, driven exercise, and body dissatisfaction.

There are two main skills to address this aspect of an eating disorder: problem-solving and behavior/urge analysis. In addition to these skills, patients are provided with information and a handout to support them in slowing down their reaction to urges and tolerating intense emotional dysregulation.

Therapist Preparation

☐ Review this chapter in advance.
☐ Review accompanying handouts and have copies available for patients.

DOI: 10.4324/9781003450849-21

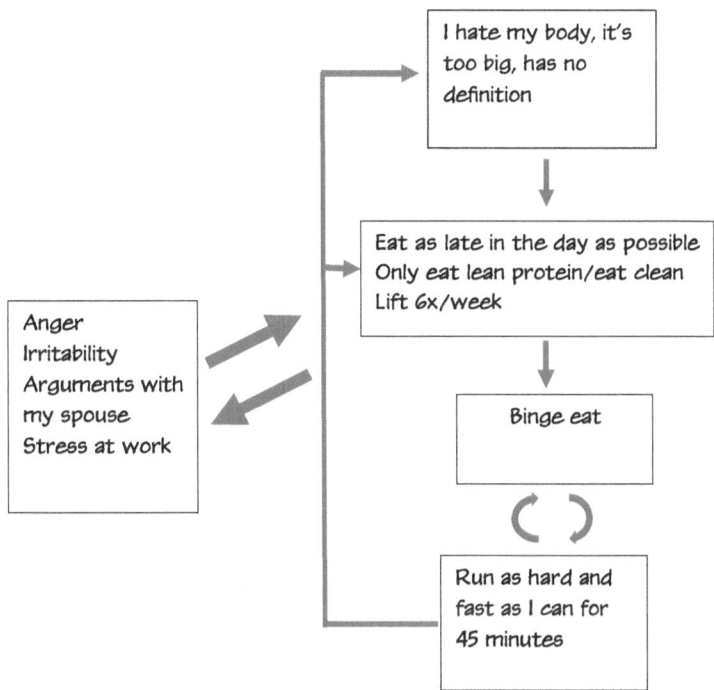

Figure 17.1 Reciprocal impact of events and emotions on eating.

Handouts

- Standard Weekly Handouts
  - *1.1 My Formulation*
  - *1.3 Self-monitoring*
  - *1.6 Between-session Work Log*
  - *12.1 Between-session Work Self-review – Session 12*

- Session-specific Handouts
  - *12.2 Problem-solving*
  - *12.3 Eating Disorder Behavior/Urge Analysis*
  - *12.4 Breaking the Emotion and Eating Disorder Behavior Connection*

Group Session Agenda

1. Setting the agenda and orienting to the session (2 minutes)
2. Between-session work self-review (5 minutes)
3. Identifying the impact of emotions and events on eating (15 minutes)
4. Addressing the impact of emotions and events on eating (35 minutes)

   a. Problem-solving
   b. Eating disorder behavior/urge analysis
   c. Slowing down and tolerating intense emotions

5. Group wrap-up (3 minutes)

1. Setting the Agenda and Orienting to the Session

Begin with a positive, encouraging welcome; share that this is Session 12 of Stage 3 with 2 sessions remaining. Clearly list the session agenda.

2. Between-session Work Self-review

Handout: *Between-session Work Self-review – Session 12*

Ask patients to complete their *Between-session Work Self-review – Session 12* handout. This review asks patients to reflect on progress with Stage 1 elements and Stage 3 interventions (dieting behaviors; diet-related rules; enhancing other areas of life; reducing body checking and avoidance; and addressing body dissatisfaction spikes). As always, the idea is to praise patients for the things that are going well; identify barriers and how to address such obstacles; and build on the existing interventions by identifying increasingly challenging ways to address eating disorder symptoms. For this session, check that everyone who shared experiencing body dissatisfaction spikes has been using the RAD Approach to address these and encourage continued use. At the end of the review, encourage patients to create updated Action Plans to reflect goals for the week, and include these on their *Between-session Work Log*.

3. Identifying the Impact of Emotions and Events on Eating

Handout: *My Formulation*

At this point in treatment, the connection between emotions and events, and how they maintain the eating disorder, has been highlighted several times, though perhaps indirectly. The personalized formulation (Session 1) included events and emotions as a maintaining mechanism. Self-monitoring records further highlight this connection, as emotions are often identified on the context and comments column as potential triggers to eating disorder behaviors.

In this session, the interaction of emotions and events on eating disorder behavior will be addressed more directly. Consistent with much of the learning throughout this treatment guide, the first step to address this mechanism is to increase awareness of these relationships and to help patients identify when emotions and events are triggering changes in their eating.

Many patients may already be aware of the connection, but others may not. For

> **Therapist Insight**
>
> For many patients, eating disorder behaviors can provide comfort and are self-soothing. As treatment works to remove these behaviors, it is essential to support patients in identifying other ways to provide themselves with comfort and alternative self-soothing techniques. Ask patients to create a list of ideas and to store this list somewhere easy to access. Frequently shared ideas include burning a scented candle, looking at pictures of loved ones, following a guided meditation, enjoying a hot drink, engaging in some joyful movement, watching a favorite show, coloring, creating/listening to a soothing playlist, and wrapping up in a comfortable blanket.

some patients, their life stressors do not have an impact on their eating habits, though this is less common in our experience. Introduce this topic in an engaging manner by asking patients to review the emotions and events box (Box E) on their personalized formulations and the role they play in maintaining their eating disorder.

Let's take a moment to review the events and emotions box on your formulations. For some of you, what happens in your life can have a very big impact on your eating. For example, binge eating or extreme food restriction can frequently be a response to a stressful life situation – such as an argument with a friend or a bad day at work. Who is aware of using food to help regulate their emotions, self-soothe, or deal with life stress or unpleasant emotions? [Have patients indicate their response.]

It looks like most, but not all, of you experience this. It makes sense that we have different responses as we know that each person's eating disorder is unique to them. Now, what about how the eating disorder impacts your life, for example, having a hard time eating out with friends? [Again, have patients indicate their response and share relevant examples.]

After highlighting how events, emotions, and eating are impacting one another, share with the group the work for the session:

Based on how many of you raised your hand, we can see that the eating disorder and emotional states are interacting a great deal. Let's move on to the skills that can help to protect against the impact emotions and events have on eating and vice versa. For those of you that do not experience or relate to this aspect of an eating disorder, I encourage you to stay alert and engaged to support your groupmates. You will likely have some ideas that will be very helpful for them, and you may potentially learn new things about your eating disorder.

4. Addressing the Impact of Emotions and Events on Eating

a. Problem-solving

Handout: *Problem-solving*

After identifying and increasing awareness of the impact of emotions and events on maintaining an eating disorder, the next step is to support patients in identifying how to break these connections and experiment with making new choices. The first skill is problem-solving. This skill is widely used in CBT at large, as it can be a highly effective, and well-liked, intervention. Problem-solving is a tool that helps in spotting potential problems before they occur, allowing someone to be prepared and have a plan in place to help handle the situation. The key is that problem-solving occurs ahead of a stressful event. This allows for advanced planning, when one is in a calm state. Planning when calm allows for well thought-out options for how one might want to handle the situation. It is much easier to plan when stress levels are low than in the middle of a highly distressing situation.

There are seven steps in problem-solving:

Step 1: Identify the problem as early as possible.

Step 2: Specify the problem.

Step 3: Consider as many solutions as possible.

Step 4: Consider the pros and cons of each possible solution.

Step 5: Choose the best option or combination of options.

Step 6: Take action! Go for it and try out the solution decided on.

Step 7: Evaluate your problem-solving skill use.

Therapist Insight

Be careful to ensure that you are slowly going through each of these steps with the patients. At times, therapists take shortcuts in this process, thinking that a more basic, nonspecific brainstorming process for how to solve problems suffices. We strongly recommend offering your patients the opportunity to learn this skill in its entirety.

Using a volunteer and the *Problem-solving* handout, illustrate the problem-solving process.

One of the ways you can avoid having events in your life cause changes to your eating or other eating disorder symptoms is by looking out for problems in advance of them occurring and thinking through ways to handle the situation. This is called problem-solving. It is a skill that you can develop and practice. Over time, it becomes a habit and something that occurs without needing to work so hard at it. Today we are going to use your Problem-solving handout to go through the problem-solving steps together. Who would like to share an upcoming event or circumstance that is likely to trigger their eating disorder?

Problem-solving works particularly well in the group setting, especially Steps 3 and 4 which often benefit from many minds thinking together. When explored as a group, we have found that potential solutions are more creative and pros and cons more developed. Present problem-solving by asking a volunteer:

• To share an anticipated problem that will occur in the next week (e.g., a stressful family function, an evening alone, a weekly staff meeting).

• To share aloud their answers for Step 1 and 2.

• To complete Steps 3 and 4 to generate solutions first, and then go back to identify the pros and cons of each solution. Ask other group members to help identify ideas. Make sure to encourage the group to be as creative as possible.

• To complete Step 5 by identifying which option(s) is best for them.

• To complete Step 6 by putting a specific plan in place (e.g., when, where, how) to take action.

• To complete Step 7 as between-session work. This is a highly valuable and important step. Evaluating the use of problem-solving for an example that has not occurred yet is impossible. Instead describe to the group how to conduct the evaluation of their problem-solving skills by saying: *The next day after you attempted problem-solving, it is important to check*

Table 17.1 Example of Problem-solving

Problem!

Step 1: Going to a family reunion tomorrow

Step 2: Worried that my family members will comment on my body shape and also pressure me with questions about who I am dating

Steps 3 and 4: Pros and cons of my options

   a. Not go
   + avoid upsetting comments and questions
   - miss out on seeing my cousins

   b. Have mom talk to everyone in advance about not commenting/asking questions
   + they will listen to mom
   - don't want to put mom in the middle

   c. Tell the family on the group chat that my body and love life are off limits
   + they will listen to me
   - someone might get offended

   d. Bring a friend with me for moral support
   + my friends always back me up and get it
   - don't want to be a burden...but don't think I will be

Step 5: Options c and d are best – and I will ask the group to help me craft the text message!

Step 6: Send text during group and call my friend after group to invite her

Step 7: I'll let you know how it goes!

---

in on your use of the skill. Assess how closely you followed the problem-solving steps, not on how successful you were in dealing with or avoiding the problem. See Table 17.1.

After the volunteer has completed their problem-solving process, ask all group members to complete their own *Problem-solving* handout with an anticipated problem that is occurring in the upcoming week. The goal is for patients to identify a plan prior to the end of the group. Give a time limit for working on this in the session to allow for completing the rest of the session agenda. If a plan is only partially finished by the end of the session, encourage patients to complete it as between-session work. If time allows, patients can share aloud areas of their problem-solving plan where they are stuck and use the group for support.

For between-session work, patients will complete the *Problem-solving* handout several times (on at least two different days). As with all skills, we recommend that patients continue to use this tool following the conclusion of the group for at least several weeks, if not longer.

b. Eating Disorder Behavior/Urge Analysis

Handout: *Eating Disorder Behavior/Urge Analysis*

Typically at this point in treatment eating disorder behaviors have likely significantly reduced. For behaviors that remain or are "residual," conducting an eating disorder behavior/urge analysis is a helpful tool. On occasions when the patient engages in, or has the urge to engage in, an eating disorder behavior, encourage curiosity. Teach the patient to examine, question, and learn from the situation by systematically reviewing what led up to the behavior or urge. Patients often believe these behaviors and urges occur without any cause. This view can be harmful as it can leave patients believing they have no ability to change these behaviors or urges. Analyzing behaviors and urges, after they occur, helps patients to monitor patterns; question what works and does not work for them; and learn from these experiences to potentially make change the next time similar situations occur.

> **Therapist Insight**
>
> It is not expected that all behaviors will have stopped at this point in treatment. Remaining behaviors let us know what areas need further practice. If a patient is no longer experiencing symptoms, ask patients to identify when they have had urges to engage in behaviors and to fill out the *Eating Disorder Behavior/Urge Analysis* handout based on these.

The aim is to help patients see the underlying causes of engaging in these behaviors. By identifying the causes, patients can then put in place the best skill to help them not engage in the eating disorder behavior in the future. Teach this skill using the *Eating Disorder Behavior/Urge Analysis* handout and engaging a volunteer.

Now that we have had the chance to think about how to scan ahead and plan for problems, let's also think about the flip side – what to do when you haven't had the chance to implement those strategies and an eating disorder behavior or strong urge to engage in a behavior has occurred. Let's use an example to think this through. Who would be willing to share a recent time when they have had an eating disorder behavior (e.g., binge eating, restricting, driven exercising) or had a strong urge? We will use this example to help us complete the components of the Eating Disorder Behavior/Urge Analysis handout.

Engage the volunteer in completing the handout aloud, while you draw the handout on a whiteboard during the discussion, and use the support of the group, when needed.

The analysis includes asking the patients to assess five likely factors that might trigger eating disorder behaviors/urges:

1. *Psychological pressure*: Breaking a diet-related rule can lead to eating disorder behaviors. Often, breaking a rule causes someone to feel that they have "given up," "been bad," or "failed" which leads to increased anxiety, shame, and guilt. Binge eating is one example of what can occur when someone feels that they have failed and disappointed in themselves that it no longer feels worth trying to resist urges to binge. This is when thoughts like "I'll start fresh again tomorrow" (meaning to diet harder) or "I've already messed up, what's the point" seem to lead to later binge eating. The discomfort in breaking a rule can also trigger other eating disorder behaviors to compensate for the food eaten (e.g., self-induced vomiting, laxative use, driven exercise, dieting).
2. *Being disinhibited*: Disinhibition could be related to any factor impacting a patient's judgment (e.g., alcohol or drug use; poor sleep). It is most often associated with binge eating, though for some it can lead to undereating.

3. *Physiological pressure*: Not eating enough puts one at physiological risk of overeating or bingeing. For some, undereating can also lead to further food restriction. The *Undereating/ Underfat* handout is a helpful resource which provides more details on this.
4. *Events or circumstances*: As discussed throughout this chapter, these can greatly impact and maintain eating disorder behaviors.
5. *Emotion dysregulation*: This can lead to a variety of eating disorder behaviors as a way to soothe or self-regulate.

After assessing all these factors, support the volunteer in completing the "What could I do differently next time?" box on the handout to identify action steps to decrease the likelihood that a residual behavior or urge will occur. Group members are often a great help in supporting the volunteer in naming action steps to protect against future eating disorder behaviors and urges. It can be useful to share with patients that the eating disorder can cause a distraction from the underlying problem.

> *This exercise helps you to think about what is triggering these behaviors. Once you can determine the triggers, you will be able to address them and decrease the eating disorder behaviors. This skill helps you to think beyond your urges/behaviors to ask yourself, "Why am I using these behaviors? What is triggering them?" and then you can address the triggers directly. For example, Naomi restricted her food intake at lunch. She started to get down on herself and think that she just needed to do "better" (diet more) the next day and started to focus a lot on food. The trigger for her missed lunch was that she was stressed about arguing with her girlfriend. If she only focuses on her food restriction as the problem, she will lose sight of the actual problem – the argument – and that problem will never be resolved through restricting. So, I want you to use these behaviors/urges as a signal to check in with yourself about what else is going on.*

For between-session work, patients will be asked to complete the *Eating Disorder Behavior/ Urge Analysis* handout when they experience eating disorder behaviors or urges over the course of the week.

c. Slowing Down and Tolerating Intense Emotions

Handout: *Breaking the Emotion and Eating Disorder Behavior Connection*

Residual Symptoms/Urges

Remember, normalize lapses for your patients! Residual behaviors are normal and expected at this point in treatment. Patients may feel disappointed that they have had a slip-up, despite working incredibly hard in treatment thus far. Support them by reminding them that they have been engaging in their eating disorder for a long time and that changing eating disorder behaviors takes time and a lot of self-compassion.

Residual symptoms offer an opportunity to begin relapse prevention work. For example, a patient may come to group upset they have binged, and you might say: *While I can see that you are disappointed that you binged and I am sorry that you feel badly, I am actually pleased (I know it is strange I am saying this) that this happened while you are still in the group. We can learn so much about your eating disorder from exploring this binge and help you to be better protected against binge eating the next time you find yourself in a similar situation. Let's think of this as an important learning opportunity.*

A third strategy is to slow down the time between experiencing an intense emotion and reacting to it. For some patients it can almost feel automatic to respond to strong emotions by engaging in an eating disorder behavior immediately. This makes sense since engaging in these behaviors is highly effective in changing or regulating emotions. However, the effect is often short-lived and keeps the eating disorder going in the long term. When used in this way, engaging in eating disorder behaviors can be viewed similarly to other maladaptive coping skills, such as drinking alcohol, taking substances, overspending, or non-suicidal self-injurious behaviors.

Remember, patients who experience intense emotional dysregulation that interferes with engaging in Group CBT-E are not suitable for the group (described in Chapter 3) and may benefit from targeted treatment for the emotional dysregulation before addressing the eating disorder. For patients who experience emotional dysregulation to a lesser extent and use eating disorder behaviors to regulate their emotional state, the *Breaking the Emotion and Eating Disorder Behavior Connection* handout may be a beneficial tool.

The main goals are to: 1) support the patients in evaluating the likelihood that engaging in an eating disorder behavior will help a situation in the long term; and 2) if not helpful in the long term, to encourage them to return to the skills of problem-solving, urge tolerating, and alternative activities. The handout provides one additional and highly valuable benefit – taking time to fill in the form is a slowing-down activity in itself. Slowing down the time between experiencing an intense emotion and reacting to it allows for the intensity to diminish somewhat and for the person to make a more informed, controlled choice about how they want to respond.

We've talked about how eating disorder behaviors provide a useful benefit of regulating emotions and decreasing anxiety, and are self-soothing. For some people, the urge or the emotional dysregulation is so intense they react quickly by engaging in a behavior. This makes sense. When we experience an intense unpleasant feeling we want it to go away quickly. Is anyone aware of reacting almost instantly to intense emotions? What behaviors do you use? [Wait to see if there are examples from the group, and then add to them.]

Examples that we often see are vomiting after a binge to reduce fear of anticipated weight change, binge eating in response to an argument, or greatly restricting eating to deal with feelings of uncertainty. Does anyone recognize any of these behaviors? It's no surprise that the eating disorder serves this additional function. To some extent, engaging in these behaviors works. Vomiting after binge eating does reduce anxiety, and binge eating after an argument can improve emotions, and likewise, calorie restriction does give some sense of control. However, the benefits are often short-lived and actually keep the eating disorder going in the long term. [Return to the formulation to highlight the arrows indicating how engaging in these behaviors maintains the eating disorder.]

Ask for a volunteer and take patients through the questions on the *Breaking the Emotion and Eating Disorder Behavior Connection* handout. As you complete the handout as a group, ask a patient to remind the group about urge tolerating- how intense urges (and in this case emotions) rise and then, with time, come back down.

For the next week, encourage patients to look out for times when they use their eating disorder behaviors to regulate their emotions. Encourage the group to look for opportunities to complete the handout between sessions in the moment when urges to use behaviors is occurring. It is essential to emphasize the importance of real-time completion. Not all patients require this work as some may not regulate emotions with eating disorder behaviors. Individualize the between-session work to each patient's needs.

5. Group Wrap-up

Session Review

In today's session we considered how life events and our emotions play a role in keeping the eating disorder going. We learned several skills today that help to deal with life events and emotions: problem-solving, eating disorder behavior analysis, and breaking the emotion and eating disorder behavior connection. The more you practice these skills, the easier in time they will become and the better you will be at not using eating disorder behaviors (e.g., binge eating, self-induced vomiting, driven exercise) to alleviate distress or regulate your emotions.

Between-session Work

Remember to encourage patients to write the between-session work on their *Between-session Work Log* handout. The between-session work for Session 12 is:

- Continue work from previous sessions:
  - *Self-monitoring* – to be completed daily, in the moment.
  - *Regular Eating* – continue to prioritize regular eating using *Planning Ahead, Alternative Activities, Urge Tolerating*, and *Feelings of Fullness* to support this work.
  - *My Breaking Food Rules Plan* – continue to plan in avoided foods and break dietary rules.
  - *Other Areas of Life* – continue to focus on the one or two new/expanded areas.
  - *Body Checking* and *Body Avoidance* – create and implement Action Plans to reduce body checking and avoidance in all its forms.
  - *Body Dissatisfaction Spikes* – create and implement Action Plans to address body dissatisfaction spikes using the RAD Approach.
  - Follow through with any Action Plans identified during the session.
- New work from Session 12:
  - *Problem-Solving; Eating Disorder Behavior/Urge Analysis; Breaking the Emotion and Eating Disorder Behavior Connection* – review these handouts and practice problem solving at least two times over the next week, and the additional skills (i.e., urge analysis, breaking the emotion/behavior connection) as needed.

Higher Level of Care Adaptations: Modular Implementation

When this session is used modularly, the following adaptations are suggested.

Events, emotions, and eating: Much of this session can be implemented as described at all HLOCs. At HLOCs, behaviors and urges will not be residual or infrequent, they are likely very active and occurring frequently. As such, modify your language when introducing the concept of the connection between events, emotions, and eating. All the interventions discussed in this session can be particularly useful at HLOCs. HLOC treatment itself, with its requirements and expectations (e.g., needing to complete meals, participate in therapy, restrict activity), can bring on many uncomfortable and intense emotions. These tools may need to be used consistently throughout a treatment day. For example, The *Breaking the Emotion and Eating Disorder Behavior Connection* handout could be carried around by patients to work through a multitude of difficult situations that may occur throughout a treatment day (e.g., mealtime, being asked by a nurse to stop exercising, feeling anxious about an upcoming family therapy session, feeling disappointed about a psychiatry meeting).

Group Session 12

Handout 12.1   *Between-session Work Self-review – Session 12*

BETWEEN-SESSION WORK SELF-REVIEW – SESSION 12

Skill/Goal	THIS IS GOING...			MY PLAN		
	Well	OK	Not Well	Make an Action Plan to address	Share with my support person for accountability	Praise myself for working hard on this!
Self-monitoring	☐	☐	☐	☐	☐	☐
Regular eating	☐	☐	☐	☐	☐	☐
Alternative activities	☐	☐	☐	☐	☐	☐
Urge tolerating	☐	☐	☐	☐	☐	☐
Addressing feelings of fullness	☐	☐	☐	☐	☐	☐
Challenging diet-related rules	☐	☐	☐	☐	☐	☐
Eating avoided foods	☐	☐	☐	☐	☐	☐
Engaging in 1–2 other areas of life activities	☐	☐	☐	☐	☐	☐
Reducing body checking overall	☐	☐	☐	☐	☐	☐
Reducing reflection checking	☐	☐	☐	☐	☐	☐
Reducing body comparisons	☐	☐	☐	☐	☐	☐
Reducing social media body checking	☐	☐	☐	☐	☐	☐
Reducing body avoidance	☐	☐	☐	☐	☐	☐
Addressing body dissatisfaction spikes	☐	☐	☐	☐	☐	☐

Which skills are going well? Which skills am I struggling to use? Do I need an **Action Plan**?

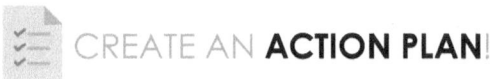

PROBLEM-SOLVING

Step 1: Identify the problem as early as possible:

_____

Step 2: Specify the problem:

_____

Step 3: Consider as many solutions as possible:

1)	4)
2)	5)
3)	6)

Step 4: Consider the pros and cons of each possible solution:

1) + −	4) + −
2) + −	5) + −
3) + −	6) + −

Step 5: Choose the best option or combination of options.

Step 6: Take action! Go for it and try out the solution you decided on.

Step 7: Evaluate your problem-solving skill use. This is best done the next day when you have had some space from practicing the skill. Ask yourself:
- How did I do with each step of problem solving?
- Did I complete all 6 steps?
- Did I praise myself?

Great work returning to evaluate your use of the skill! Remember you are not evaluating whether or not it worked. You are evaluating how well you worked through the steps.

SELF-CHECK: How many of the steps did you complete?

☐ Completed all   ☐ Completed half   ☐ Completed less than half

Handout 12.3   *Eating Disorder Behavior/Urge Analysis*

EATING DISORDER BEHAVIOR/URGE ANALYSIS

Psychological Pressure
(Did I break a diet-related rule? Am I denying myself foods I would enjoy eating?)

_____

_____

_____

Physiological Pressure
(Am I feeding my body the amount of food it needs?)

_____

_____

_____

Name the **Behavior/Urge**
(Binge, vomit, etc.)

_____

Being Disinhibited
(Did I drink alcohol or take any substances? Am I too tired?)

_____

_____

Events or Circumstances
(Did anything happen in my life that could have triggered this urge/behavior?)

_____

_____

_____

Emotion Dysregulation
(How was my mood leading up to the urge or behavior? Was I feeling regulated?)

_____

_____

What could I do differently next time?

_____

_____

_____

_____

_____

BREAKING THE EMOTION AND
EATING DISORDER BEHAVIOR CONNECTION

Step 1: Name the situation. What is happening?

_____

Step 2: Which eating disorder behavior(s) do I feel the urge to engage in?

_____

Step 3: Will using this behavior help me to feel better/more regulated in the short term?

_____

Step 4: Will using this behavior help me to feel better/more regulated in the long term?

_____

Step 5: Is using this behavior aligned with my recovery goals?

_____

Step 6: If 'no' for any questions (3–5): **Do not do the behavior**!

Step 7: Instead, return to **problem-solving**, use your **alternate activities** list, and practice **urge tolerating**.

Remember these skills take time to master. It will likely take many times of practice for them to become habits. You have relied on your eating disorder for a long time in stressful situations and so it will take time for these new behaviors to become automatic. Keep practicing – you can do this!

Ending Well

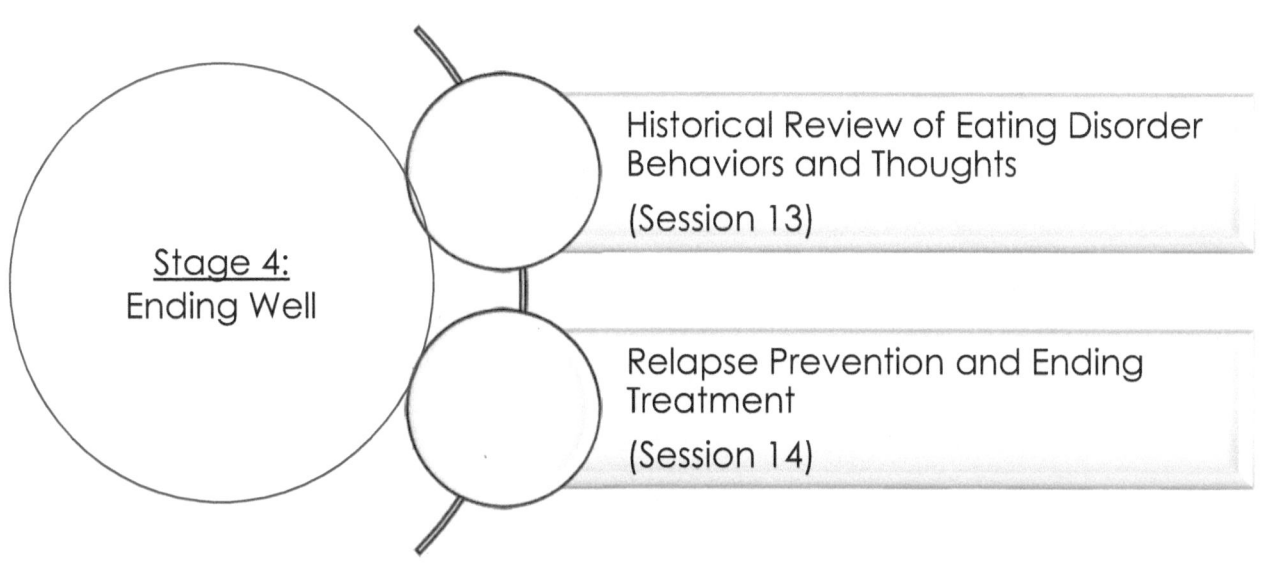

Chapter 18

Group Session 13

Historical Review of Eating Disorder Behaviors and Thoughts

Stage 4 of Group CBT-E focuses on ending well. This includes patients considering letting their eating disorder go, making plans for staying on track with recovery, and addressing thoughts and feelings related to treatment ending. By the end of Stage 4, patients' progress and discharge status is assessed, follow-up treatment recommendations are made, and therapist self-reflection is conducted.

Overview

Much of CBT-E, like all cognitive behavior therapy, is both present and future focused. CBT-E focuses on understanding and addressing what is keeping the disorder going currently, as well as planning for the future. In this session only, the treatment focus shifts to the past, exploring the origins of the patient's eating disorder behaviors and thoughts. By exploring these origins, CBT-E seeks to enhance patients' insight into the historical influences that may have sensitized them to shape, weight, and eating behaviors over time. This process often fosters self-empathy and compassion, as patients reflect on the specific factors, events, and situations that potentially contributed to the development of their eating disorder.

This *historical review* explores the effect of stressful life events and acknowledges that the eating disorder may have served a beneficial function initially, providing comfort or a sense of control over these events. The review also explores the ongoing impact of the eating disorder and unwanted consequences. Patients are offered the opportunity to reassess whether these behaviors continue to serve a constructive purpose in their present lives. Through this exploration, patients may move toward letting some of these perspectives go or leaving them in the past to better shape their current and future lives.

The historical review explores 4 timepoints (Fairburn et al., 2008):

1. Before any eating disorder behaviors or symptoms occurred (life up to 12 months before the start of eating disorder behaviors/symptoms)
2. The 12 months immediately prior to the onset of the eating disorder
3. The 6–12 months after the eating disorder behaviors started
4. Since then

DOI: 10.4324/9781003450849-23

Note that in cases where patients have experienced trauma, the content of this group may be inappropriate. Use your clinical judgment, knowledge of the patient, and patient preferences to determine the appropriateness of attending this group. If relevant, speak with patients in advance to determine if they would like to attend the group or if they would prefer to miss it. An individual session to review the material may be useful or it may be better to leave out this intervention completely.

Therapist Preparation

☐ Review this chapter in advance.
☐ Review accompanying handouts and have copies available for patients, including a final blank copy of the EDE-Q and CIA.

Handouts

* Standard Weekly Handouts
  ○ *1.3 Self-monitoring*
  ○ *1.6 Between-session Work Log*
  ○ *13.1 Between-session Work Self-review – Session 13*

* Session-specific Handouts
  ○ *EDE-Q and CIA (available at www.cbte.co)*
  ○ *13.2 Historical Review*

Group Session Agenda

1. Setting the agenda and orienting to the session (2 minutes)
2. Between-session work self-review (5 minutes)
3. Exploring the historical review of eating disorder behaviors and thoughts (25 minutes)
4. Reflecting on the historical review of eating disorder behaviors and thoughts (20 minutes)
5. Preparation for Session 14 (5 minutes)
6. Group wrap-up (3 minutes)

1. Setting the Agenda and Orienting to the Session

Begin with a positive, encouraging welcome; share that this is Session 13 and the first session of Stage 4 with 1 session remaining; and clearly list the session agenda.

2. Between-session Work Self-review

Handout: *Between-session Work Self-review – Session 13*

Ask patients to complete their *Between-session Work Self-review – Session 13* handout. This review asks patients to reflect on progress with Stage 1 elements and Stage 3 interventions (dieting behaviors; diet-related rules; enhancing other areas of life; reducing body checking and avoidance; addressing body dissatisfaction spikes; and addressing events, emotions, and eating). As always, the idea is to celebrate the things that are going well; identify barriers and how to address such obstacles; and build on the existing interventions by identifying increasingly challenging ways to tackle eating disorder symptoms. For this session, check in on patients' attempts at problem-solving, monitoring any eating disorder behaviors/urges and their triggers, and challenging how emotions can impact eating. These three skills can be highly beneficial for patients who report changes in their eating related to their emotional state or events. Each of these skills takes time and a good amount of practice to create meaningful change and should be continued after the conclusion of Group CBT-E. At the end of the review, encourage patients to create updated Action Plans to reflect goals for the week, and include these on their *Between-session Work Log*.

At the end of this review, let patients know that it is now time to stop completing the self-monitoring records. They have served their purpose of highlighting eating patterns, supporting regular eating, and were used as tools to identify body dissatisfaction spikes and other treatment interventions. Some patients are relieved to hear this, some may have already stopped completing them, and others may be reluctant to stop monitoring as they have found them to be a highly useful intervention. In this latter case, patients are encouraged to continue to use them and to add them as a tool on their staying well plan, completed in the next session. These patients are further encouraged to review on an ongoing basis the usefulness of continuing with the forms and to stop using them when they are no longer helpful or are only partly completed. The goal is to stop monitoring eventually. Resuming monitoring can be an option in the future, if helpful during a setback.

3. Exploring the Historical Review of Eating Disorder Behaviors and Thoughts

Handout: *Historical Review*

As you lead patients through completing the *Historical Review* handout, keep in mind the main aims of this session:

1. To engage in a process to identify aspects of life (at particular time periods) which have sensitized a patient to eating disorder behaviors and thoughts.
2. To increase the patient's self-empathy related to how their relationship with their body and eating has developed and has been functional at times.
3. To support patients in recognizing that despite the potentially helpful function of eating disorder behaviors in the past, these may no longer be behaviors that patients want to engage in.

Therapist Insight

Often discussing this timeline can be emotionally difficult for patients as it can bring up past traumatic experiences and other vulnerabilities. Be careful to create a safe and comfortable environment, with enough time to allow patients to fully engage in this exercise.

Begin by introducing the rationale for the group:

As you know, we have primarily focused on how your eating disorder impacts you currently and could impact you in the future. Today we are going to spend a session looking at the past to better understand how your life has been shaped in ways to make you more sensitized to shape, weight, body, food, eating, appearance, and any other eating disorder behaviors and thoughts. These events may have impacted your perspective on how the world looks around you and the way in which you evaluate your self-worth. For some of you, this may have started at a very young age and may have almost "primed" you for thinking about your body in a particular way. It is important to understand how your thoughts and behaviors related to shape and weight may have served a function early in life, and also consider the consequences of developing the eating disorder. Eating disorder thoughts or behaviors may have been useful in situations that felt out of control, or impossible to understand, particularly when appraising situations in childhood through a child's mind. To make meaning of these situations, or to feel in control, the eating disorder may have served a purpose. But likely, it is now no longer serving you well. Today we will explore this using your Historical Review handout.

Start by giving the group some time (10 minutes or so) to enter initial thoughts on the *Historical Review* handout. Then ask patients to share their reflections and make a composite list from the group on the whiteboard for the four timepoints listed. Table 18.1 shows how the final version of the composite group list might look.

While patients are working on the handout, walk around the group (or send individual chat messages if the group is virtual) to check in with patients about whether they are comfortable engaging in this exercise. If any patient reports that reviewing the past is too challenging for them, allow them to take a break from the group and check in with them immediately following the group.

Keep in mind the following common clinical points to highlight while completing the handout and in the group discussion:

Timepoint 1: Before Any Eating Disorder Thoughts or Symptoms Occurred

- We exist in a diet-(and exercise-)positive culture, with body ideal messaging everywhere (see Session 6). Many patients will describe specific diet culture messaging they recall from childhood. Add these specific messages on the whiteboard and encourage them to be added to the handout.
- Additionally, patients will often have experienced significant personal early life events that sensitized them to body, weight, shape, appearance, or eating. Examples of these events are vast and can be directly related to someone's appearance or can seem more circuitous. Some examples that we have heard about are bullying; sexual abuse or trauma; negative comments made about the patient's body; negative comments made by parents about their own bodies or food; fear related to parental health issues; personal health issues; and weight-stigmatizing messages received from medical providers about body size and weight.

Table 18.1 Sample Whiteboard – Composite Historical Review

Before any eating disorder thoughts or symptoms occurred:	– Mom and dad were always dieting – Teased for being tall – My sister went on a diet for prom – Lots of social media about exercise, dieting, summer body – My dad always talked about needing to be buff to be good at sports – Diet culture! Thinness = goodness!
The 12 months immediately prior to the onset:	– Parents got divorced – Moved to a new house – Gained weight and grandma told me to "watch what you eat" (I now know this was related to puberty – and normal!) – COVID-19 hit – school went virtual
The 6–12 months after its onset:	– Started weighing myself every day – Felt in control – Took some of my sister's diet pills – Tried laxatives for the first time – Made myself throw up – Was happy – Had to work out 7 days a week at the gym
Since then:	– Binge eating daily – Vomiting weekly – Dieting every day – Not allowing myself foods I enjoy – Getting ready for my wedding – Not really being present for my kids

Timepoint 2: The 12 Months Immediately Prior to the Onset of Eating Disorder

- About 12 months prior to the onset of the eating disorder patients often describe an experience or life event that was highly disruptive or stressful such as moving, changing schools, starting puberty, parental separation, questioning one's sexuality, transitioning to college/independent living, feeling lonely, or feeling sad. Other patients share experiences that are more clearly shape and weight related, for example, losing weight due to a stomach flu or surgery and finding that people reacted highly positively to this; starting a new sport or moving to more competitive levels of sports; becoming pregnant; starting a new sexual relationship; or trying the latest dieting trend with a friend.

> **Therapist Insight**
>
> Ask patients to consider how the introduction of social media use falls onto their timeline and how this usage may or may not have sensitized them to shape, weight, and eating.

- Though not always the case, sometimes when someone has been sensitized to shape and weight at a younger age, they may respond to stressful life transitions with negative body image cognitions (e.g., "If only I lost weight, my parents wouldn't be so angry at each other because they would be proud of me," "If I had the body I want, I wouldn't have to worry that I am doing so poorly in school"). If patients have knowledge from their past that their shape and weight matter, during a major life transition, this knowledge is relied on to cope with those situations.

Timepoint 3: The 6–12 Months after the Eating Disorder Behaviors Started

- Often, the first months of the eating disorder is a time when the behaviors appear to be "working" with few negative consequences. For some patients (whose clinical presentation includes food restriction or other weight control behaviors) this may be a time of weight loss, achieving desired weight goals, receiving complements and encouragement from people around them, feeling happier, and/or being more social. These patients are usually following many dietary rules and see this positively. For other patients (where there is less food restriction), initial experiences of binge eating can also be viewed with pleasure and as an effective tool for self-soothing with few negative consequences. Many patients share a longing to return to this initial time period and view their inability to maintain this level of dieting or to "control" their binge eating as an indicator of their lack of willpower.
- Many patients will share that as time progressed, they started to engage in other eating disorder behaviors, like binge eating, self-induced vomiting, or laxative abuse. They also report starting to notice other unwanted consequences of the disorder including increased irritability, difficulty socializing, and negative impacts on school or work performance.

Timepoint 4: Since Then

- For many patients, the "since then" timepoint is filled with negative consequences caused by the eating disorder – further binge eating, vomiting, loneliness, poor sleep, etc.- and a worsening of the negative impacts on one's social life, relationships, and school/work performance. This period may also include factors that have continued to sensitize a patient to shape, weight, and eating behaviors (e.g., having one's body labeled a certain way, engaging in a school/work challenge related to exercise/weight loss, going into an HLOC eating disorder treatment).

4. Reflecting on the Historical Review of Eating Disorder Behaviors and Thoughts

Once the group has completed the four sections of the handout, begin a group discussion to reflect on the exercise. The questions below can be used as a guide:

- *What thoughts/feelings came up for you when thinking back to these times in life?*
- *How do you think diet culture plays into the development of some of your experiences?*
- *What surprised you about what you remembered?*
- *What specific factors did you notice that impacted your focus on shape, weight, and eating?*
- *What do you notice about how transitions have played a role in the development of your eating disorder behaviors and thoughts?*
- *How do you think having an eating disorder was "helpful" in your past?*

- *Do you think it is still helpful?*
- *If you could go back to that young child who was experiencing all the shape- and weight-focused messaging, what would you want to say to them now?*

Where appropriate, take time to highlight that a patient's early over-evaluation of shape, weight, and eating behaviors may have been helpful to better function in their environment at that time. For example, controlling eating (e.g., counting calories, weighing food, cutting out food categories) can provide a general sense of control and calm during times when life feels out of control. An example of this was seen during the COVID-19 pandemic. Many patients found life to feel out of control during this time for a variety of reasons, including fears about getting ill, inability to see loved ones, death of loved ones, changes in routine, loneliness, and navigating remote school or work. For some, turning to controlling eating provided a sense of stability. For others, binge eating provided soothing. In these ways, the behaviors were "helpful." Unfortunately these practices often started, worsened, or re-started eating disorder symptoms and quickly became unhelpful. As another example, it can be "functional" to believe that losing weight is "good" if one grows up in a household where there is a strong emphasis on dieting and exercise. It is understandable that when an individual is sensitized to dieting in this way and then experiences weight gain (e.g., related to puberty or medication use), they could react by viewing this weight change as "bad" and desperately act to control their body size.

With distance from the initial experiences, and having completed most of Group CBT-E, often patients begin to recognize that these beliefs are no longer functional or helping them reach their goals. Encourage patients to consider how they would like to think about themselves and their bodies now, what messages they want to believe, and what behaviors and thoughts are aligned with their values.

Suggest that patients consider two steps for applying their learning from the historical review:

1. Offer themselves grace and compassion for the experiences that made them vulnerable to an eating disorder.
2. Mentally let go of the eating disorder with the knowledge that it is no longer serving them well. Ideas for how to do this include:

> **Therapist Insight**
>
> Be clear that the factors on the historical review that sensitized patients to shape, weight, and eating are not a comprehensive list of causes of their eating disorder. For example, many children grow up in households that are focused on dieting and exercise and many of these individuals do not develop eating disorders. It seems that some of these factors, in combination with other factors (e.g., biology, chemistry, temperament, culture, gender, early learning experiences, coping style) make an individual vulnerable to developing an eating disorder.

- Write a goodbye letter to the eating disorder
- Write a letter to their younger self
- Make a commitment, on paper, to a support person letting them know that they are ready to leave the eating disorder behind
- Create a piece of artwork that symbolizes the illness and a piece representing recovery

- Sail a leaf boat that represents their eating disorder in some way (e.g., words, images) down a stream

Some patients express sadness in letting go of the eating disorder. For many individuals, the disorder represents something familiar and has provided some sense of control in life. Normalize this feeling with understanding.

It is not uncommon to have feelings of sadness or loss at the idea of letting go of the eating disorder. For some of you, the eating disorder has been a constant in life and provided a sense of control when other aspects of life felt out of control or offered a way to soothe yourself. If you feel this way, allow yourself to grieve the loss of your eating disorder. It is OK to simultaneously feel sad and relieved as you move away from the eating disorder and in the direction of your recovery goals.

5. Preparation for Session 14: Reviewing Progress

In the last few minutes of this group ask patients to complete the EDE-Q and CIA. As in session 4, patients completing these at the end of the session will allow you time to review their scores and compare them to timepoint 1 (pre-session) and timepoint 2 (Session 4). Having this knowledge in advance will guide you to which areas require focusing on in the next group, and importantly will inform discharge planning. Provide a brief reminder of the purpose of these measures and how to complete them.

Before we end, I'd like to ask everyone to complete the same two assessment measures we completed at the end of Session 4 and prior to the start of Group CBT-E. You may remember that these two measures include questions about how things have been going for you over the past month. These measures help to give an idea of the progress you are making in treatment and will be used as part of our relapse prevention session next week.

6. Group Wrap-up

Session Summary

In today's session, we thought about where your eating disorder behaviors and thoughts started, or originated, for each of you. We looked at various timepoints in your life and considered how your life circumstances, and perhaps some of the messages you received about shape, weight, and eating behaviors, may have initiated a focus on your body. We considered how eating disorder behaviors can make sense initially and can offer a way to cope with life, but how this may no longer be serving you well.

Between-session Work

Remember to encourage patients to write the between-session work on their *Between-session Work Log* handout. The between-session work for Session 13 is:

- Continue work from previous sessions:
  - *Regular Eating* – continue to prioritize regular eating.
  - *My Breaking Food Rules Plan* – continue to plan in avoided foods and break dietary rules.
  - *Other Areas of Life* – continue to focus on the one or two new/expanded areas.
  - *Body Checking* and *Body Avoidance* – create and implement Action Plans to reduce body checking and avoidance in all its forms.
  - *Body Dissatisfaction Spikes* – create and implement Action Plans to address body dissatisfaction spikes using the RAD Approach.
  - *Problem-Solving; Eating Disorder Behavior/Urge Analysis; Breaking the Emotion and Eating Disorder Behavior Connection* – continue to practice these skills and implement as needed.
  - Follow through with any Action Plans identified during the session.

- New work from Session 13:
  - *Self-monitoring* – remind patients to stop completing these forms.
  - *Historical Review* – encourage patients to create plans related to offering themselves compassion for developing the eating disorder and for letting the eating disorder go.

Higher Level of Care Adaptations: Modular Implementation

When this session is used modularly, the following adaptations are suggested.

Exploring the historical review of eating disorder behaviors and thoughts: This session can be implemented as described at all HLOCs. Be mindful when deciding which patients to include in this group as it is more likely for patients at HLOCs to have experienced trauma and this group may not be appropriate for them. Additionally, in the early stages of treatment, the idea of letting go of the eating disorder may feel distant or unrealistic, or even unwanted by the patient, and it could be inappropriate, depending on their level of motivation. Many HLOC settings have creative arts therapy groups, or scheduled time to engage in creative or reflection activities. If available, consider using a piece of this time to follow through with some of the ideas for how to mentally let go of the eating disorder (e.g., writing a letter, creating an art project).

Group Session 13

Handout 13.1   *Between-session Work Self-review – Session 13*

BETWEEN-SESSION WORK SELF-REVIEW – SESSION 13

Skill/Goal	THIS IS GOING...			MY PLAN		
	Well	OK	Not Well	Make an Action Plan to address	Share with my support person for accountability	Praise myself for working hard on this!
Self-monitoring	☐	☐	☐	☐	☐	☐
Regular eating	☐	☐	☐	☐	☐	☐
Alternative activities	☐	☐	☐	☐	☐	☐
Urge tolerating	☐	☐	☐	☐	☐	☐
Addressing feelings of fullness	☐	☐	☐	☐	☐	☐
Challenging diet-related rules	☐	☐	☐	☐	☐	☐
Eating avoided foods	☐	☐	☐	☐	☐	☐
Engaging in 1–2 other areas of life activities	☐	☐	☐	☐	☐	☐
Reducing body checking overall	☐	☐	☐	☐	☐	☐
Reducing reflection checking	☐	☐	☐	☐	☐	☐
Reducing body comparisons	☐	☐	☐	☐	☐	☐
Reducing social media body checking	☐	☐	☐	☐	☐	☐
Reducing body avoidance	☐	☐	☐	☐	☐	☐
Addressing body dissatisfaction spikes	☐	☐	☐	☐	☐	☐
Using problem-solving	☐	☐	☐	☐	☐	☐
Using behavior/urge analysis	☐	☐	☐	☐	☐	☐
Reducing the emotion and ED connection	☐	☐	☐	☐	☐	☐

Which skills are going well? Which skills am I struggling to use? Do I need an **Action Plan**?

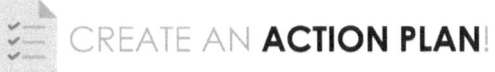 CREATE AN **ACTION PLAN**!

Handout 13.2   *Historical Review*

HISTORICAL REVIEW

In this activity, you will think back about how different experiences and events in your life contributed, or may have contributed, to the development of your eating disorder. You will also consider the consequences of the development of the eating disorder. At time points 1 and 2 below, list **events and circumstances that may have sensitized you to over-evaluating your shape, weight and eating behaviors.** At points 3 and 4, also list any specific eating disorder behaviors and related consequences.

This exercise may bring up a variety of feelings. If at any point you find this to be too distressing to complete, please stop working on it and let your group leader know.

1. Prior to 12 months before the eating disorder (Age:_____)	2. 12 months before the eating disorder (Age:_____)
3. 6–12 months after the eating disorder started (Age:_____)	**4.** Since then (Age:_____)

THOUGHTS AND REFLECTIONS

1. Are there any clear ways your life circumstances and events primed you to develop an eating disorder?

2. Does it seem like the eating disorder behaviors initially "helped" you to cope with life in some way?

3. Do you still need the eating disorder behaviors to help cope in life? Do you feel ready to let them go?

4. Are you able to offer yourself understanding and compassion about developing the eating disorder?

MY PLAN

1. Give myself **grace** and **compassion**! There are reasons why I was vulnerable to an eating disorder.

2. Mentally let go of my eating disorder. It is no longer serving me! I will:

☐	Write a goodbye letter to my eating disorder
☐	Create a piece of art work about my eating disorder and recovery
☐	Write a letter to my younger self
☐	Make a commitment and share with a support person
☐	Sail a leaf boat (symbolic of my eating disorder) and let it go
☐	
☐	
☐	

Chapter 19

Group Session 14
Relapse Prevention and Ending Treatment

Overview

Session 14 is the final session of the group. This session focuses on ending treatment well and summarizing relapse prevention skills. Relapse prevention is a key component of CBT-E and most of the skills introduced already in the group are designed to prevent relapse. This session is reserved to review these skills with the goals of:

1. highlighting individual progress made in treatment
2. identifying how to reduce setbacks
3. increasing awareness of circumstances that are likely to trigger a relapse
4. creating steps for getting back on track following a setback or relapse.

Following the conclusion of Group CBT-E, patients are likely to experience many more additional benefits of the treatment. Their recovery status at this final session will strengthen as they continue to further solidify their skills independently outside the group in the months ahead. It is essential to emphasize the importance of continued practice to stay well. One of the primary goals of this session is that each patient will create an individualized maintenance plan (*My Staying Well Plan*) that they will use to help stay on track with their recovery. Patients are asked to commit to weekly self-check-ins where they will review their *My Staying Well Plan*, as well as monitor their overall progress, for several months following the conclusion of group.

At this point, eating disorder behaviors are likely reduced, but some remain. This is completely expected and it is equally expected that improvements will continue with further practice, highlighting the importance of patients prioritizing weekly self-check-ins. Many therapists report their own feelings of anxiety or worry about ending treatment with patients who remain symptomatic. If you are feeling this way, remember that continued change and improvement is expected. However, some patients will require additional treatment following the conclusion of Group CBT-E. Guidance on this appears at the end of the chapter.

DOI: 10.4324/9781003450849-24

Therapist Preparation

☐ Review this chapter in advance.

☐ Review accompanying handouts and have copies available for patients.

☐ Score and compare patients' EDE-Q and CIA measures from timepoint 1 (pre-group administration), to timepoint 2 (Session 4), to timepoint 3 (the final administration completed in Session 13). Have copies of these forms available for patients to review in the session.

☐ Consider EDE-Q and CIA scores, as well as clinical impression, to determine individualized discharge plan needs (see the Discharge Planning textbox at the end of this chapter).

Handouts

- Standard Weekly Handouts
  - *14.1 Between-session Work Self-review – Session 14*

- Session-specific Handouts
  - *EDE-Q and CIA from timepoint 1, timepoint 2, and timepoint 3*
  - *14.2 My Staying Well Plan*
  - *14.3 Staying Well Weekly Self-check-in*

Group Session Agenda

1. Setting the agenda and orienting to the session (2 minutes)
2. Between-session work self-review (5 minutes)
3. Exploring feelings about group ending (5 minutes)
4. Reviewing scores on EDE-Q and CIA (10 minutes)
5. Highlighting progress (5 minutes)
6. Setbacks (25 minutes)

   a. Setting realistic expectations
   b. Reducing the risk of setbacks
   c. Identifying what triggers setbacks
   d. Identifying (early) warning signs of a setback
   e. Dealing with triggers and setbacks
   f. When to ask for more help

7. Using the *My Staying Well Plan* and *Staying Well Weekly Self-check-in* (5 minutes)
8. Final group wrap-up (3 minutes)

1. Setting the Agenda and Orienting to the Session

As you have with all sessions, begin this final group with a positive, encouraging welcome; share that this is Session 14, the final session of Group CBT-E. Clearly list the session agenda.

2. Between-session Work Self-review

Handout: *Between-session Work Self-review – Session 14*

This is the final between-session work self-review. Ask the group how they did with stopping monitoring records and their ongoing progress with all treatment interventions. Specifically, check in on any efforts to accept self-compassion this week and/or engage in an activity to say good-bye to the eating disorder. All skills take time and a good amount of practice to create meaningful change. Encourage group members to prioritize consistent use of skills in the coming weeks of all interventions learned in treatment.

3. Exploring Feelings About Group Ending

Patients view the ending of a group in all sorts of ways. Some patients are happy that the group is over. They may feel a sense of accomplishment or relief in getting the time back in their week. Some patients are sad that the group is ending. They may have formed solid peer relationships or feel connected to the group leader. Some patients feel worried. They are uneasy about what will happen to their eating disorder behaviors in the future. Most patients feel a mix of emotions, and some don't feel much at all. All of these feelings are normal. Begin this final group by acknowledging, validating, and normalizing any feelings that ending may bring up.

Before we get into the main agenda items for our group today, let's begin by checking in about your feelings about the group ending. [Go around the group giving patients the opportunity to share any thoughts or feelings they have regarding the end of group.]

4. Reviewing Scores on the EDE-Q and CIA

Provide patients with all three timepoints of their completed EDE-Q and CIA.

Take a few minutes to review your most recent EDE-Q and CIA scores. What are your overall impressions? Have you seen further changes? Are there areas that have remained quite problematic?

Typically by the end of treatment scores will be improving, with many patients no longer having scores indicating an eating disorder. It is not expected that scores will be zero, and be sure to let patients know that many people without eating disorders score above zero on some of the questions. Use the information gathered from the measures to help inform the next sections of this group.

Now we are going to move on to think more about treatment and how you have done. Please keep in mind the information from the measurements to help you with this discussion.

In cases where someone's scores indicate little or no improvement, use the guidelines below related to discharge planning to guide next steps in the patient's treatment.

5. Highlighting Progress

Handout: *My Staying Well Plan*

Next, encourage the group to reflect specifically on the progress they have made throughout treatment. Highlighting progress allows patients to consider the positive changes they have made and also helps in identifying areas to continue to work on after the group is over. It is usually a highly positive and enjoyable finish to the group program. Ask patients to complete Section 1 of their *My Staying Well Plan* handout. It is important to make sure that patients complete the handout as it will become their relapse prevention plan.

Let's now think about all of the progress each of you has made during this group. Working through a treatment like CBT-E is challenging and hard work. I'd like to start by congratulating each of you for being here and making it to the final session. Well done! Let's now take a few moments to think about specific achievements you made during the group, some of which you may have noticed on the assessment measures. Please fill out Section 1 of your My Staying Well Plan handout. There are some example achievements you can check off and also be sure to add some of your own. Once you are done, I am going to ask you to share what you have noticed in yourself or in others in the group.

6. Setbacks

a. Setting Realistic Expectations

Providing brief relapse prevention education to the group helps to foster a realistic understanding of relapse prevention, set appropriate expectations, and normalize the idea of setbacks. It is important to emphasize to patients that eating disorder thinking is likely to return or "pop up" during times of stress. Much of this session is focused on learning ways to protect against this stress or vulnerability, which can lead to a setback, and how to get back on track when a setback occurs.

In a moment we will talk about some strategies for staying well. Before we do, I want to first talk about what to expect in your recovery. Though today is the last day of our group together, this is not the last day that you will use the skills that you learned in group, and it is not the last day that you will have symptoms. Group CBT-E is designed to help you reduce eating disorder symptoms while you are in active treatment, and also to help you continue to make progress through continued practice, for at least another 6 months following the end of treatment. That means that though you may still be struggling with some symptoms today, you will likely experience some continued benefit the more you practice the skills you learned in treatment. It takes time for brains to get into a habit after introducing new skills (e.g., regular eating, urge tolerating, reducing body checking), so continued practice is essential.

It is also quite likely that some symptoms will pop up or return in the future. This is normal and to be expected. Rather than a straight line, staying well can be bumpy [draw

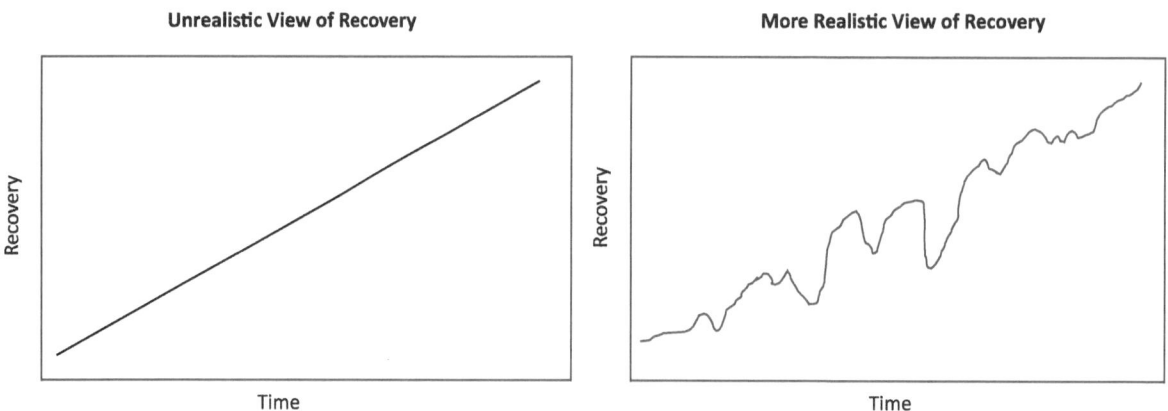

Figure 19.1 Illustration of unrealistic and realistic recovery.

out Figure 19.1 on a whiteboard]. *You have been using eating disorder behaviors for a long time and it would be unrealistic (and unfair to you) to think that all of your symptoms would go away completely, without any difficulties in the future. Having a clear plan of how to respond to these expected setbacks can help prevent you from feeling like you are failing and protect you from a setback causing a full-blown relapse. Spotting setbacks early is one of the best ways to prevent relapses. Today we are going to create plans so that you feel better prepared when setbacks happen and to help avoid setbacks from happening altogether. Be careful if you notice any unrealistic expectations about your recovery, all-or-nothing thinking about recovery, or self-judgment about symptoms popping up. Remember, setbacks are normal!*

b. Reducing the Risk of Setbacks

The best way to prevent a full relapse is to reduce the risk of setbacks. Support patients to reduce setbacks by 1) identifying the skills they learned in group that helped them to reduce eating disorder behaviors and symptoms – these are the skills they should keep using, and 2) identifying any upcoming circumstances or life events that may trigger a setback – and problem-solve how to handle them (Figure 19.2).

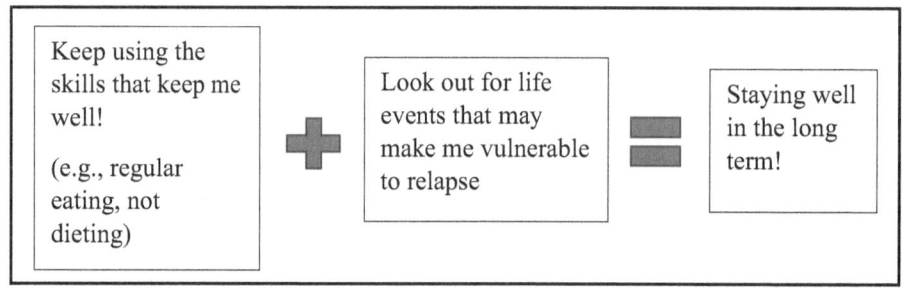

Figure 19.2 Staying well in the long term.

Step 1: Identifying which Skills Learned in the Group are Important to Continue to Use

Emphasize that continued practice of the skills that have helped is essential to ongoing recovery.

> *Let's create a list together as a group of the skills you have learned that are likely to keep you well. These are skills that I want to encourage you to continue to practice for at least the next six months – the goal being that they will eventually become habit. Once we are done completing this list, I want you to record on Section 2 of your My Staying Well Plan handout the skills that you want to keep practicing to protect against setbacks and to keep you well.*

Using Table 19.1 as an example, record responses on a whiteboard. Take time to understand and discuss each item. Ask patients to add these skills in Section 2 of their *My Staying Well Plan*.

Table 19.1 Sample Whiteboard – Skills to Keep Practicing to Protect Against Setbacks and Stay Well

1 Eat regularly – meals and snacks every day, no skipping!
2 Eat enough – avoid undereating.
3 Remember to sit down when eating.
4 Avoid dieting and following diet rules.
5 Continue to use the bathroom before meals.
6 Remember to use my support person – this is really helpful for me.
7 Keep in place all my reflection checking strategies (don't add mirrors, keep off the video in virtual meetings, no more selfie checking).
8 Keep wearing summer clothes, even if I start to feel anxious about it.
9 Use the RAD Approach when I have those negative body image spikes – it works!
10 Remember to give myself grace – there is a reason that this has happened to me and I am doing the best I can to stay on track.
11 Weekly weighing helps me.

c. Identifying What Triggers Setbacks

Step 2: Identifying Potential Triggers of Setbacks

Some setbacks will be triggered when one stops using the skills learned in treatment. For example, eating regularly is a skill that helps patients to stay well and therefore not eating regularly can trigger a setback. Triggers can also be any upcoming potential stressful life event or circumstance that may possibly lead to a return of eating disorder behavior, for example starting a new job. Just as the group did with creating a skills list, now the group will create a list of setback triggers. Remind patients that spotting potential triggers to setbacks early is similar to the "scanning ahead" skill they learned during the problem-solving group (Session 12). The skills of problem-solving can be used once a potential trigger is spotted.

Let's now create a list together [using a whiteboard] *of any events or circumstances in your life that are likely to trigger a setback and record these in Section 3 of your handout. Remember your eating disorder served an important role and acted as a coping mechanism (albeit not a completely helpful one), so it is understandable that in times of stress you are vulnerable to returning to it. Recognizing potentially upsetting events ahead of time will allow you to better be able to problem-solve in advance. Doing so will help you to use other coping skills and tolerate the associated distress without using eating disorder behaviors.*

Take time to understand and discuss each item. Common triggers to include are listed in Table 19.2.

Table 19.2 Sample Whiteboard – Triggers of Setbacks

- Going on a diet
- Going on vacation/the start of summer
- Starting or ending a relationship
- Stress about school exams
- Feeling stressed in general
- Starting college
- Seeing my cousin
- Moving
- Seeing others that I haven't seen since I have had shape/weight changes
- Meeting with a medical provider who comments on my weight
- Attending a formal gathering (e.g., wedding, graduation)
- Holidays that focus on food

At the end of jointly listing potential triggers, ask patients to complete Section 3 on their *My Staying Well Plan*.

d. Identifying (Early) Warning Signs of a Setback

It is also important to ensure that patients are skilled at noticing their personal early warning signs that a setback may be about to occur or is already occurring. Sharing these early warning signs with a support person in advance is encouraged. Support people often notice when the eating disorder thoughts and behaviors are returning before an individual may be aware of them. When appropriate for an individual's circumstances, we ask patients to give their support person permission to tell them if they notice a return to any behaviors on their list. Having a complete list allows support people and patients to be aware of what to look out for.

For the fourth list on your My Staying Well Plan, let's identify any behaviors or thoughts that indicate you might be starting to experience a setback or a return to eating disorder behaviors. Setbacks are not uncommon and the sooner you catch them, the sooner you can act to reverse them. The best way to catch them early is to know what they look like. Each of you will have different signs, though there is likely to be some overlap. I am going to ask that you share this list with a support person following the group, if possible. I would ask that you consider thinking about what these signs might look like to another person. For example, if I came to your home to check in on you (which I am not going to be doing), how would I know that a setback is occurring?

As you did with the skills above, take time to understand and discuss each item. At the end of jointly listing some early warning signs [see Table 19.3], ask patients to complete Section 4 on their *My Staying Well Plan*.

Table 19.3 Sample Whiteboard – Signs that I am Experiencing a Setback

- Eliminating certain foods, following particular diet-related rules, reading about dieting strategies.
- Skipping meals and snacks.
- Increased urges to binge and/or engaging in binge eating/eating secretively/hiding food.
- Increased urges to exercise too much (e.g., exercising daily, going to the gym even if I am tired or sick, working out instead of doing other things that are important to me).
- Noticing that I am thinking a lot more about my weight and shape (e.g., asking others if they think I am fat, increased distraction).
- Noticing that my mood is worse (e.g., increased depressed behaviors, increased anxious behaviors).
- Feeling more irritable (e.g., "snappy" with my partner, decreased patience when things are different than I expect).
- Isolating myself (e.g., avoiding eating out with friends, avoiding doing activities that I love).

e. Dealing with Triggers and Setbacks

Once the signs of a setback are identified, group members need to know what to do to get back on track when they experience them (see Figure 19.3). Getting back on track means restarting any skills that were helping and have since been stopped, while at the same time reducing unhelpful behaviors that may have restarted or increased in frequency. Teach group members the importance of making firm plans and a commitment to get back on track. Sharing this commitment with a support person makes it more likely that the patient will stick with it. Setting phone alarms or email notifications with the title of the alarm stating the skill is another helpful tool. The following example can be shared to highlight how one does this:

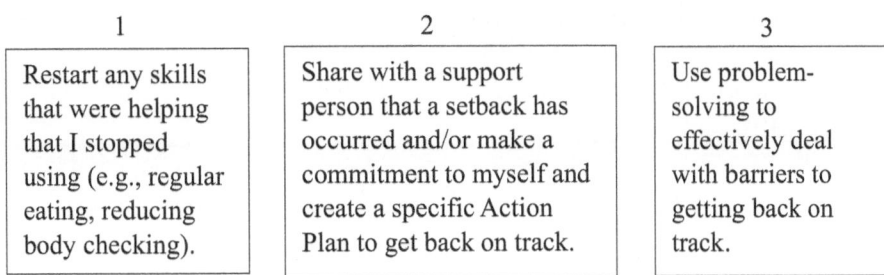

1	2	3
Restart any skills that were helping that I stopped using (e.g., regular eating, reducing body checking).	Share with a support person that a setback has occurred and/or make a commitment to myself and create a specific Action Plan to get back on track.	Use problem-solving to effectively deal with barriers to getting back on track.

Figure 19.3 How to get back on track after a setback.

About 4 weeks after the end of Group CBT-E, Ayla starts to notice that they are skipping snacks and are starting to think more often about how they are unhappy with their body. During a weekly self-check-in, Ayla looks back at their My Staying Well Plan and feels that restarting regular eating and reducing body checking will be helpful (in particular reducing checking in the mirror and looking at old photographs of themself). Ayla's best friend and roommate, whom they shared their My Staying Well Plan with, has started to notice some of these behaviors and the two of them talk about how best to get back on track. Ayla adds reminders in their phone for snack time, decides to delete social media apps from their phone, and adds a timer when using the mirror.

Using the handout, ask patients to record their plan in Section 5 of their *My Staying Well Plan*.

Therapist Insight

We often share with patients that it is important to look at and evaluate setbacks, as opposed to letting them happen without much reflection and trying to "just do better next time." When setbacks are addressed in an exploratory way, they can become learning experiences that can help a patient to move even further along in recovery.

f. When to Ask for More Help

In the ideal situation, completing the group provides patients with the skills to stay well long term. Ongoing practice and spotting setbacks early will help to further solidify changes. Unfortunately, for some, eating disorder behaviors may slip back into place more significantly, causing a full-blown relapse.

Give clear advice on when to seek more help for a return or worsening of eating disorder behaviors. You also want to help patients identify future life events that may be known to be associated with eating disorder relapse (e.g., the postpartum period, major life stressors, other life transitions). See Table 19.4 for additional examples.

> Encourage using the *My Staying Well Plan* as soon as a setback is noticed. It is much easier to get back on track when symptoms have been in place for 3 days (or 3 hours), rather than 3 weeks (or 3 months).

> Setback = The start of eating disorder symptoms in low frequency/intensity/duration that can be one step toward relapse.
>
> Relapse = More significant eating disorder symptoms consistently engaged in over time that are negatively impacting functioning, and which patients feel they have no control over.

By continuing to practice the skills learned in group and getting back on track when you notice setbacks, you have every possibility of staying well from your eating disorder in the long term. Sometimes though, the eating disorder is too strong to overcome on our own and I want to encourage you to reach out for help during these times. I often find that a one-off check-in with a provider can be enough to help you get back on track. And if you need more,

Table 19.4 Sample Whiteboard – When to Ask for More Help

I am engaging in eating disorder behaviors and cannot stop.
I have restarted body checking or body avoidance and cannot stop.
I am experiencing physical symptoms of my eating disorder (e.g., dizziness, constipation, blood in vomit).
I am planning to get pregnant/I am pregnant/I am in the postpartum period.
I am clinically depressed.
I have encountered a huge life stress (e.g., divorce).

I can help you identify the best next steps for accessing treatment going forward. Let's create a whiteboard list of the signs that indicate when to call a provider for more support or a check-in. Add the items that match your experience to Section 6 of your My Staying Well Plan.

7. Using the My Staying Well Plan and the Weekly Self-check-in

Handout: *Staying Well Weekly Self-check-in*

At the end of this group, patients will have a completed *My Staying Well Plan*. It is important to provide guidance on how to use this plan going forward. Encouraging patients to plan to have a session with themselves to review their plan on a weekly basis is a helpful tool for at least the next few months. These sessions are guided by the *Staying Well Weekly Self-check-in* handout and cover four topics:

1. Completing a symptom check
2. Reviewing their *My Staying Well Plan*
3. Making Action Plans on which skills to focus on for the following week (and which corresponding handouts need to be reviewed or recompleted)
4. Writing in a specific date and time for the next self-check-in session.

The *Staying Well Weekly Self-check-in* also has space for naming an identified support person for continued support. When possible, it is best to share this plan with a support person soon after group finishes. In group, review a blank *Staying Well Weekly Self-check-in* handout and provide guidance on how to use it. Be sure to also provide patients with clear guidance on how best to structure the session with themselves. Let patients know that these sessions do not need to be long – 10 dedicated minutes is often sufficient.

You can use the Staying Well Weekly Self-check-in handout to guide your self-check-ins. During your check-in, review your My Staying Well Plan. Read the various sections and check to see if there is anything you need to focus your attention on for the coming week. Perhaps you are experiencing some early warning signs of a setback and need to put certain skills back into place. Be sure to make a solid plan for the week ahead. Bring out old handouts to review or recomplete, set reminders if helpful, and talk with your support person. And don't forget to praise yourself for having the check-in session! I want to ask you now to identify a time and day about a week from now when you will schedule your first self-check-in and include that at the bottom of your My Staying Well Plan. If it is useful, go ahead and put that in your calendar now.

Encouraging group members to schedule the first self-check-in session in the moment helps to prevent forgetting to plan the first session and increases the likelihood of the session occurring. Encourage patients to prioritize these sessions and pick a quiet, private time when they can focus on themselves.

8. Final Group Wrap-up

As with other sessions, you will provide a brief summary of what was covered in group. We also standardly offer a good-bye and good luck to patients. There is no between-session work distributed as this is the final group.

To summarize, today is our final session. In group we talked about ways to stay well for the future, focusing on identifying triggers to setbacks and proactively problem-solving when they occur. I emphasized how useful weekly self-check-ins can be, and encouraged you to prioritize them (and yourself!) over the next few months. Also, don't forget to use the support of your loved ones, as needed, to educate them about your My Staying Well Plan.

Well done on completing Group CBT-E! It has been a pleasure to get to know, and work with, each of you. I wish you the best of luck as you continue on your eating disorder recovery journey.

Discharge Planning

Appropriate discharge planning following completion of the outpatient/sequential form of Group CBT-E is best made through combining your clinical judgment, the desires of the patient, and their objective outcome measures.

We tend to see four main outcomes when this group is delivered on an outpatient basis:

1. *Patients who have done well and experienced a reduction in their symptoms.* The recommended discharge in this case is to encourage patients to continue to have weekly self-check-ins and to graduate from treatment (i.e., stop therapy).

2. *Patients who have done well and experienced a reduction in their symptoms, but have a comorbid disorder that they would like to focus on.* In this case there can be several options.
   a. Encourage them to consider having a period of time (3–5 months) where they further practice the skills learned in treatment before starting treatment for the comorbid condition. Doing so increases the likelihood that they will be quite well from their eating disorder and therefore able to fully engage in therapy for a comorbid disorder. They may also experience a reduction in comorbid symptoms as their eating disorder continues to improve.
   b. Depending on the comorbidity, consider referring for a medication evaluation, if appropriate.
   c. Assist them in finding evidence-based treatment to treat the comorbid disorder.

3. *Patients who have made little progress and remain highly symptomatic.* If this is the case, be sure to review your input on this individual case throughout the group. Were their symptoms missed throughout? Did they suddenly worsen at the end? Have they made progress, but it has been at a slower rate and the pace of the group did not match this? Where possible, it is important to catch someone who remains highly symptomatic as early as possible while they are in the group and move them into more supportive treatment (e.g., a HLOC, Individual CBT-E, or another individual treatment) well before the final session. Sometimes a therapist misses the fact that symptoms are not improving or are worsening, while other times, there are no other treatment options available other than Group CBT-E. In these cases, consider with the patient at the end of treatment next steps based on your clinical judgment and their particular needs. Consider if they are eligible for more intensive treatment or may benefit from a different treatment approach or format.

4. *Patients who have done well and experience a reduction in their symptoms but would like general counseling to discuss day-to-day life challenges or to explore other related issues.* In these cases, we encourage patients to first have a period of no input (i.e., a follow-up period of 3–5 months) to continue to practice the skills learned in treatment. At the end of this period, we recommend offering an individual psychotherapy check-in session and then assist them in finding supportive general counseling if recommended.

Therapist Self-reflection

At the end of the group it can be useful to debrief with yourself and your supervisor, if available. In the same way you encouraged the group members to recognize their progress you can do this for yourself. You have successfully facilitated Group CBT-E! In doing so, you have provided evidence-informed treatment to individuals with eating disorders and moved them closer to recovery. By offering this therapy in a group setting you provided treatment to far more patients than you might otherwise have been able to reach – thus expanding access to care. Similar to what you have just done in this session with the patients, consider the elements of the group that went well (and what you want to keep doing more of next time) and the areas that were more of a struggle. Problem-solve how to handle struggles differently next time. Congratulations on all your hard work!

Higher Level of Care Adaptations: Modular Implementation

When this session is used modularly, the following adaptations are suggested.

Maintenance and continued progress: The title of this session differs for modular implementation. This is because when delivered at HLOC it is not expected that patients have completed treatment. A session devoted to maintaining progress – in whatever form this takes – remains essential at all levels of care. The main elements are the same across all levels of care: highlight positive changes; encourage patients to continue to practice these changes; support them in identifying how they will do this when they return home or step down in care; and support them in identifying factors that will support them in their recovery journey. As well as creating group lists using a whiteboard, encourage patients to write down their plans so they can take them home to share with support people and their next treatment team.

Group Session 14

Handout 14.1   *Between-session Work Self-review – Session 14*

BETWEEN-SESSION WORK SELF-REVIEW – SESSION 14

Skill/Goal	THIS IS GOING...			MY PLAN		
	Well	OK	Not Well	Make an Action Plan to address	Share with my support person for accountability	Praise myself for working hard on this!
Regular eating	☐	☐	☐	☐	☐	☐
Alternative activities	☐	☐	☐	☐	☐	☐
Urge tolerating	☐	☐	☐	☐	☐	☐
Addressing feelings of fullness	☐	☐	☐	☐	☐	☐
Challenging diet-related rules	☐	☐	☐	☐	☐	☐
Eating avoided foods	☐	☐	☐	☐	☐	☐
Engaging in 1–2 other areas of life activities	☐	☐	☐	☐	☐	☐
Reducing body checking overall	☐	☐	☐	☐	☐	☐
Reducing reflection checking	☐	☐	☐	☐	☐	☐
Reducing body comparisons	☐	☐	☐	☐	☐	☐
Reducing social media body checking	☐	☐	☐	☐	☐	☐
Reducing body avoidance	☐	☐	☐	☐	☐	☐
Addressing body dissatisfaction spikes	☐	☐	☐	☐	☐	☐
Using problem-solving	☐	☐	☐	☐	☐	☐
Using behavior/urge analysis	☐	☐	☐	☐	☐	☐
Reducing the emotion and ED connection	☐	☐	☐	☐	☐	☐
Having self-compassion and letting the ED go	☐	☐	☐	☐	☐	☐

Well done on completing all of the between session work self-reviews! This is the last one. As always, add any Action Plans that might be needed.

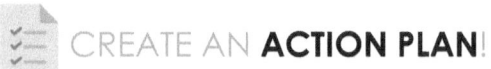

CREATE AN **ACTION PLAN**!

Handout 14.2   *My Staying Well Plan*

MY STAYING WELL PLAN

1. Praise yourself (check all that apply and add some more).

☐ I attended all/most of the group sessions. ☐ I completed all/most of the between-session work. ☐ I made time for a review session with myself. ☐ I used regular eating. ☐ I used alternative activities and/or urge tolerating. ☐ I started eating avoided foods and/or breaking diet rules. ☐ I am engaging in new areas of life.	☐ I have decreased my focus on shape/weight. ☐ I am practicing new ways of dealing with emotions and stressful events. ☐ I have been able to do weekly weighing. Other things I am proud of in terms of my treatment:

2. These are the skills I need to keep practicing to stay well:

☐ Eating regularly each day (3 meals, 2–3 snacks) ☐ Giving my body the amount of food it needs (not under-eating and eating foods I enjoy) ☐ Eating in a balanced way (carbs, fats, proteins, including fruits and vegetables) ☐ Using alternative activities ☐ Practicing urge tolerating ☐ Using the RAD Approach for feelings of fullness ☐ Not going on a weight loss diet ☐ Eating foods I am fearful of ☐ Not having rules about eating ☐ Engaging in other areas of life ☐ Reducing body checking behaviors	☐ Reducing body avoidance behaviors ☐ Practicing the RAD Approach for body dissatisfaction spikes ☐ Understanding how my emotions impact my eating (and vice versa) ☐ Giving myself compassion for developing an eating disorder ☐ Allowing my eating disorder to go ☐ Weekly weighing for _____ number of weeks Other skills to practice (be specific):

3. What might trigger a setback for me?

☐ Going on a weight loss diet ☐ Going on vacation ☐ Starting or ending a relationship ☐ Arguments with loved ones ☐ Starting a new school year or job ☐ Comments about my weight ☐ Being weighed at medical appointments	☐ Not receiving affirming care ☐ Not sleeping well ☐ Moving Other triggers (be specific):

4. Signs I am starting a setback/ returning to eating disorder behaviors:

☐ Not feeding my body enough food ☐ Avoiding foods I enjoy eating ☐ Feeling more irritable, depressed, and/or anxious ☐ Starting to binge eat more ☐ Using compensatory behaviors	☐ Isolating Other (add in as many of your 'signs' as you can):

5. Getting back on track. List the specific skills in treatment that you will use to get back on track (e.g., return to self-monitoring, restart regular eating, tell my support person).

6. When to ask for more help. Sometimes it is difficult to get back on track on our own and it is important to know when to ask for more help. This usually means contacting your current/previous treatment team. Below are some signs when it is time to ask for more help. You know yourself best – so be sure to add your own ideas.

I need to ask for more help when:

- ☐ I am using eating disorder behaviors and can't stop.
- ☐ I am thinking about eating/dieting/my shape and weight all day long.
- ☐ My weight is changing quickly.
- ☐ My medical providers are concerned about my health.
- ☐ I am pregnant, planning to get pregnant, or am in the postpartum period.
- ☐ I am feeling hopeless.
- ☐ I feel like hurting myself or ending my life.
- ☐
- ☐
- ☐
- ☐

Review sessions with yourself are a key to staying well! **My next session is:**_____

Handout 14.3   *Staying Well Weekly Self-Check-in*

STAYING WELL WEEKLY SELF-CHECK-IN

Taking time to have a weekly self-check-in is one of the most important ways you can maintain your progress. It is time well spent - you are worth it! Use the template to guide your review. You will need your My Staying Well Plan for the check-in. Ask yourself the questions for each section.

Step one: Quick symptom check

Did you experience any of the following in the past week?

- ☐ Dieting (food restriction, not allowing myself to eat certain foods)
- ☐ Binge eating
- ☐ Self-induced vomiting, laxative/diuretic/diet pill use
- ☐ Driven exercise

Step two: Review My Staying Well Plan

- Did I give myself praise for areas I worked hard on?
- Which skills are currently helping me?
- Which skills do I need to work on?
- Did I experience any triggers?
- Are any triggers coming up?
- Am I noticing any signs that I am starting to lapse?

Step three: Make an Action Plan for areas to work on and think about relevant handouts that might be worthwhile to review/complete again.

ACTION PLAN		DATE:
PROBLEM:		
CURRENT FREQUENCY (IF APPLICABLE):		
GOAL FOR UPCOMING WEEK:		
SPECIFIC PLAN:	MY PLAN:	MY SUPPORT:

Step four: Schedule a specific time and date for my next check-in: _____

For continued support, my support person is: _____

Appendix A

List of Handouts

Session 1

1.1 *My Formulation*
1.2 *My Formulation Information Tool*
1.3 *Self-monitoring Form*
1.4 *Self-monitoring Example*
1.5 *Self-monitoring Instructions*
1.6 *Between-session Work Log*

Session 2

2.1 *Between-session Work Self-review – Session 2*
2.2 *Self-monitoring Review*
2.3 *Regular Eating*
2.4 *Planning Ahead*
2.5 *Dieting*
2.6 *Binge Eating*
2.7 *Underweight/Underfat*
2.8 *Self-induced Vomiting and Medication Misuse*
2.9 *Driven Exercise*

Session 3

3.1 *Between-session Work Self-review – Session 3*
3.2 *Regular Eating Review*
3.3 *Alternative Activities*

Session 4

4.1 *Between-session Work Self-review – Session 4*
4.2 *Urge Tolerating*
4.3 *Feelings of Fullness*

Session 5

5.1 *Between-session Work Self-review – Session 5*
5.2 *Progress Review – Treatment Components*
5.3 *General Barriers to Change*
5.4 *Ways to Overcome Barriers to Change*
5.5 *Therapist Self-review*

Session 6

6.1 *Between-session Work Self-review – Session 6*
6.2 *Resetting My Thinking About Dieting*
6.3 *My Avoided Foods List*
6.4 *My Food Rules*
6.5 *Exposure*
6.6 *My Breaking Food Rules Plan*

Session 7

7.1 *Between-session Work Self-review – Session 7*
7.2 *Self-evaluation*
7.3 *Over-evaluation of Shape and Weight – Extended Formulation*
7.4 *Other Areas of Life*
7.5 *Body Shape and Weight Checking Self-monitoring*
7.6 *Body Shape and Wight Checking Self-monitoring Example*

Session 8

8.1 *Between-session Work Self-review – Session 8*
8.2 *Body Checking*
8.3 *Weighing*

Session 9

9.1 *Between-session Work Self-review – Session 9*
9.2 *Reflection Checking*
9.3 *Body Comparisons*
9.4 *Social Media Body Checking*

Session 10

10.1 *Between-session Work Self-review – Session 10*
10.2 *Body Avoidance*
10.3 *Body Dissatisfaction Spikes Self-monitoring*

Session 11

Session 12

Session 13

Session 14

Appendix C

Appendix E Welcome Packet and Additional Materials

Appendix B

In-depth Exploration of the Transdiagnostic CBT-E Formulation

The Transdiagnostic Formulation

Creating a personalized formulation or case conceptualization is an essential component of CBT-E. It provides a blueprint for treatment and, when done well, is highly engaging for patients. To better understand the transdiagnostic formulation, review Figure 2.1 in Chapter 2. This example of a CBT-E formulation highlights clinical concepts using technical terms for eating disorder features. Using Figures 21.1 and 21.2 as a patient illustration, this appendix provides a detailed description of both the maintaining mechanisms and the associated eating disorder features typically encountered.

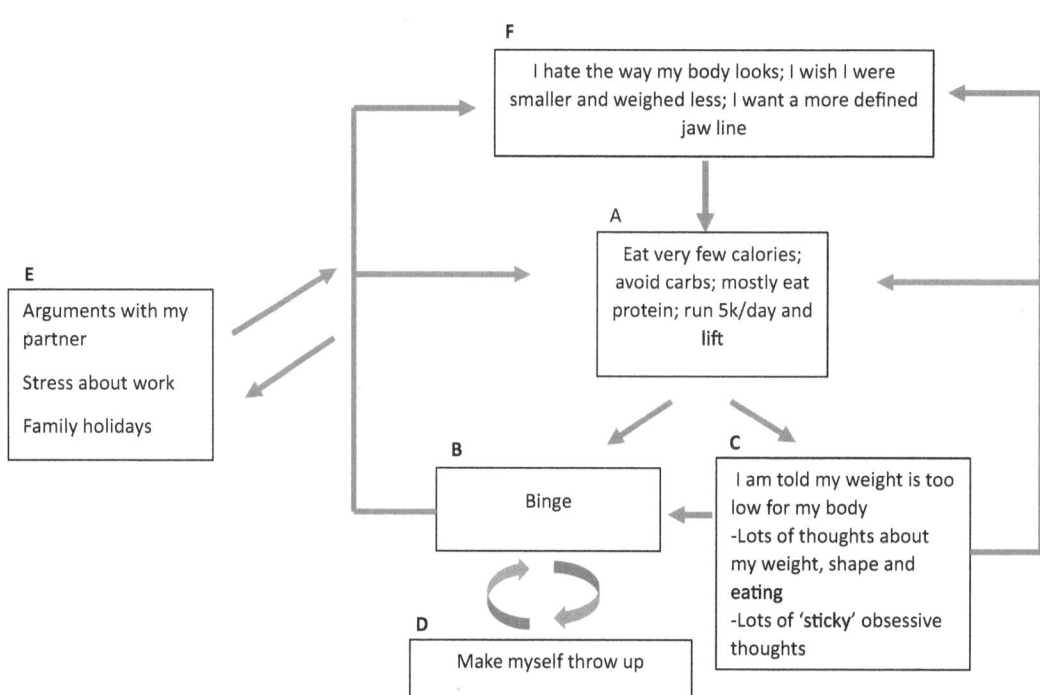

Figure 21.1 Sample formulation – Eating disorder features (boxes).

Eating Disorder Features

Eating disorder features are contained in the boxes on the formulation. The box content will be personal to each patient and how their eating disorder presents. When supporting a patient in creating their formulation, the aim is for it to be highly personalized to the individual. This is achieved by using the patient's own words and adding as much individualized detail about the feature as possible. For example, instead of simply recording "dieting" in Box A, you would encourage the patient to list all their specific dieting behaviors. While wanting the formulation to accurately capture the individual patient, you also want to ensure that certain aspects that appear to be present, but are not acknowledged by the patient, are not missed. The nature of the disorder itself can impact awareness and insight, causing a patient to minimize features of their eating disorder. In these cases, if you are noticing a feature that the patient is not including, we recommend using a box with a dashed line around it, adding a question mark, writing the box content in a different color, or adding in words to indicate that the patient is not yet sure about a certain feature.

Below is a description of the content for each box. The box letters match onto the letters used in the *My Formulation* handout (1.1). Review the *Personalized Formulation Information Tool* handout (1.2) in tandem with this appendix for additional specific examples of symptoms that may fit into each box.

Box A

Box A contains any behaviors that may be used to change one's shape, weight, and appearance in an effort to respond to the beliefs in Box F. This includes a variety of dieting behaviors related to food intake (e.g., eating low calorie amounts; avoiding certain types of foods; avoiding entire macronutrient food groups such as carbohydrates or fats); and any non-compensatory weight control behaviors (e.g., diet pill use and driven exercise). It is important to note that the behaviors in Box A do not need to be practiced regularly, consistently, or at a high intensity. Patients' attempts or plans to eat very few calories, or to avoid certain types of foods, would also go into this box.

Box B

Box B includes all forms of binge eating. Most patients use the term binge eating, while others may use "eating out of control," "losing control over my eating," "emotional eating," or "compulsive overeating." Be sure that patients use their own words on the formulation. Both subjective and objective binge eating behaviors go into this box.

Box C

Box C includes symptoms related to weight loss or maintaining a weight lower than one's body needs. Being "underfat," or eating in a restrictive way that results in not having enough body fat, also goes into this box. (We will refer to these three states as: "weight loss/maintaining a weight too low for one's body/being underfat" throughout this appendix.) The more personalized these symptoms are, the more likely they will resonate with the patient. As you can see in Figure 21.1, this patient was not ready to agree that their weight was likely too low for their body so added the "I am told" to indicate this. It is important to use the patient's words and what they are comfortable with, so "I am told my weight is too low for my body" works fine at this stage of treatment.

Box D

Box D includes compensatory behaviors which are any behaviors used to counteract binge eating. These typically include self-induced vomiting; laxative, diuretic, and diet pill misuse; and driven exercise. Less typically, these behaviors include misuse of insulin and breast/chest-feeding/pumping. Remember some of these behaviors may fall into Box A if they are used as a consistent form of dieting, as opposed to a response to binge eating. For example, running 6 days a week to try to lose weight as an overall diet strategy is considered non-compensatory and would go in Box A. Running before or after a binge to get rid of the binge calories would go in Box D.

Box E

Box E contains any life events or emotional dysregulation that interact with the eating disorder. Sometimes these life events or emotions can trigger eating disorder behaviors (e.g., binge eating following a stressful day as a way to self-soothe) and other times, the eating disorder behaviors can worsen emotions or events (e.g., rigid and inflexible diet rules causing increased social isolation and loneliness).

Box F

Box F contains the "core psychopathology," or dysfunctional self-evaluation scheme, in which there is an over-evaluation of shape, weight, and their control to define self-worth. As can be seen in Figure 21.1, the sample patient has included in this box, "I hate the way my body looks" and then expanded on this belief using more details. These negative views of one's shape and weight are often highly influenced by the intense diet culture that we live in, which perpetuates the myth that it is possible to achieve one's ideal body.

Eating Disorder Maintenance Pathways

Eating disorder maintenance pathways are represented by various lines and arrows on the formulation. The arrow direction highlights the direction of the relationship. In the same way as in the eating disorder feature boxes, the arrows will be personalized to fit the individual patient's experience. And as with the boxes, sometimes the eating disorder limits one's awareness or insight. In these cases, it is recommended to use a dashed line or arrow, or some other way, to indicate that a pathway may be present but the patient is not yet sure of this.

Pathway 1

The over-evaluation of shape and weight pushes a patient to engage in a number of dieting behaviors that are often highly rigid and inflexible. In many ways this makes sense. If someone focuses extensively on shape and weight to evaluate themselves and determines that they are not doing well in this area (having a body shape or weight they do not like), engaging in dieting behaviors to change their shape and weight (as promised by diet culture) is a logical decision.

Pathway 2

Eating in this highly restrictive way, or attempting to do so, can lead to binge eating. Sometimes eating in a highly restrictive way can lead to weight loss/maintaining a weight too low for one's body/being underfat. Many patients, cycle back and forth between binge eating and weight loss/maintaining a weight too low for one's body/being underfat.

Binge eating: Binges are often caused by both undereating and depriving oneself of foods that may otherwise be liked. Not consuming enough calories puts physiological pressure on a patient to eat, often in an out-of-control way due to the body's need to restore balance (i.e., sugar/glucose levels and the release of appetite-stimulating hormones). Undereating, and attempting to undereat, also causes psychological deprivation. Following, or attempting to follow, multiple, inflexible rules drives this psychological deprivation. It is impossible to follow such strict rules all the time and when a rule is broken or seems impossible to achieve, a thought of "I've failed, I may as well continue eating now" can follow, which can result in a binge.

Weight loss/maintaining a weight too low for one's body/being underfat: Following diet-related rules often does, for the short term, lead to weight loss. For some, it leads to ongoing maintenance of a weight that is too low for their body or maintaining a body fat percentage that is too low. Because of the physical and psychological impacts of this state, it can lead to increased thinking about food, shape, and weight, increased social isolation, and increased obsessionality.

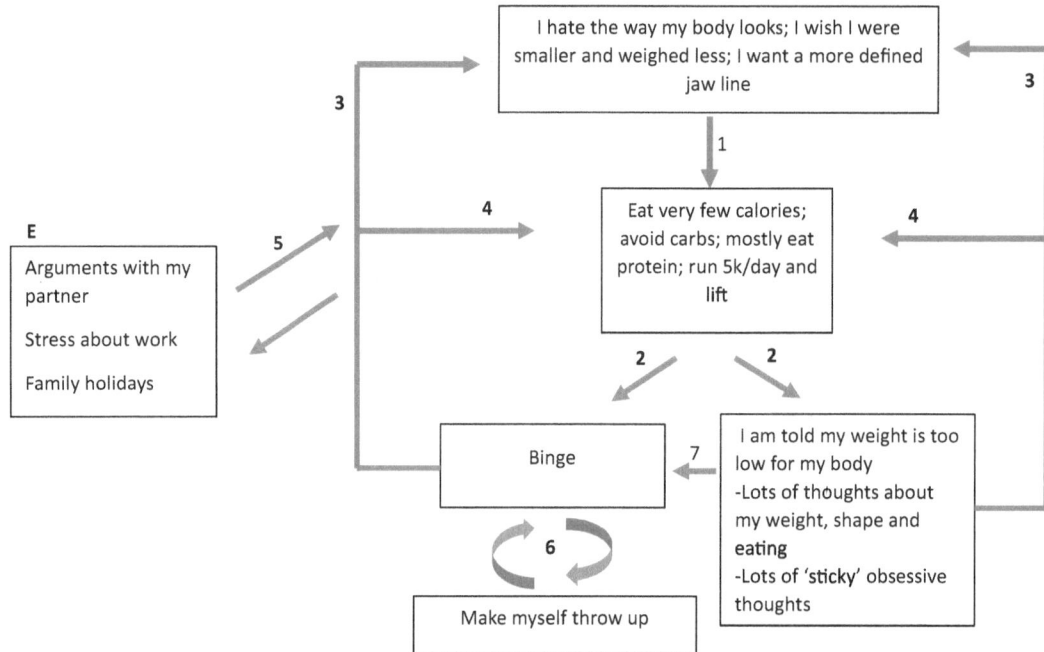

Figure 21.2 Sample formulation – Eating disorder maintenance pathways (arrows).

Pathway 3

Both binge eating and weight loss/maintaining a weight too low for one's body/being underfat loop back and reinforce the over-evaluation of shape and weight.

Binge eating: When someone experiences a binge, this almost always activates a negative appraisal of their self-worth, shape, and weight (the top box, Box F). To highlight this loop, when drawing out the formulation with a patient it can be helpful to ask: "*And when you binge eat, how does this impact your thoughts and feelings about your shape and weight?*" Patients often respond: "*It makes me feel so much worse and makes me worry about my shape and weight even more.*" For patients with BED, it is suggested that some patients will have an over-evaluation of shape and weight, while others do not. In our clinical experience, we very rarely encounter patients with BED who do not have an over-evaluation of shape and weight. In cases where a patient does not endorse an over-evaluation of shape and weight, Box F would not be included.

Weight loss/maintaining a weight too low for one's body/being underfat: As described above, a side-effect of this state is a preoccupation of thinking about eating, food, weight, and shape.

Pathway 4

Similarly to Pathway 3, both binge eating and weight loss/maintaining a weight too low for one's body/being underfat loop back and reinforce engaging in strict and inflexible eating.

Binge eating: Most patients who experience a binge attempt to follow their diet-related rules even more strongly after the binge. It is not uncommon to hear a patient state, "*I was out of control with my eating that night and felt terrible. When I woke up the next morning, I tried to be good, so I skipped breakfast and had a light lunch.*" In combination, Pathways 2 and 4 illustrate the vicious and repetitive cycle between binge eating and dieting, in that one leads to the other, back to the other, and so forth.

Weight loss/maintaining a weight too low for one's body/being underfat: Patients who find that they are "successful" in underfeeding their body make commitments to continue to engage in strict, and sometimes stricter, diet-related rules.

Pathway 5

Life events and emotional dysregulation have a reciprocal interaction with all aspects of the eating disorder formulation. The areas of the eating disorder that impact Box E, and vice versa, will be individual to each patient. Some patients, for example, may find that feelings of sadness and low mood lead to binge eating. The binge may be self-soothing and temporarily lead to an improvement in mood, but later lead to worsening mood and negative feelings. Other patients describe how extreme control and rigidity with their eating "calms" them; however, this style of eating is often ultimately associated with further mood lability. Patients often describe feelings of shame and guilt as a result of the core psychopathology, and that low mood worsens negative thoughts about shape and weight, leading back to the core psychopathology.

Pathway 6

For many patients there is a vicious cycle between binge eating and compensatory behavior(s) (e.g., vomiting, laxative misuse, etc.). This cycle can be difficult to break as often the more someone binges, the more they use a compensatory behavior, and the more they use a compensatory behavior, the more likely it is for a binge to occur again. For patients who engage in compensatory behaviors following binge eating, many will not binge if they know in advance that they will not be able to engage in these behaviors. To highlight this cycle, in CBT-E we often ask: "*If you knew that right after a binge someone was coming for a surprise visit to your home, which would prevent you from vomiting, what do you think would happen?"* The response is often along the lines of: *"I definitely would not binge if I knew there was no way to get rid of the food."* By asking this question, we can help highlight to patients how continuing to engage in compensatory behaviors reinforces binge eating. If we can help the patient to stop the compensatory behavior, we have a good chance of reducing the binge eating.

Pathway 7

Weight loss/maintaining a weight too low for one's body/being underfat can put great pressure on the person to binge eat. This mechanism works similarly to Pathway 2 whereas undereating leads to binge eating. Binges along Pathway 7 are primarily caused by the physiological pressure of undereating, though feelings of deprivation caused by rigid and inflexible food rules (described above), applies here too, depending on the patient.

Not all eating disorder presentations will require all these boxes to be filled in. The transdiagnostic formulation emphasizes that given the shared underlying core psychopathology, some components of the formulation will fit most eating disorders. The majority of patients will have a top box regarding dissatisfaction with shape, weight, and appearance leading to some form of dieting behaviors or diet-related rules. Most patients will also describe an interaction between life events, emotional dysregulation, and eating disorder symptoms. For example, a patient with AN-restrictive subtype would likely complete Box A (dieting), Box C (symptoms of weight loss and being at a body weight too low for one's body), Box E (events and moods), and Box F (core psychopathology), but would skip Box B (binge eating) and possibly Box D (compensatory behaviors).

In Session 1 of Group CBT-E, it is suggested to follow the steps starting with Box A – dieting behaviors and diet-related rules. As you gain comfort and skill in creating formulations with a group, you will be able to flexibly implement this intervention, building up a formulation step by step with the ordering guided by the patient. The ideal starting place is often an aspect that the patient most wants to change about their eating disorder or current state. Some patients may start with thoughts, while others start with behaviors. Sometimes it can make sense to first identify all the content that would go into the boxes and save the arrows (maintaining mechanisms) to be completed together once the boxes are created. Other times, arrows can be added in as the patient describes the connections. At first, however, we recommend completing the formulations in a standard way (described in Session 1), taking all group members through the steps in the same order.

Appendix C

Pre-treatment Assessment Tool

Pretreatment screening can take a variety of different forms, depending on the structure of the program and the timing of the screening. For example, some screenings are a part of a more comprehensive assessment, while others are brief phone screenings distinct from more thorough evaluations. Be sure to include parents/guardians if screening an adolescent and consider including information from support people (if clinically indicated) when screening an adult. Often, collateral information from support people, along with treatment providers, can help to make the screen more complete.

Therapist Style

During a screening, the therapist style is nonjudgmental, understanding, and direct. Ask direct questions about eating disorder behaviors in a gentle way that displays both compassion and your knowledge of eating disorder symptoms. You may be the first person to ask about these behaviors and many patients experience a sense of shame related to their eating disorder. Keep in mind how challenging contacting you about treatment may be for them. We often start our screenings with the following:

> *I need to ask you some questions about your eating difficulties so that I can best help you. Some of the questions may be difficult to answer as often disordered eating can be hard to talk about. If you find the questions upsetting, or hard to answer, please let me know so that I can best support you.*

Throughout the assessment, let the patient guide you. Some patients are comfortable speaking about their eating difficulties and others are less so. Again, use clear, direct, and neutral language to help build trust that you know about eating disorders and are not going to be surprised by what you hear. Frequently, we have found that patients visibly relax seeing our comfort and knowledge in asking about things they initially feel uncomfortable talking about (e.g., self-induced vomiting, binge eating, or laxative misuse).

Patient Goals

- Why did you schedule this brief evaluation today?

Eating Disorder-Related Behaviors

- What are the concerns you have about your eating behaviors? <u>Frequency</u>? <u>Duration</u>? <u>Intensity</u>?

- Food restriction and food intake

    - Can you tell me <u>what you typically eat and drink in a day</u>? *Make sure to ask the patient to slow down to provide specific information, including portion sizes, types of food (diet vs. non-diet), and eating times.*

    - How typical is this food and drink intake for you? Do you have some days where you eat more or less than this? If so, what do you eat on those days? What does a "good" day look like? What does a "bad" day look like?

    - How long have you been eating/drinking this way?

    - Are there certain types of foods that you avoid eating?

    - Are you dieting?

- Binge eating

    - Do you have days when you eat a large amount of food and feel out of control when eating, like you can't stop?

    - On these days, do you experience any of the following:
        - Eating larger portions than others?
        - Eating rapidly?
        - Eating until uncomfortably full?
        - Eating when not hungry?
        - Eating alone?
        - Experiencing guilt or shame after eating this way?

    - When was the last time one of these eating episodes happened and what did you eat?

    - How often does this occur?

    - How long has this been happening?

Figure 16.1 **Pre-treatment screening tool.**

- Vomiting

  - Do you ever make yourself throw up after eating in an effort to get rid of calories or to prevent weight changes?

  - How often does this occur?

  - How long has this been happening?

- Medication (e.g., laxative, diuretic, diet pill, insulin) misuse

  - Do you ever use laxatives, diuretics, diet pills, or any other substances in an effort to prevent weight changes?

  - How often does this occur and how much do you use at a time?

  - How long has this been happening?

- Exercise

  - Do you exercise? What do you do? How many days per week? How long is each session?

  - Do you exercise before or after eating in an effort to prevent weight changes?

  - On days when you cannot exercise, do you change your eating and/or does missing exercise cause anxiety/worry?

  - Do you exercise when sick or injured?

  - Does prioritizing exercise negatively impact other aspects of life?

Body Image Thoughts and Behaviors

- Do you often think about your shape, weight, and eating?

  - What kinds of thoughts or worries do you have?

  - What percentage of your day (i.e., how often) is taken up with these thoughts?

  - How distressed by these thoughts are you?

- Are you afraid of gaining weight? On a scale of 1-10 (10 being extremely worried), how worried are you about gaining weight?

- Do you have body checking behaviors (e.g., frequently weighing, scrutinizing your reflection, comparing your shape to others)?

- Do you have body avoidance behaviors (e.g., avoiding weighing, avoiding wearing certain types of clothing, avoiding activities that will show off your body)?

Physical Symptoms

- Are you experiencing any of the following symptoms:
    - menstrual irregularities or lack of menstruation (if applicable)
    - fatigue/low energy
    - poor sleep
    - bone aches and pains
    - feeling cold much of the time
    - gastrointestinal distress: constipation, watery stool, acid reflux, pain
    - muscle pain
    - dizziness, lightheadedness, fainting
    - chest pain/pressure
    - heart palpitations
    - blood in vomit
    - edema
    - dental cavities if current or historical vomiting
    - low blood pressure
    - issues with heart rate
    - throat issues
    - weakness
    - issues with concentration/memory
    - hair loss

Physical Characteristics

- <u>Height and weight</u>
    - Current height
    - Current weight
    - Highest lifetime weight? When?
    - Lowest lifetime weight? When?
    - Highest weight in the last 12 months? When?
    - Lowest weight in the last 12 months? When?
    - Have you had a period of time without eating disorder symptoms (e.g., dieting, binge eating, vomiting) and what was your weight at that time?

Diagnoses and Medication

- Do you have any current or past medical or psychiatric diagnoses? If yes, what are they?

Use your clinical judgment to further evaluate other psychiatric conditions. There should be a particular focus placed on ruling out other psychiatric presentations that may be the cause of the patient's disordered eating. Assess the patient's readiness and appropriateness for eating disorder treatment and if there are other significant concerns (e.g., clinical depression, active psychosis) that would suggest that Group CBT-E may not be the best fit for them at the moment.

- Have you ever received higher level of care treatment for a psychiatric reason, including eating disorder treatment?

- <u>Current medication list</u>
    - Do you take any psychiatric medication(s)? Yes/No
        - What are they?
    - Do you take any other medication(s), including weight loss medication(s)? Yes/No
        - What are they?

Some safety concerns may warrant additional assessment and safety planning.

- Suicidal ideation
    - Do you have, or have ever had, thoughts of killing yourself? Yes/No

    - On a scale of 0-10 (10 being severe hopelessness), how hopeless do you feel?

    - Do you have a history of attempting suicide? Yes/No
        - If yes, date(s) of suicide attempt(s):

- Self-harm
    - Do you have, or have you ever had, thoughts of harming yourself? Yes/No
        - If yes, date of most recent thoughts:

    - Do you have a history of engaging in self-injurious behaviors (e.g., cutting, scratching, burning, hitting yourself)? Yes/No
        - If yes, when was the last time that you harmed yourself?
        - What happened?
        - What did you use to harm yourself? Do you still have access to what you used to harm yourself?
        - How often does this occur and for how long?

- Substance Use
    - Do you use substances (including alcohol and nicotine)?
    - If yes:
        - What substance(s)?
        - Frequency?
        - Duration?
        - Amount?
        - Any current or historical concerns about substance use?

Neurodivergence

- Do you identify as neurodivergent (e.g., autistic; /dyslexic person)?

Food Insecurity

- Within the past 12 months, have you worried whether your food would run out before you had money to buy more?

- Within the past 12 months, did you have the experience that the food you bought did not last and you did not have money to get more?

- Prior to the last 12 months (i.e., when you were growing up or other time points), did you worry whether your food would run out or that the food you had would not last and you did not have money to get more ?

- Do you receive government-funded nutritional assistance (SNAP, etc.)?

Consent to Speak with Other Providers

- <u>Primary care provider and consent</u>
    - In order to ensure your medical safety, we require that your PCP provides their assessment of your medical stability. Do I have your consent to speak with them?
        - Name?
        - Contact information?
        - Recent lab work (interpreted by PCP for non-medical therapists)?
        - Recent EKG, if indicated?

- <u>Outpatient provider (e.g., therapist, psychiatric provider, dietitian) and consent</u>
    - In order to provide the most comprehensive treatment, we collaborate with other outpatient providers. Do you have outpatient providers and do I have your consent to speak with them?
        - Name?
        - Contact information?

Motivation and Engagement

- <u>This treatment is a short-term group therapy lasting 14 sessions.</u> Is this in line with the kind of therapy you are seeking?

- What are your thoughts about working on these eating difficulties in a group setting?

Attendance

- <u>Regular attendance is essential</u> to help you get the most out of group. Do you have any long breaks, vacations, or other reasons that attending the groups on the scheduled dates would be impossible for you? Yes/No
    - When?
    - Are there options to rearrange any of these plans?

Preferences and Other Considerations

- Is there anything else about you that would be helpful for me to know in terms of making sure Group CBT-E is the most effective form of treatment for you?

Use clinical judgment to assess if there is anything else that would be helpful to know in making a determination about Group CBT-E treatment appropriateness.

Appendix D

Additional Considerations Prior to Implementing Group CBT-E

In addition to reviewing this entire guide in advance of offering Group CBT-E, this Appendix contains some important additional practical matters to consider for first-time application.

Session Length and Frequency

Outpatient

In an outpatient level of care, Group CBT-E is designed to be 14 one-hour sessions delivered once a week. We have found that one-hour groups are more acceptable to patients and satisfy insurance regulations regarding billing reimbursement. We strongly advise following this format closely and carefully. There are occasions when extending the group beyond the 14 sessions is appropriate, but one must have a high threshold for doing so. Some possible reasons to extend the group include: the therapist had an unexpected absence and momentum was lost, and/or the therapist believes that all group members could benefit from a refresher of a certain treatment element.

Higher Levels of Care

At HLOC, there are many considerations related to session length and frequency. In many situations, CBT-E groups may need to be offered more than once a week and depending on the program and group size, some groups may be longer than 60 minutes. See Chapter 4 for additional HLOC considerations.

Age of Group Members

Outpatient

In the outpatient setting, Group CBT-E can be used with both adolescents and adults. When adapting the treatment to younger patients, be careful to assess the needs of an adolescent patient's parents/ guardians. In most situations, we recommend that adolescents are encouraged to share, following each session, their *Between-session Work Log*, Action Plans, and a summary of the group content with their parents/guardians. Some parents/guardians may need additional assistance in how best to support the patient's recovery efforts. For example, some may benefit from being offered education related to Group CBT-E, either through providing a packet of all of the Group CBT-E handouts, or recommending reading a CBT-E parent guide, such as *Cognitive Behaviour Therapy for Eating Disorders in Young People: A Parents' Guide* (Dalle Grave and el Khazen, 2021). Other parents/guardians may benefit from an individual session with a focus on describing the treatment, patient's progress, and treatment goals; answering questions; and identifying ways that the parent/guardian can be supportive of the patient's treatment goals. If this is a need for all of the adolescents in the group, consider adding a multifamily therapy group session or parent/guardian session to accomplish the same agenda. Less frequently, parents/guardians may need more support and may benefit from adding a family therapy intervention while the patient is in Group CBT-E.

We recognize that there will be exclusions of who is appropriate for the group related to factors such as developmental level, insight, judgment, self-drive, and motivation, all of which can be impacted by age. We recommend that therapists use their clinical judgment to determine what is the best fit for the needs of the patient. We strongly recommend that all therapists are sensitive to comprehension differences based on age, as well as other factors, and are careful to accommodate for such needs when running the group.

Regarding the ages within a particular group, we have observed a unique mutual learning process within mixed age groups. We also recognize that for many environments, mixed age interventions are critical from a practical standpoint to serve as many patients as possible at once. In some instances, there are patients who feel uncomfortable receiving treatment with others that are much younger or older than themselves. This should be addressed collaboratively and respectfully, perhaps offering to have the patient try the group for a certain number of sessions to see if the age difference is as meaningful as anticipated. It is our experience that once starting in the group, patients often become more comfortable. If administering a mixed age group, we recommend you are careful to ensure that group material is appropriate for all ages and communicate this clearly to group members. Some programs and practices are designed to separate treatment by age, which works fine for Group CBT-E.

Higher Levels of Care

Group CBT-E can be used modularly with both adolescents and adults. It is important to follow the guidelines set out by your governing/licensing organizations. In some hospitals, for example, mixed age groups are not allowed.

Group Size

Outpatient

Outpatient groups are best run with a minimum of four, and a maximum of eight, patients. In practice, this is not always possible. While groups can be run with as few as two patients, more than 10 patients can be challenging in ensuring all members are able to fully participate and share. In situations where group size is above 10 patients, a longer 90-minute group therapy session may be needed to allow for adequate time to fully deliver the content.

Higher Levels of Care

Smaller groups (10 patients or less) seem to be most ideal; however, this is not always possible at HLOCs. If there are more group participants, consider an option to have longer Group CBT-E therapy sessions, break a group session down into two doses, and/or have two therapists.

Closed versus Open Groups

Outpatient

Ideally, Group CBT-E is administered as a closed group with all patients starting together in Session 1 and working through the sessions sequentially. The outpatient version is designed in this way.

Higher Levels of Care

At HLOC, closed groups are not possible and the modular, or non-sequential, application is best.

Transdiagnostic

Group CBT-E, like Individual CBT-E, focuses on treating shared eating disorder "core psychopathology." By doing so, the treatment is not diagnosis specific and is transdiagnostic (see Chapter 2). As a result, groups will likely have patients with differing eating disorder presentations and diagnoses.

Gender-specific versus Gender-inclusive Groups

It is our experience that Group CBT-E can be administered to patients of all genders simultaneously and that there is nothing specific about this treatment that would warrant a separation based on gender. Individual patients may have views and preferences on this, so do let patients know this aspect of the group before they start, to allow patients to make an informed decision. Some material can be more uncomfortable for patients to discuss with someone of a different gender (e.g., body avoidance, trauma-related responses to body or food, historical review of eating disorder behaviors and thoughts) and we recommend using the group process to help support a patient with this anxiety. Therapists should be attuned to this and talk openly about how to create a safe space in the group.

Number of Group Therapists

In an effort to increase treatment availability, Group CBT-E is designed to be led by one group leader. The use of handouts and the patient-led aspects of Group CBT-E enable one therapist to successfully lead the group. That said, if resources allow, and there is good clinical justification, it can be led by two group leaders, which is traditional in many group therapies.

Virtual and In-person Formats

This treatment is designed to lend itself well to either virtual or in-person group administration.

Virtual Formats

Telehealth sessions have revolutionized access to behavioral healthcare. Virtual delivery of Group CBT-E is well liked by patients and has allowed for far easier scheduling compared to in person. Virtual sessions increase access to specialized care and are especially important for patients living in rural areas and/or those with other restraints related to traveling to appointments (e.g., physical disabilities or associated travel costs). Virtual Group CBT-E sessions require considerations, similar to applying other virtual therapies, including privacy and confidentiality, technology literacy, technology reliability, cost of technology, and the need to establish emergency safety plans.

Specific tips include:

- Have a system in place to easily share group materials and handouts electronically with group participants. Appendix A lists all handouts in this book. Creating a single document with all handouts to share with patients at the start of the group can be helpful.
- Get comfortable using a virtual whiteboard to effectively engage patients in group-based activities.
- Encourage patients to close out any other material on their computer, turn off cellphones, join group in a private setting without distractions, and commit to sitting on screen throughout the length of the session.
- Offer stretch breaks to help with attention and focus.
- Have a keen sense of how the group is working together in the virtual space and engage patients in such a way as to strengthen group cohesion when necessary.
- Encourage patients to be prepared for the group by setting up the area they use for therapy a few minutes in advance. Ask patients to take time to transition from their day into the treatment, check that all technology is working, and take out between-session work.

In-Person Formats

For in-person Group CBT-E, the following tips may be beneficial:

- Ask participants to arrive about 5 minutes early to prepare. If this is not possible or appropriate at HLOCs, provide patients with a moment to transition into the group.
- Have handouts printed ahead of time.
- Ensure the room is set up well with:
  - Easy access to a whiteboard that all patients can see.
  - A large table for the patients to sit around (e.g., a conference room) so that the patients can actively complete handouts and take notes during the session.

- Set expectations for the period of time directly following the group. In-person group therapists should consider how accessible they want to be at the end of a group. Sometimes patients can use that time to engage in processing individual thoughts and feelings with the therapist that are outside of the bounds of the group treatment. Reminding patients that clinical concerns need to be addressed during the group session can be helpful in these circumstances. At times, an individual session may need to be scheduled, if clinically appropriate.

Appendix E

Welcome Packet and Additional Materials

Many different psychological therapies exist. These therapies are researched by therapists and scientists to determine their effectiveness in addressing specific mental health conditions. When a treatment consistently demonstrates its efficacy for a particular condition through extensive, high-quality research, it is considered an evidence-based treatment. For eating disorders, cognitive behavior therapy is one such evidence-based treatment. **Enhanced Cognitive Behavior Therapy (CBT-E)** is a specialized version of cognitive behavior therapy that is tailored to individuals with a range of eating disorder symptoms. Group CBT-E expands upon this evidence-based protocol by adapting it to a group format, enhancing accessibility to treatment and facilitating mutual learning and support within a group environment.

It has been shown that roughly 2/3rds of individuals who complete well-implemented Individual CBT-E have an excellent response. Factors impacting whether or not someone will respond to CBT-E are still unknown; however, committing to treatment sessions, completing work between sessions, engaging in therapy sessions, and allowing oneself to do hard work (i.e., getting uncomfortable) is often reported by patients as having a helpful impact on their recovery.

GROUP CBT-E is...
• **14** sessions and each session is **60** minutes long.
• an active treatment which primarily addresses the **present** and **future** and is less focused on the past.
• a treatment that **focuses on eating disorder symptoms**. Other topics that do not relate to treatment goals will not take priority. This can be challenging because you may arrive to a session with life stressors that have occurred over the previous week (or could have occurred just prior to stepping into group). Despite this, group will continue to focus on the CBT-E agenda for that week. At times, this may mean that you will be redirected by your therapist back to the agenda.
• committed to making **change**. Though making change can be incredibly uncomfortable and difficult, it is in that change that you will start to see recovery happen.

GROUP GUIDELINES

Group guidelines help to create a safe and comfortable group environment for all.

CONFIDENTIALITY

- Please do not share any content that is discussed in the group outside of the group. Everyone must feel that they can talk openly about very personal and vulnerable topics and members need to agree that this can happen in a confidential space. Keep in mind:
  - If you run into another group member outside of the session, please do not acknowledge one another's connection when in public, limit conversation, and move on.
  - Your group therapist has limits of confidentiality, including their need to break confidentiality in the event that you are reporting that you are a danger to yourself or others, that you report abuse, or that your records are subpoenaed by a court system.
  - If you have signed consent for the group therapist to be in touch with another member of your treatment team, that allows the therapist to openly share information about your care with that provider.
  - If you are not yet 18 years old, check with your therapist about confidentiality as it pertains to your parent(s)/guardian(s).

RESPECT

- Respect means upholding respectful behaviors, including using "I" statements and treating others as you would want to be treated.

INCLUSIVITY

- Regardless of age, race, gender, gender identity, sexual orientation, economic status, class, religion, weight, size, and ability, all are welcome in this group. Inclusivity includes asking others what their names and pronouns are.

SAFETY

- If you are feeling unsafe in any way – in the group or at home – it is essential that you let the group therapist know.

ATTENDANCE

- Please avoid missing any group therapy sessions. As the group sessions will continue moving ahead, it puts you at risk for missing important material, and it can impact behavior change momentum. Your group therapist will review specific cancellation and lateness policies for their practice.

ARRIVAL AND GROUP SESSION PREPARATION

- In order to maximize the time spent in the sessions, it is recommended that you take a short period of time (about 5 minutes) just prior to the session to shift your focus to therapy, and review material from the previous week and between-session work.

BETWEEN-SESSION WORK

- You will have specific between-session work each week that will be summarized and written down at the end of each session. It cannot be underscored enough that **work done outside of group is key to how well you will respond to treatment.** The vast majority of the therapeutic work that you will do will happen outside of the group therapy sessions. In fact, a weekly group therapy session is one hour a week of your life, as opposed to the rest of the 167 hours a week that you live. That said, what is done between sessions will dictate your treatment response. The more you put in, both in and out of sessions, the more you will get out.

CONVERSATIONS ABOUT NUMBERS

- Avoid conversation that includes specific numbers related to weight, calories, exercise repetitions, sizes, etc. These types of numbers can be distracting and distressing for group members.

PARTICIPATION

- We find that group members typically have the best response to group if they participate to the best of their ability. This includes avoiding any distractions; coming prepared for treatment with your handouts and a writing utensil; and participating in treatment as much as possible, while respecting/balancing the needs for others to contribute. You will never be forced to participate, but are encouraged to challenge yourself to engage in the group and tolerate any participation discomfort. It is often the case that patients who were initially hesitant to participate in group sessions find that once they do start to participate, they are able to get more out of the treatment.

DISTRACTIONS

- Please turn off and put away all cellphones, and minimize other distractions, so that you can fully immerse yourself in this treatment during the 1 hour group time. If you are struggling to minimize distractions around you, please bring this to the group to utilize group support. If you find using a tool (e.g., fidget toy) helpful for your engagement with the group, please let the therapist know and bring this to session with you. Likewise, if taking a moment to stand or stretch helps with your attention, please let the therapist know so that these can be incorporated into group.

WORKING AS A TEAM

- In this group, we work together as a team to overcome everyone's eating disorder. We agree as a group to help support one another, while in session, with the successes and challenges of treatment, while upholding the long-term goal of recovery.

GROUP SESSION CONTENT

To give you an overview of what you will be learning in group, here are the topics for each session. The items below are the main content for the sessions. Each session will also include time for reviewing between-session work from the previous week and summarizing new work for the upcoming week.

Session 1	Understanding what keeps your eating disorder going
	Monitoring eating, thoughts, emotions, and other behaviors
Session 2	Adopting a supportive eating pattern
Session 3	Replacing eating disorder behaviors with alternative activities
Session 4	Tolerating urges to engage in eating disorder behaviors
	Understanding feelings of fullness
Session 5	Reviewing progress in treatment so far
Session 6	Exploring dieting behaviors and diet-related rules
Session 7	Understanding what it means to have an over-evaluation of shape and weight
	Adding in other areas of life

Session 8	Understanding and changing body shape and weight checking (Part 1)
Session 9	Understanding and changing body shape and weight checking (Part 2)
Session 10	Understanding and changing body shape and weight avoidance
Session 11	Reviewing Progress
Session 12	Learning to problem solve
	Analyzing eating disorder behaviors and urges
Session 13	Exploring the origins of the eating disorder
Session 14	Ending well

GETTING TO KNOW ME

Everyone is different. We think differently, have different perspectives on the world, learn differently, have different cultural contexts, and have different needs. Our differences are what makes for a rich and diverse world. Knowing these differences before the group will allow your group therapist to make adaptations to how they deliver certain interventions and better meet your needs. Please take a moment to complete the following form and return it to your group therapist. If something is missing that is important for your therapist to know about you, please be sure to add it in the space provided.

I like to be called/my name is:	
My pronouns are:	
Recovery from my eating disorder looks like:	
My goals for this group are:	
I may struggle with the following in group:	
Things to help me engage better in group include:	
Specific cultural needs I have include:	
Apart from eating disorder behaviors, I cope by:	
I have the following sensory needs:	
My special interests are:	
Other things about me that I would like to share:	

General Group Overview

This group offers enhanced Cognitive Behavior Therapy (CBT-E) in a group format to individuals with eating disorder diagnoses that do not require significant weight regain (e.g., binge eating disorder, bulimia nervosa, and otherwise specified feeding or eating disorder, excluding all forms of anorexia nervosa). If your patient has decided to start in this treatment then they:

- have met criteria for the group based on a specialized eating disorder screening assessment
- are interested in actively modifying eating disorder symptoms
- are open to a group-based treatment
- are agreeable to the Group CBT-E approach, knowing that Individual CBT-E is one of the leading treatments for eating disorders
- are not currently pursing weight loss treatments

Group CBT-E consists of 14 one-hour weekly sessions. The group is structured with each session following an agenda. Individualized between-session work (i.e., therapy homework/goals), and a suite of handouts allows for a more patient-led approach.

Do I need to continue to see my patient while they are in Group CBT-E?

Group CBT-E is intended to be a standalone psychological treatment.

For current medical treatment (primary care provider):
As a psychological treatment, Group CBT-E does not take the place of standard medical care. Collaboration with the Group CBT-E therapist is recommended, particularly if there are medical concerns that may warrant a more intensive treatment or may impact the patient's ability to respond to Group CBT-E. Again, this treatment is not meant for patients who require significant amounts of weight regain. If you have concerns that your patient falls into this category, please consult with the Group CBT-E therapist as soon as possible. The Group CBT-E therapist will encourage the patient to contact you if they are reporting medical symptoms.

For current psychological or psychiatric treatment (individual therapist, family therapist, psychiatric provider):
Group CBT-E is designed to be the start of eating disorder treatment for a patient new to outpatient care. For patients that are currently in outpatient therapy, it is recommended to pause or terminate the psychological treatment for the eating disorder, if the patient is not responding to that intervention. If the patient is responding, then Group CBT-E is likely not needed. If the patient is treated for another mental health condition, the recommendation is to consult with the Group CBT-E therapist to determine the best treatment plan (e.g., continuing with the current treatment and supplementing with Group CBT-E, pausing the current treatment). For patients that require psychiatric

medication management, it is expected that they continue to work with their psychiatry provider throughout the group.

For current nutritional treatment (dietitian):

Group CBT-E does not require dietitian-based interventions. Similar to psychological treatment, it is recommended to pause dietitian interventions unless there are certain circumstances that require treatment under the care of a dietitian. These include an initial nutritional assessment to determine if a patient is maintaining a weight too low for their body or are not eating in a fully balanced way (e.g., undereating certain nutrients or food categories such as carbohydrates or fats). This also includes nutritional therapy for patients requiring specific nutritional advice (e.g., certain health conditions including diabetes mellitus, celiac disease, food allergies, osteopenia/porosis; patients who have undergone any form of bariatric surgery; patients with low levels of nutritional knowledge). Again, consultation with the group therapist is important in these situations to identify a collaborative treatment plan.

I will continue to see the patient regularly; how can I support them in Group CBT-E?

If you will be seeing the patient regularly while they are enrolled in Group CBT-E, there are many ways in which you can support a patient to receive the full benefits of the group:

- Holding the patient **accountable for therapeutic homework assignments** can be useful. All Group CBT-E patients have two primary types of homework assignments following each session:

  - Self-monitoring: All patients are asked to self-monitor their eating and eating disorder behaviors (and sometimes body image behaviors and thoughts) following the first group session through to the end of group. Self-monitoring forms are meant to be completed each day and in real time. The completion of these forms is crucial for participation in group (as working toward a regular pattern of eating is an initial and primary treatment intervention); therefore, if a patient does not complete these forms regularly, they may not be an ideal candidate for group.
  - Between-session Work: Work that all group members are working on individually throughout the week (e.g. working toward regular eating patterns, applying a new strategy, following through with behavior goals related to an Action Plan). When goals are identified, they are meant to be realistic (in that they can be accomplished in the course of a week), measurable, and related to the eating disorder. Goals are then reviewed each week and updated goals identified.

- Supporting the patient to understand that to fully benefit from the treatment, their **anxiety and discomfort will likely increase**. This is a part of the difficult task of behavior change. It is important for the patient to work toward experiencing this anxiety and tolerating it in order to work past fears related to change. Staying too comfortable in Group CBT-E often means that work is not being accomplished.

- Supporting the patient to **fully commit to the group**. At the start of each group series, each patient agrees to commit to the group. Patients agree to come each and every week unless there are extenuating circumstances, which should be minimal. Each patient agrees to complete the between-session work and goals identified each week and commit to identifying a system where they apply, review, and maintain skills and goals addressed in group outside of group on a regular basis.

- **Identify patient-specific goals that could be practiced in group**. Often group can be a place to practice particular social skills and to test out cognitions, hypotheses, and expectations related to assumptions. The group can also be used as a place to find out other perspectives on what the patient is struggling with and ideas for change.

What is addressed in each session?

The group follows a structured group protocol with specific topics and skills to address in each session, as well as skills to practice in between the sessions. The protocol is a group adaptation of the Individual CBT-E protocol: Fairburn, C. G. (2008). *Cognitive behavior therapy and eating disorders*. The Guilford Press.

Session 1. Personalized Formulations & Self-Monitoring
Session 2. Regular Eating
Session 3. Alternative Activities
Session 4. Urge Tolerating & Feelings of Fullness
Session 5. Progress Review
Session 6. Dieting & Diet-Related Rules
Session 7. Over-evaluation of Shape & Weight

Session 8. Shape/Weight Checking- Part 1
Session 9. Shape/Weight Checking- Part 2
Session 10. Shape/Weight Avoidance
Session 11. Check-in & Body Dissatisfaction Spikes
Session 12. Events, Emotions, & Eating
Session 13. Historical Review of the Eating Disorder
Session 14. Relapse Prevention & Ending Treatment

Who can I contact if I have additional questions about group?

Please do be in touch with the Group CBT-E therapist throughout the patient's treatment to coordinate care.

Group CBT-E Therapist Name and Contact Details: _____

EXTRA ACTION PLAN TEMPLATES

ACTION PLAN	DATE:

PROBLEM:	
CURRENT FREQUENCY (IF APPLICABLE):	
GOAL FOR UPCOMING WEEK:	

	MY PLAN:	MY SUPPORT:
SPECIFIC PLAN:		

ACTION PLAN	DATE:

PROBLEM:	
CURRENT FREQUENCY (IF APPLICABLE):	
GOAL FOR UPCOMING WEEK:	

	MY PLAN:	MY SUPPORT:
SPECIFIC PLAN:		

GROUP CBT-E COMPONENTS CHECKLIST

COMPONENT (include both introducing and reviewing skills)	Pre	1	2	3	4	5	6	7	8	9	10	11	12	13	14
Pre-group screening (including EDE-Q, CIA)															
Treatment description provided															
Getting to Know Me handout completed															
Stage 1															
Personalized formulation (including reviewing/updating throughout treatment)															
Self-monitoring															
Regular eating															
Education about eating disorders (informational handouts)															
Alternative activities															
Urge tolerating															
Feelings of fullness															
Stage 2															
Progress review (including EDE-Q, CIA)															
Describing Stage 3															
(Therapist self-review)															
Stage 3															
Dieting behaviors and diet-related rules															
Self-evaluation pie chart															
Extended formulation															
Increasing focus on other areas of life															
Shape and weight checking															
Shape and weight avoidance															
Body dissatisfaction spikes															
Problem-solving															
Behavior/urge analysis															
Slowing down reacting to urges/tolerating emotions															
Stage 4															
Historical review															
Stopping self-monitoring															
Review of progress (including EDE-Q, CIA)															
Relapse prevention															

Adapted from © Bailey-Straebler, Calugi, Cooper, Dalle Grave & Murphy 2022. *The CBT-E Components Checklist (CBT-E CC)*.

Optional Session Material: In-session Food Exposures

In-session food exposures can be helpful for patients to address particularly challenging foods in a therapeutic environment. This intervention allows patients to work together as a group to confront their fears. In-session food exposures are an optional component of Group CBT-E, since they are not always feasible. Not all therapists are set up to implement an in-session exposure or it may not seem like an appropriate fit for the particular group (e.g., based on the time of day the group is offered). When this in-session intervention is not possible, the group can still be a useful tool in supporting breaking food rules. For example, patients can eat an avoided food just prior to group and then utilize the support of the group as they tolerate urges.

Introducing In-session Food Exposures

At the end of Session 6, prepare patients for the in-session food exposure intervention. Let them know that to support them in breaking their diet-related food rules, all future sessions will include bringing in a food item to be eaten in the group. Ask patients to choose a food from their avoided foods list to bring to Session 7.

> *Breaking diet-related rules can be a challenging task. To support your work with this, I will ask you next week to bring in one of your avoided foods to the group session to eat during group. This is something we will continue in all sessions moving forward. This likely will feel scary. As we talked about, exposure to things that are avoided often causes fear. Anxiety/fear during exposure is often a sign that you are doing exactly what you need to do to address your eating disorder. Eating an avoided food alongside other group members can often be very useful as you will be supported by everyone else who will also be completing their avoided foods. I hope that the support of the group will help you to reach your goals.*

Then provide the following guidance:

> *Choose a food that is tricky, but doable for you, from your avoided foods list. Be brave! Remember, you will have the support of the group to push yourself a little further than you might be able to do otherwise, so use this as an opportunity.*
>
> *If your rule is to not eat in front of others, likely any food you choose will break this rule, but again be brave and pick the most challenging food that you can tolerate.*
>
> *Take a moment to write the food you intend to bring for next time on your Between-session Work Log.*

Implementing the In-session Food Exposures

At the start of Sessions 7–14, ask patients to start eating their snack while they complete the between-session work self-review.

At the end of the between-session work self-review, go around the room and ask patients to briefly share:

> Joining the patients and eating a snack with them can be beneficial to role model comfort in eating. For this to be successful, choose balanced, non-diet type foods.
>
> If treatment is in person, if possible, have a few back-up snacks for patients to choose from if they forget to bring their snack.

1. the progress they have made with eating their food
2. any related feelings, thoughts, or urges that are occurring for them
3. what skill (e.g., urge tolerating, alternative activities) they will practice throughout group (and potentially after) to address negative thoughts or urges to engage in behaviors.

For the first in-session food exposure, provide the following guidance to patients about what to expect during the exposure:

- *Resist safety behaviors! A safety behavior is anything you do to attempt to decrease your anxiety about eating the food (e.g., do not take teeny bites or wipe oil off).* [Look out for these behaviors and help to redirect when you are noticing them.]

- [Introduce food comparisons as a potential and common behavior.] *If you find yourself engaging in food comparisons (looking at what others are eating and calorie comparing, etc.), catch yourself, label it as comparison making, move your eyes to something else, and re-engage with the group content. Consider sharing this in group. Food comparisons are common and it is best to openly voice when this is happening.*

- *Sometimes the thoughts and emotions that come up as a result of eating this food item can be distracting from the group content. If this is happening, please let the group know so that you don't miss any important material.*

- *If breaking your rule triggers urges to engage in an eating disorder behavior (binge eating, vomiting, skipping your next meal), bring this up in group. Again, this feeling is normal when breaking diet-related rules. In fact, this is part of why we want you to practice breaking rules – to see that even when the urge occurs you have the tools to ride it out and tolerate it.*

- *Sometimes eating disorder behaviors do happen to compensate for breaking a diet-related rule. You know what to do: get back on track at the next meal or snack. Each eating experience is another opportunity to put your skills back in action. When you are more settled on track again, think about what may have led to you using an eating disorder behavior – is there something to learn for the next time you break a food rule?*

This intervention can be difficult for some patients. If the intervention is seemingly too difficult for the patient to complete, support the patient by suggesting that they try a less anxiety-provoking food in the next in-session food exposure or that they consider bringing in a food to the session that they have had some practice eating at home. Some patients find it most difficult to eat around others so eating both a new food and eating socially is too feared. In these situations, suggest that the patient brings in a food that they are currently eating, but face their fears around eating that item around others. Over time, they can slowly choose more difficult foods to try.

Remember that whatever food is eaten in the session will need to be added to the patient's *Between-session Work Log* to be completed regularly following the session. It is important that a food is not only eaten in the session, but is then practiced consistently outside of the session to generalize the learning.

Index

[Terms in **bold** indicate the main treatment interventions; page numbers in *italics* refer to handouts]